Fitness
and Wellness
The Physical Connection

Fitness and Wellness

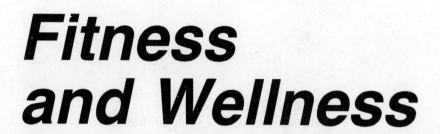

The Physical Connection

Frank D. Rosato
Memphis State University

West Publishing Company
St. Paul   New York   Los Angeles   San Francisco

Art: Charles R. Schroeder
Composition: Carlisle Communications
Copyediting: Tage Publishing Services
Cover Design: John Edeen
Text Design: John Edeen

Library of Congress Cataloging-in-Publication Data

Rosato, Frank D.
  Fitness and wellness: the physical connection / Frank D. Rosato.
    2nd ed.
        p.   cm.
    Includes bibliographical references.
    ISBN 0-314-66786-5
    1. Health.   2. Physical fitness.   3. Exercise.   4. Nutrition.   I. Title.
RA776.R728   1990
  613—dc20   89-70440
                                                                     CIP

This text is dedicated to my wife Pat for her continuing patience and support during this and all of my professional endeavors.

Contents

8 *Developing the Muscular Component*   *195*

11 *The Reduction Equation:*
Exercise + Sensible Eating = Weight Control 285

12 *Fitness for Life* 317

Preface

The aim of the second edition of this text is the same as the first—to establish through contemporary evidence the connection between physical fitness and wellness. The fact that this is a second edition attests to the interest in fitness and wellness by college and university instructors and their students.

There has been an explosion of new information since the first edition appeared in 1986. The massive research effort in this exciting field of study is manifestly evident as a host of researchers submit the results of their work to medical, exercise science, and nutritional science journals for publication. The stream of new information has been continuous and prolific. It clearly indicated that a revision was in order, and it presented several important challenges.

The first of these challenges involved filtering this new information and deciding what should be included in an introductory text of this type and what would have to be excluded. A second challenge was deciding what would be deleted from the first edition. These difficult decisions had to be made in order to keep the text within manageable proportions, yet expansive enough in scope and depth to convey the nature of the relationship between physical fitness and wellness as it is scientifically observed at this writing. Every chapter in this new edition has been significantly upgraded by the addition of new information and the deletion of outdated material. As a result, this edition is current, while approximately 30 percent larger than the first—a growth that reflects the research explosion in the field.

A third challenge to writing this edition involved the selection of specific references, and the decision upon the sheer number of references that would be used for documentation. Although the references that have been cited represent a fraction of those that were read in preparation for writing this manuscript, the number finally selected is greater than the number found in other introductory physical fitness texts. This is so for several reasons, but to fully comprehend the rationale for the need of a rich research emphasis, one must examine the major goals of the text. First, the primary objective is to inform and educate college-age students regarding physical fitness and wellness through strong documentation and the presentation of current and accurate information. Second, college and university instructors can also benefit from this text because it pulls together current research data from exercise science, medicine, and the allied health professions. This text is heavily referenced not only to validate the information it contains, but also to provide a convenient and handy source for those who are interested in gaining knowledge beyond its scope.

This edition, like its predecessor, does not utilize an exercise-by-the-numbers approach to physical fitness. Instead, through its content, it attempts to establish a sound base for lifetime participation in physical fitness activities and an active way of living. The "why" of exercise is emphasized, but the "how" is certainly not neglected.

Many changes have occurred in the second edition. The text has been expanded from eight to twelve chapters. There are more self-assessment tests, and these appear at the ends of chapters in which they belong as opposed to all appearing in an appendix. The adopters of this edition will receive an updated instructor's manual with a test bank and transparency masters. Also, a newsletter will be generated and periodically sent to adopters for the purpose of keeping them current. This newsletter will include new and interesting information, and adopters should feel free to make as many copies of the newsletter as they wish for class handouts or for other purposes.

Chapter 1 has been expanded, and a wellness self-inventory has been included. Chapter 2 from the first edition (The Fitness/Wellness Connection) has become Chapters 2, 3, and 4 in the current edition. This reorganization was necessary in order to accommodate the proliferation of new information intrinsic to these chapters, and secondly to partition the contents in such a way as to have homogeneous material in each chapter. Chapter 5, entitled "Motivation" is larger than its predecessor (Chapter 3), covering exercise adherence more fully, and adding more techniques for keeping people active. Chapters 6 and 7 in this edition have grown from the first edition Chapter 4 (Developing The Cardiorespiratory Component). Both Chapter 6 and Chapter 7 are concerned with cardiorespiratory fitness, but Chapter 6 presents the guidelines (or the "how") associated with the accomplishment of this goal, while Chapter 7 examines the various bodily adaptations that accrue from participation in activities of a cardiorespiratory nature. Chapter 8, Developing The Muscular Component, has been substantially updated. Chapter 9, Developing The Flexibility Component, was least affected by the revision, but some changes have occured. Chapters 10 and 11 in this edition grew from the first edition Chapter 7 (Developing The Body Composition Component). Significant additions and some deletions have occurred with this material. Chapter 10 presents the basics of nutrition, while Chapter 11 emphasizes the role of exercise and nutrition in weight management. Chapter 12 deals with lifetime fitness, and it too has been expanded and updated.

Chapter 12 is the only chapter which does not have a mini-glossary of important terms, but it, like all other chapters, features questions and statements that summarize major points (*Points to Ponder*), and margin notes that provide interesting tidbits of information on salient and timely topics. Self-assessment tests are included where appropriate at the ends of chapters. These can be administered and supervised by instructors, or students may take them as outside assignments by following the accompanying instructions. Norms or standards are presented as a frame of reference for interpretation of the results.

A textbook is usually not the work of one person, and this effort is no exception. The ideas of many people are represented here. The contributions begin with the data generated by all of the researchers whose works provide the cognitive base for this text, and extend from there to the reviewers whose ideas and suggestions helped to refine the finished product, to the young models who contributed to the aesthetics of the text, and to the professional staff of

West Publishing Company—Jerry Westby, Managing Editor, and Tom Hilt, Assistant Production Editor, who kept me on track in terms of direction and meeting deadlines.

Many thanks to my good friend Sheri Seiser who took the photographs that have substantially enhanced the written word. Thanks also to the attractive people who were willing to serve as models for this edition. Their names are: Angela Anton, P.J. Gardner, Raymond Hoffman Jr., Susan Hunter, Barbara McClanahan, Renee Melton, and Angela Rosato. Special thanks also go out to Tresa Holt and Brenda Johnson. Tresa spent several hours in various libraries digging out references, and Brenda typed and cut-and-pasted the entire manuscript.

As mentioned previously, the reviewers for this text were instrumental in refining the final product. Their strong contributions deserve both praise and appreciation. These individuals are:

Ralph Barclay	Division of Health and Physical Education Wayne State College
Loren Cordain	Sports Science Department Colorado State University
Tom Crum	Department of Physical Education Triton College
Sandra Flood	Department of Physical Education Northern Illinois University
Art Gilbert	Department of Physical Activities and Recreation University of California—Santa Barbara
Steven G. Gregg	Department of Physical Education University of California—Berkeley
Lenny R. Klaver	Division of Health and Physical Education Wayne State College
Dorothy Kozeluh	Department of Health and Physical Education Chicago State University
Richard W. Latin	School of Health, Physical Education, and Recreation University of Nebraska/Omaha
Katie P. McLeod	Physical Education Department Pensacola Junior College
Frank G. Micale	Department of Health, Physical Education, and Recreation Ithaca College
Lynette Silvestri	Department of Health and Physical Education University of New Orleans
Sherman K. Sowby	Department of Health Science California State University—Fresno
Ray Webster	Mabee Center William Jewell College
Jerry White	Department of Health and Physical Education Oxnard College

–Frank D. Rosato, Ed. D.

1

Introduction to Fitness and Wellness

Chapter Outline

Mini Glossary

Acute (or communicable) disease: a severe disease of short duration.

Agility: the ability to rapidly change direction while maintaining dynamic balance.

Balance: involves the maintenance of a desired body position either statically or dynamically. Also referred to as equilibrium.

Body composition: the amount of lean versus fat tissue.

Cardiovascular disease: a complex of diseases of the heart and circulatory system.

Cardiovascular endurance: the ability to take in, deliver, and extract oxygen for physical work.

Chronic disease: a long-lasting and/or frequently occurring disease.

Chronological age: an individual's calendar age.

Coordination: the integration of body parts resulting in smooth, fluid motion.

Flexibility: range of motion around a specific joint.

Health age: an individual's biological age.

Health-related fitness: a type of fitness that enhances one's health status by modifying many of the risks associated with lifestyle diseases.

Muscular endurance: the capacity to exert repetitive muscular force.

Muscular strength: the maximum amount of force that a muscle can exert in a single contraction.

Performance-related fitness: a type of fitness that allows one to perform physical skills with a high degree of proficiency.

Power: a function of work divided by the time that it takes to perform the work.

Reaction time: the elapsed time between the presentation of a stimulus and its response. Also called response latency.

Risk-factor profile: an objective representation of risk factors for a selected disease, with a probability statement regarding how and when death may occur based upon lifestyle habits.

Speed: performance of a movement in the shortest amount of time. Also known as velocity.

Wellness: a dynamic and multifaceted approach to optimal health that centers upon individuals taking responsibility for their health status.

Introduction

Wellness involves optimal development of the physical self, the constructive use and management of stress energy, effectiveness in communicating and dealing with emotions, positive use of the mind, environmental sensitivity, and the development of productive relations with other people. Wellness is a perpetual quest. It is characterized by individuals who take the responsibility for striving for optimal functioning by mitigating the negatives and building on the positives in their lives. The choices that we make influence our state of health and well-being.

Disease care is very expensive in our country. Most of the dollars spent for health care are really spent for disease care with few resources devoted to preventing disease.

Physical fitness, one of the supporting structures of wellness, is comprised of health- and performance-related components. An overview of the relationship between physical fitness and wellness is presented. Data from surveys that indicate the approximate number of Americans who exercise as well as the types of activities in which they participate are examined. A short chronology delineating the events having an impact on physical fitness during this century with particular reference to the development and continuance of the present movement is presented.

We must stop trying to buy health with our dollars and start earning it with our behaviors.
—Don Ardell
Planning for Wellness

Wellness Defined

Wellness embodies a characteristic lifestyle—a mind-set that personifies a positive approach to health. It is the antithesis of our present health care system which many have more accurately labeled a "disease care" system.

Health Care or Disease Care?

Wellness goes beyond prevention in that it initiates a whole new way to conceive of health: not simply as the absence of disease, as most of us have been led to believe, but as a continual process of attaining greater and greater personal well-being. Wellness does not describe dos and don'ts; it's much more than that.

Health promotion is the fiber of wellness. These two words may have a familiar ring to them, since they have indeed been part of our vocabulary for years. In fact, they have long been drowned out by organized medicine's traditional orientation not toward health, but toward illness.

To understand this orientation, it may help to call to mind a legendary Cornish test of sanity. Imagine a running faucet, beneath which sits a bucket rapidly filling with water. Handed a ladle, you are instructed to empty the bucket. As Cornish legend has it, if you fail to shut off the water before you start ladling, you may find yourself declared insane.

So it goes, say many critics, with our current health-care system, a system that ladles frantically—removing cancerous lungs, bypassing blocked coronary arteries, prescribing all manner of pills—with hardly a glance at the still-running faucet. In name, we speak of our health-care system. In truth, we have built a multi-billion-dollar disease care system, which according to many estimates, allocates up to 96 percent of these dollars for treatment and only 4 percent or less for prevention and education. Ergo, we ladle with 96 percent of our resources and expend only 4 percent of our efforts trying to slow the flow from the faucet. The wellness movement seeks to bring these numbers considerably closer together.

It does so in the belief that significant society-wide gains in health can no longer be expected from fancier hospitals, more sophisticated surgical procedures and more potent drugs.

Grossman, John, "Inside the Wellness Movement," *Health*, Family Media, Inc., Nov./Dec. 1981. Reprinted by permission.

The World Health Organization has defined health as "a state of complete physical, mental, and social well-being, and not merely the absence of disease or infirmity." The generic correctness of this definition is irrefutable, but its lack of specificity renders it meaningless in the practical sense.

High-level wellness is a process of growth, evolving, and changing which includes:

1. being free from symptoms of disease and pain as much as possible
2. being able to be active—able to do what you want and what you must at the appropriate time
3. being in good spirits most of the time.

These characteristics indicate that good health is not something that is suddenly achieved at a specific time, such as getting a college degree. Rather, health is an ongoing process—indeed, a way of life—through which you develop and encourage every aspect of your body, mind, and feelings to interrelate harmoniously as much of the time as possible.[1] It involves optimal development of the physical self, the constructive use and management of stress energy, effectiveness in communicating and dealing with emotions, positive use of the mind, environmental sensitivity, and the development of productive relations with other people.[2] From this description, it is quite clear that the quality of one's health and the quest for total well-being is primarily the responsibility of each individual—it is not the responsibility of physicians nor the conventional medical care and delivery system, it is not the responsibility of government, and it is not the responsibility of society. It is not our intention to denigrate this country's medical care system; it is currently the best in the world. Medical training focuses upon treating diseases rather than preventing them, and there will always be a critical need for these skills. Even if medicine shifted its priorities toward prevention (and this entails considerable resources), the fact remains that we are to a large extent the masters of our own destinies. We ultimately make the choices that influence our health.

Health: A Matter of Choice

We make choices, both positive and negative, about smoking cigarettes, wearing seat belts, exercise, weight control, nutrition, alcohol intake, frequency of medical examinations, and so on. These choices and the ensuing behavior patterns profoundly affect the state of our health.

Some people make seemingly inappropriate choices and live to a ripe old age, but these are the exceptions rather than the rule. They have beaten the odds and make headlines as a result. Winston Churchill was an example of one who defied the principles of good health and lived more than eighty years. But one must wonder how much longer he might have lived if he were less indulgent when it came to the harmful excesses in his life. Genetically, he was probably well-endowed for longevity, but his lifestyle practices seemed to detract from his biological potential. The majority of those who follow similar lifestyles die early and become mere statistics in some esoteric piece of research. These people do not make headlines because their fate is the norm: it is expected and it is not newsworthy. By featuring these exceptions, the media inadvertently promotes a cavalier attitude toward good health practices.

Figure 1.1 graphically emphasizes the importance of self-responsibility in a wellness lifestyle by ascribing to it the predominant position among all factors.

Living in accordance with this model fosters an attitude of responsibility for our actions and removes the compulsion to blame others or to make excuses for our predicament. During the last 20 years, many Americans have positively altered their daily habits and accepted responsibility for their own health. Unfortunately, this group still represents a minority of the population. The notion that good health is represented by the absence of disease and the avoidance of disability has outlived its usefulness, but it continues to persist. Consequently, high-level wellness escapes most Americans, since many will continue to rely upon the annual or biannual medical exam in the hope that they will receive a "clean bill of health." If they do, the old lifestyle is reinforced, regardless of the healthy or unhealthy practices that characterize it. If the old lifestyle includes cigarette smoking, a diet high in fat and cholesterol, sedentary habits, and an inability to effectively cope with stress, then it is virtually certain to lead to premature disease. In fact, the **chronic diseases** (cardiovascular diseases, cancer,

You the individual can do more for your own health and well-being than any doctor, any hospital, any drug, any exotic medical device.
—Joseph Califano

To a greater extent than most of us are willing to accept, today's disorders of overweight, heart disease, cancer, blood pressure, and diabetes are by-and-large preventable. In this light, true health insurance is not what one carries on a plastic card, but what one does for oneself.
—Lawrence Power, M.D.

FIGURE 1.1

A Constellation of Selected Wellness Factors.

Adapted from D. Ardell, *Planning for Wellness*, Dubuque, Iowa: Kendall/Hunt Publishing Co., 1982.

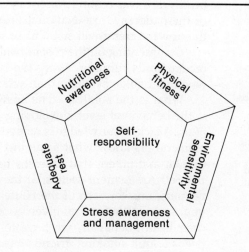

Nutritional awareness

Physical fitness

Self-responsibility

Adequate rest

Environmental sensitivity

Stress awareness and management

diabetes, etc.) that have replaced the **acute or communicable diseases** as the leading causes of death in the past four to five decades, are the result of such a lifestyle. The chronic diseases are not transmitted from person to person through contact; rather, they are voluntary or self-inflicted. The tendency for developing a few of the chronic diseases appears to run in some families. Whether or when these diseases manifest themselves is influenced substantially by the living habits of those who are involved. The chronic diseases are not prevented by innoculation nor can they be cured with antibiotics; instead, they are the calamitous results of the choices we have made. Consider the following:

1. Seven of the ten leading causes of death can be substantially reduced by controlling blood pressure, quitting the cigarette habit, eating more wisely, getting regular exercise, and reducing alcohol consumption.
2. The heart attack risk is doubled in men who are cigarette smokers.
3. Ten percent of all deaths in the United States are alcohol-related.
4. Occupational hazards are responsible for approximately 20 percent of cancer mortality.
5. Highway accidents are responsible for nearly 50,000 deaths annually. A significant number of these can be prevented with seat belts, shoulder harnesses, and sobriety.
6. High-blood pressure, a precursor of 500,000 strokes and 1,500,000 heart attacks per year, afflicts approximately 17 percent of Americans.
7. Suicide is steadily rising as a leading cause of death among teenagers and young adults.[3]
8. Eighty million Americans are overweight; 70 million have arthritis.
9. Premature employee deaths account for the loss of $20 billion per year.[4]

"Americans annually lose 15 million years of living from preventable causes."
—*Surgeon General's Report*[5]

The difference in the health status of any two Americans is primarily determined by factors beyond a physician's control.[4] By following reasonable rules for healthy living, we can reduce the rate of premature morbidity and mortality. This has become imperative as the cost of disease care rises to a staggering and disproportionate amount of the gross national product. In 1979, the nation's total health care bill was $212.2 billion;[6] by 1984, it had risen to $400 billion,[7] and in 1986, health care was costing Americans $458.2 billion. This represented 10.9 percent of the nation's Gross National Product (GNP), and there is no indication that the upward trend will stabilize or reverse itself in the near future.[8]

Health has become one of America's biggest businesses. It is the nation's second largest employer, after education, and third largest industry in consumer spending, behind only food and housing.
—Joseph Califano

Commenting on the cost of health care, George Sheehan, a cardiologist who recommends running, says "the rules of health require less monetary outlay when you abide by them than when you break them."[9]

What is the solution? The answer is obvious when we think about it, but, at the behavioral level, developing good health habits is very difficult for many of us. A lack of knowledge is responsible for some people's poor health practices, while others know what to do but find it too easy to slip back into bad habits.

An instrument that assesses health and wellness behavior is presented in the Self-Assessment section at the end of this chapter (page 18). Read the directions, answer each of the 60 items honestly and then read how to interpret your scores. We have all given good advice to our friends and family regarding their health behavior, we have told Dad that he needs to lose weight, Mom needs to quit smoking, friends need to eat more wisely, others need to use seat belts, and so on. This inventory will assist us to define our own behaviors. The test is: Can we take our own advice?

Contributing to the Solution

The importance of living a healthy life was demonstrated and quantified in several studies that were produced in California.[10] More than 6000 residents of Alameda County were randomly selected and followed for five years. A definite relationship was observed between selected health practices and longevity. The following positively influenced length of life:

1. eat breakfast regularly
2. eat moderately with no snacking between meals
3. maintain normal body weight
4. never smoke cigarettes
5. drink no alcohol or only drink moderately
6. exercise regularly
7. sleep 7 to 8 hours per night

The data indicated that people who lived in accordance with these health principles lived longer than those who did not. For example, 45-year-old men who followed six of these practices lived, on the average, eleven years longer than 45-year-old men who followed three or less. The data for 45-year-old women who followed similar health patterns as the males in this study was less dramatic but still highly significant. The healthful living group showed a seven-year advantage in longevity. These convincing data prompted the researchers to conclude that "the daily health habits of people have a great deal more to do with what makes them sick and when they die than all the influences of medicine." This is a powerful statement, but one that seems to be consistent with research and authoritative opinion.

A nine-year followup of this study showed that five of the seven health habits (the maintenance of normal weight, having never smoked cigarettes, use of alcohol in moderation, regular exercise, and sleeping 7 to 8 hours) were associated with lower mortality from all causes.[11] Eating breakfast regularly and not snacking between meals were not related to lower mortality. This very sophisticated study essentially reconfirmed the results of the original study. The evidence inexorably continues to accumulate, confirming what knowledgeable people already knew: We are the chief determiners of our own health. We are not hapless victims of disease; instead, we set our course and chart our destiny. We are victims only in the sense that we have been victimized by our lifestyle choices. As George Sheehan remarks, "we have come to an era in which aberrant life-style can no longer be ignored."[12]

A recent questionnaire study in Massachusetts examined the prevalence of four risk factors among the state's inhabitants.[13] The results showed that 43.3 percent of the respondents were at least 10 percent heavier than their ideal weight, 33 percent smoked, 28.3 percent did not exercise, and 11.7 percent drank four or more alcoholic drinks on at least two occasions per week. Men drank more alcohol than women, but women reported more high-risk behavior in the other three categories. Older people exercised less and were more overweight, but smoked and drank alcohol less than younger people. Older people who exercised preferred walking, while younger people preferred jogging. Higher educational and socioeconomic levels were significantly related to positive health practices.

Health Habits: What Do the Doctors Do?

Where difficult decisions are concerned—about surgery, risky procedures, or medicines with side effects—people often ask physicians: "What would YOU do, doctor?"

Less often do we ask what decisions our doctors make on a daily basis about matters that are long-term and not crisis-oriented but still critical to their own health.

Recently, a survey of Harvard Medical School clinical faculty did just that. A total of 595 members responded to these and other questions:

- Do you smoke cigarettes? Ninety-two percent do not. But 38 percent of the non-smokers were former smokers. This is consistent with surveys in this country and Britain showing that more doctors have quit smoking than any other professional group.

    Doctors routinely confront the ravages of smoking in cases of heart disease, lung cancer, and other respiratory disease. They may be more continually aware than the average person not only that smoking is responsible for 350,000 premature deaths every year but that it is also the cause of a great deal of lingering, long-term suffering and disability.
- Do you use sleeping pills more than three times a week? Ninety-eight percent said no. Doctors probably have as much stress and worry as anybody, yet they know that sleeping pills interfere with normal healthy sleep and that prolonged use results in less, not more sleep. Answers to other questions also indicated reluctance to take medicines without real necessity.
- Do you use seat belts routinely? Seventy-three percent answered yes. This is far better than usage shown by studies of other groups. Doctors, especially those in emergency rooms, may be more aware that most traffic and highway deaths occur when victims are thrown from cars at impact. Very good, well documented studies from many countries have consistently shown that 60 percent of all deaths and serious injury from automobile accidents could have been prevented by seat belts.
- Do you take antibiotics for a cold? Ninety-seven percent said no. Colds are caused by viruses, which are not affected by antibiotics. Rest and chicken soup remain the best treatments.

■ Do you jog or take equivalent aerobic exercise 20 minutes or more at least three times a week? Forty-nine percent take the kind of exercise that improves heart fitness, again higher than the national average.

■ If practicing contraception, do you or your partner use contraceptive pills? Ninety-five percent do not.

■ Do you weigh more than 10 pounds above what you'd like to? Seventy-one percent answered no.

■ Do you take more than two alcoholic drinks a day? Ninety-three percent do not. Medical studies have shown that more alcohol than this can be harmful to health in many ways.

Forty-four percent restrict consumption of red meat, 79 percent eat three or fewer eggs per week, and 69 percent use margarine instead of butter—probably to control consumption of saturated fat and cholesterol.

Forty-one percent eat a high fiber diet. Good evidence shows that vegetable fiber not only aids elimination but also protects against colon cancer and other bowel diseases. Ninety-seven percent do not take laxatives for constipation.

Kirk, B., "Health Habits: What Do The Doctors Do?" *House Call*, University of Tennessee College of Medicine, Feb. 6, 1983. Reprinted by permission.

Far from being simply the absence of disease, health is a dynamic and harmonious equilibrium of all the elements and forces making up and surrounding a human being.
—Andrew Weil, M.D.

For optimal health, we need to integrate our knowledge, attitudes, and behaviors into a balanced approach that avoids excesses and extremes. This approach can and should be extended beyond health into all other areas of our lives. We should channel our energies toward continued growth as fully functioning human beings living in a manner that enhances health and minimizes the risk of illness.

The following vignette summarizes quite nicely what may be accomplished when one's actions, thoughts, feelings, and values are in congruence. Mahatma Gandhi, long-time spiritual and political leader of India, appeared before the British government on behalf of Indian sovereignty. He spoke for three hours without notecards or other aids. Members of the British press were awed by Gandhi's eloquent performance and as the speech concluded, they descended upon his press secretary demanding to know how he could speak so persuasively and cogently for that length of time. "It's simple," replied his secretary. "What Gandhi thinks, says, and does are one. You British think one thing, say a second, and do a third. That's why you need notecards to keep track."[14]

POINTS TO PONDER

1. *How would you define and/or describe wellness?*
2. *What is the role of the individual in developing and maintaining optimal wellness?*
3. *What are the components of a wellness lifestyle?*

Physical Fitness Defined

Humans have been intrigued with the concept and applications of physical fitness for centuries. Many cultures, both past and present, have been concerned with the development of fit people for the utilitarian purposes of war and conquest. During the Golden Age of Greece, fitness was elevated from the level of necessity to a lofty goal along with the development of the mind as individuals attempted to achieve their full potential. The Greeks were truly ahead of their time. Twenty-five centuries later, we have finally come full circle by resurrecting this worthy concept.

The Harvard Fatigue Laboratory, which was initiated during the early years of the twentieth century, began a systematic and scientific investigation of physical fitness. Some 60 years and a cadre of exercise scientists have not produced a definition of physical fitness that satisfies all conditions and all authoritative factions. A panel of experts charged to develop an acceptable definition of physical fitness was convened in 1968. With time running out and unable to agree on specifics, a generic definition finally emerged after seven frustrating attempts. As defined by the panel, fitness is "the ability to perform muscular work satisfactorily under specified conditions."[15] This definition was too general, providing little direction and no criteria by which to judge the attainment of physical fitness. Other definitions from different people and groups have been developed, but none has been accepted universally. More recently, fitness has been dichotomized into health-related components and performance-related components. This dual emphasis has provided new directions for the development of fitness definitions. This model, which serves as the conceptual basis for fitness in this text, has been well received by the community of exercise scientists and physical educators.

Health-Related Fitness

Falls defines **health-related fitness** as "those aspects of physiological and psychological functioning which are believed to offer some protection against degenerative-type diseases such as coronary heart disease, obesity, and various musculoskeletal disorders."[16] Cundiff's definition is "the state of complete well-being including the absence of disease and the possession of specific physical attributes that will reduce chances of disease and add enjoyment to life."[17]

Most authorities agree that health-related fitness consists of cardiovascular endurance, muscular strength, muscular endurance, flexibility, and body composition.[18] **Cardiovascular endurance** refers to the ability of the body to take in, deliver, and extract oxygen for physical work. It is the best physiological index of total body endurance. **Muscular strength** is the maximal force that a muscle can exert in a single contraction. **Muscular endurance** is the capacity to exert repetitive muscular force. **Flexibility** refers to the range of motion around specific joints. **Body composition** refers to the amount of lean versus fat tissue. There is some question regarding the validity of muscular strength, muscular endurance, and flexibility as genuine aspects of health fitness and there is some concern that these might be categorized better as components of performance-related fitness. This point of view can be defended, but this writer believes that all five components are important. In this text, the effect of physical fitness upon wellness or the quality of life and the possibility of warding off premature death is emphasized. In light of both objectives, it seems reasonable to assume (and this writer will attempt to show) that all five components can contribute to health-related fitness.

Understandably, the contribution of each component to health and wellness is one of degree. Cardiovascular endurance is undoubtedly the most important of the components. This will be fully explored later, along with the development of a rationale for the other components.

Performance-Related Fitness

Performance-related fitness, though not essential for health, is necessary for the execution of sports skills. Speed, power, balance, coordination, agility, and reaction time are the components of performance-related fitness. **Speed** refers to velocity or the ability to perform a movement in the shortest amount of time. **Power** refers to work divided by time; the faster the completion of work the greater the power. **Balance,** or equilibrium, refers to the ability to maintain a desired body position either statically or dynamically. **Coordination** is the ability to integrate the body parts to produce smooth fluid motion. **Agility** is the ability to rapidly change direction while maintaining dynamic balance. **Reaction time** represents the time that it takes to respond physically to a given stimulus. It is usually measured in fractions of a second.

Highly skilled athletes possess these abilities in a highly refined state. The sports in which they participate may also require one or more of the health-related components, because there is not mutual exclusivity between the two types of fitness. The primary objective for noncompetitors may be health-related fitness, but the activities they use to achieve this goal may also require some or all of the performance related components. In fact, some people prefer the challenge of developing skill and fitness concurrently. These people are usually athletic and enjoy athletic competition. Their principal mode of developing and maintaining fitness is through athletic games. There are literally millions of people participating in racquetball, handball, tennis, and other games that combine both types of fitness. But it is important for people to understand that the attainment of health-related fitness does not depend upon athletic ability or physical activities that are high in the performance-related components. Health-related fitness can be achieved with minimal psychomotor ability. Almost anyone, even those with varying degrees of physical disability, can participate in such natural activities as walking and jogging. Other activities such as biking (including use of a stationary bike), hiking, backpacking, orienteering, swimming, rope jumping, and so on, require minimal cognitive and psychomotor abilities when one participates for physical fitness purposes rather than for skill development. Health-related fitness training differs from competitive training because the objectives of each program differ. The adage that most of us grew up with "no pain, no gain," while probably necessary for competitive athletes is inappropriate for the purpose of health-related fitness.

How Fitness Fits

Physical fitness is an integral part of a multifaceted wellness lifestyle. It can only be developed and maintained through persistent and progressively increasing effort, but the payoff includes an impressive array of predictable physiological, emotional, social, and health benefits. Participation in a vigorous physical fitness program, one which attempts to develop all of the components of health-related fitness, has far-reaching effects upon the quality and quantity of life. Practitioners of this lifestyle present physical profiles that are synonymous with vibrant and robust health. There are significant differences in health status between them and sedentary people matched for age and sex. In general, active people are leaner, have lower levels of blood fats, lower blood pressure, handle stress more effectively, and smoke less.

Comparisons made between active and inactive groups using Health Risk Appraisal analyses indicate that the **health age** (or biological age) of the active group is generally lower than their **chronological age.** That is, an active 52-year-old is likely to be the equivalent of a 45-year-old with regard to health. We often see the converse when people enter our Fitness and Wellness Center. The health age of our entry-level clients is likely to be higher than their chronological age. This is an undesirable situation, but there are some positives associated with it: one being that it acts as a powerful motivator for change. We usually see favorable changes when people participate in our programs for several months.

Health Risk Appraisals are questionnaires used to assess lifestyle habits. Respondents react to questions which inquire into such behaviors as tobacco and alcohol usage, exercise habits, dietary habits, use of seat belts, frequency of self-exams and medical evaluations, blood pressure and blood lipid values, and so on. These instruments also project, on the basis of heredity and lifestyle habits, each individual's likely age at death. Of course, the prediction is only as good as the data base upon which it is conceived, the respondent's honesty, and the built-in error associated with laws of probability. None of these instruments predict infallibly, but they are educational tools that graphically identify negative and positive health behaviors while providing suggestions for improving health status and longevity. Regardless of their shortcomings, the predictions for active people are generally more favorable than for sedentary people.

The attainment of physical fitness seems to act as a catalyst for change in other facets of our life. The evidence in this regard is anecdotal, but there are literally thousands of people who have capitalized upon fitness as a springboard for successfully changing nutritional, smoking, alcohol, and rest habits. In effect, they are maximizing the health benefits that were acquired initially through regular exercise. Exercise as a change agent certainly requires more investigation, but it is considered to be one of the vehicles for altering some unhealthy behaviors.

Is Fitness A Fad?

Nations have passed away and left no traces, and history gives the naked cause of it. One single, simple reason in all cases—they fell because their people were not fit.
— Rudyard Kipling

The fitness movement began in the 1960s. Since its inception, skeptics have proclaimed it a passing fancy—a fad akin to streaking and the hula hoop. Thus far, it has survived both and continues to grow. A number of probability surveys by the Gallup and Harris organization as well as other privately generated and government sponsored polls have indicated that the number of Americans who exercise has generally increased steadily since 1961.[19, 20, 21] A national survey conducted by Lieberman Research Inc. for *Sports Illustrated* in 1986 revealed some interesting characteristics of the present fitness movement.[22] Seven out of ten respondents reported that they participated in sports or fitness activities during the past twelve months. On the surface, this is indeed impressive but closer inspection of the data indicated that the respondents participated an average of only 53.2 times per year, or about once a week. This frequency of exercise is definitely well below the threshold required for the development of physical fitness. Only one out of ten respondents reported participating four or more times per week and 27 percent of all respondents indicated that they never participate in sports or physical fitness activities.

The *Sports Illustrated* pollsters provided a list of 34 activities ranging from very light energy expenditure to very vigorous. Table 1.1 illustrates those activities and the percentage of respondents reporting to have participated in each.

Plausible conclusions from all of the surveys dating back to the 1960s indicate that there has been a relative and consistent upward trend in the number of adults participating in sports and fitness activities in the last two decades. The fitness movement was spearheaded and continues to be led by persons classified as being in the middle and upper socioeconomic strata.[23] There are more men than women involved in vigorous activity and participation declines steadily with age.[22]

It is also obvious that most Americans are unaware of the proper intensity, frequency, and duration of exercise needed for the development of cardiorespiratory endurance. Furthermore, many respondents participate in activities that are perceived by them as being fitness activities but which in reality, contribute either minimally or not at all to the components of fitness, such as fishing, softball, bowling, pool, and billiards.[24] In fact, only 10 percent of those who exercise "meet the requirements believed to prevent heart disease."[25]

The jogging/running craze has moderated to some extent in the last couple of years. The number of active joggers is estimated at approximately 25 million people.[26] The Brook's study showed jogging to be the third most popular fitness activity following swimming and cycling.[27] However, when all activities were compared on the basis of frequency of participation, jogging ranked number one.

TABLE 1.1.   Frequency of Participation by Activity/Sport for a 12-Month Period

Activity	Percent of Respondents Participating	Activity	Percent of Respondents Participating
Swimming	48%	Tennis	11%
Bicycling	37	Water skiing	10
Fishing	35	Snow skiing	9
Jogging	30	Horseback riding	9
Calisthenics/ Aerobics	30	Roller skating	9
Using exercise machines	30	Squash/Racquetball	7
Baseball/ Softball	28	Ice skating	
Bowling	23	Sailing	5
Hiking/Backpacking	23	Soccer	4
Pool/Billiards	22	Wrestling	4
Weight lifting	21	Snorkeling/Scuba diving	3
Boating (except sailing)	20	Auto racing	3
Hunting	18	Boxing	3
Volleyball	16	Track and Field meet	2
Basketball	15	Ice hockey	2
Golf	14	Handball	2
Football	13	Marathon running	1

Sports Illustrated, "Sports Poll '86," Time Inc: 1986.

Several popular fitness activities have decreased in the total number of participants from 1984 to 1987 as indicated by Table 1.2.[26] These figures represent shifts in activities believed made by the same people who continue to exercise but change activities frequently. You will observe that aerobics, the fastest growing activity just a couple of years ago, has experienced a decrease of more than a million participants. Racquetball, running, swimming and tennis are all down.

This decline has been offset by increasing participation in other activities. Exercise walking claims to have 58 million devotees, volleyball has increased by 20 percent, basketball is up by 18 percent, and golf is up by 7 percent.

Race directors have indicated that participation in marathon races has declined but this has been neutralized by the increased popularity of 10k races (6.2 miles). This change has no doubt been influenced by the fact that running/jogging injuries increase in prevalence as training mileage increases.[28],[29] Also contributing to the popularity of the 10k races is that less time is required for training and therefore more time can be devoted to family and other interests. In addition, the training mileage required for the 10k race is certainly enough to enhance cardiorespiratory health. Most adults participate in jogging for health enhancement reasons anyway—primarily to prevent heart attack or for weight loss—regardless of whether or not they compete.[23] Race competition is not a prerequisite for health enhancement for fitness, it is simply an option for those who enjoy such pursuits.

The fitness movement is evident everywhere in America. Fitness devotees are ubiquitous as people participate in jogging, swimming, cycling, aerobic dancing, roller and ice skating, skiing, racquetball, tennis, and a variety of other sports and activities. In 1986, Americans spent $1.2 billion for exercise equipment.[30] According to the National Sporting Goods Association, in 1986 Americans spent $424 million on stationary bikes, $217 million on rowing machines, $83 million on treadmills, and $231 million on multipurpose gyms (weight training machines).[30] Accompanying the sale of exercise equipment was the purchase of athletic and sports clothing. We spent a staggering $4 billion dollars on these

TABLE 1.2   Activity Participation 1984–1987

Activity	Participants (in millions)				Percent change 1984–1987
	1984	1985	1986	1987	
Aerobics	24,412	23,925	21,853	23,126	−5.3%
Exercise walking			53,504	58,065	
Exercise with equipment	34,748	32,101	31,996	34,775	0.1
Golf	18,990	18,853	20,022	20,258	6.7
Racquetball	9,987	7,897	7,820	7,867	−21.2
Running	29,539	26,267	23,148	24,832	−15.9
Swimming	74,379	73,266	72,649	66,068	−11.2
Tennis	19,456	18,951	18,017	16,911	−13.1
Basketball	21,194	19,498	21,176	25,065	18.3
Volleyball	19,732	20,127	20,736	23,616	19.7

Adapted from J. Feld, "NSGA Sports Survey," *Club Industry*, 4, no. 12, (Aug. 1988): 20.

sport-related items. In addition, we spent another $3.2 billion on athletic footwear. Outdoor bicycles reached $1.3 billion in sales and this did not include cycling paraphernalia such as shorts, cleated shoes, gloves, helmet, and shirt.

Pulse meters of different types and degrees of sophistication have been developed to monitor the intensity of exercise. Pedometers measure distance telling us how far we have travelled, and skinfold calipers measure the thickness of skin telling us how much fat we have lost.

The interest in physical fitness is also reflected in the increasing amount of literature devoted to promoting health/wellness and physical fitness. Books featuring exercise of all types for fitness purposes have regularly appeared on the best-seller list. Every month popular magazines feature articles on some aspect of exercise and health. Exercise videos have become very popular regardless of the credentials and expertise of the producers of these items.

Sports drinks touted to replace the exercising body's lost nutrients are heavily advertised. It is not uncommon to see athletic teams consuming such beverages during television coverage of their games. Certain foods are hawked as energy foods and vitamin and mineral supplements are sold in large quantities with the promise of enhancing performance.

Some advertising agencies have gone to the extreme in affiliating with the fitness movement. Products that have nothing to do with fitness are advertised using a fitness motif. This is an eloquent commentary by those advertisers who recognize the importance of associating their products, however marginally, with the public's generally positive attitude toward fitness. The object, of course, is to transfer that positive attitude from fitness to the product which is being promoted. Whole new industries have developed around the fitness movement while others have been revitalized. Memberships in health clubs, spas, YMCAs, and so on, have increased or remained steady over the last decade.

In an effort to cut escalating health care costs, many businesses and corporations have turned to fitness and wellness programs. According to the Association for Fitness in Business, American businesses paid out more than $70 billion in health care costs in 1986 and 500 million workdays were lost to illness and disability.[31] To the average person, these numbers are so large that they are incomprehensible.

To better understand the scope of these costs, we may need to look at them from the following perspective: "Ten percent of a company's payroll goes to health insurance, and the health-related expenses of a typical Fortune 500 corporation are equal to 24 percent of its profits.[31] These are significant expenditures which are in need of reduction.

Many companies have instituted fitness and wellness programs in an effort to lower health care costs, and the early data are indeed encouraging. Containing the spiraling cost of health care seems to be worth the effort and the initial expense of developing and implementing the program.

The effects of wellness programs of which physical fitness constitutes but one component cannot be measured overnight. It takes time, effort, and an educational emphasis to change long-standing behavior patterns such as cigarette smoking, overeating, eating a high-fat diet, and following a sedentary lifestyle. However, corporations who have implemented wellness programs have found that health care costs have been reduced, there is less worker absenteeism, there is greater productivity, less worker turnover, and less on-the-job accidents.[32] Having a wellness program with fitness facilities is often used as a perk by corporations to recruit and keep key personnel.

The medical profession has become aware of the importance of regular exercise and the development and maintenance of physical fitness. A growing number of medical schools are offering courses in the physiology of exercise and a number of physicians have expressed the opinion that physicians should be able to prescribe exercise with as much skill as they prescribe medicine.

The attitude of the American public toward exercise is generally positive. Most people feel that exercise is "good for you," although many are not quite sure why or how it is good for you. This is probably one of the reasons why only 10 to 20 percent of the exercisers are working hard enough and often enough to become physically fit. Although the exercise surveys indicate that increasing numbers of people are exercising—and this is a positive trend—a large segment of our society does not participate and a larger segment exercise at a level below that which is required to promote health and fitness. We need to continue to educate the people regarding the importance of an active lifestyle and regular exercise.

The Mechanization of America

The health of nations is more important than the wealth of nations.
—Will Durant

The fitness movement was largely a reaction to developments in science and technology and their relationship to the changing disease and death patterns in the nation. The communicable diseases (tuberculosis, pneumonia, typhoid fever, smallpox, scarlet fever, etc.) were the leading causes of death during the early years of this century. Advances in medical science have virtually eradicated these maladies and threats to life, but they have been replaced by chronic and degenerative diseases such as heart disease, stroke, cancer, diabetes, and so on. This group of diseases is largely lifestyle-induced and has reached epidemic proportions.

Cardiovascular disease accounts for approximately 50 percent of all deaths in the United States.[33] Atherosclerosis, a progressive degenerative disease resulting in narrowed blood vessels, is responsible for most of the heart attack and stroke deaths. The risk factors connected with heart disease were identified by the landmark Framingham Study which began in 1949.[34]

As the risk factors were identified there evolved the realization that heart disease was not the inevitable consequence of aging but an acquired disease that was potentially preventable. Cigarette smoking, high blood pressure, elevated levels of blood fats, diabetes, overweight, stress, lack of exercise, and a family history of heart disease were found to be positively related to heart attack and stroke. Fortunately, most of these risk factors can be modified by the way we live.

Progress and growth are impossible if you always do things the way you've always done things.
—Wayne Dyer

We have within our locus of control the opportunity and the right to choose what to eat and how much, whether or not to smoke cigarettes, whether or not to exercise, and how we control stress. We can choose when to be screened for blood pressure and blood fats and we can choose whether or not to act upon that information. During the last two decades, millions of Americans have changed eating, smoking, and exercise habits and concomitantly deaths from cardiovascular disease declined by approximately 35 percent during this time. Other factors are involved in this favorable trend, but modifications in lifestyle have made their contribution.

Our lives today are considerably different from life in the early years of this century. Scientific and technological advances have made us functionally mechanized. Labor saving devices proliferate all phases of life—our occupations, home life, and leisure time pursuits—always with the promise of more and better to come. Each new invention helped foster a receptive attitude toward a life of ease and we have become enamoured with the easy way of doing things. The mechanized way is generally the most expedient way and in our time-oriented society, this became another stimulus for us to indulge in the sedentary life.

Today, exercise for fitness is contrived; it is programmed into our lives as an entity separate from our other functions. On the other hand, the energy expenditures of our forefathers was integrated and inextricably interwoven into their work, play, and home life. Physical fitness was a necessary commodity and fit people were the rule rather than the exception. Tilling the soil, digging ditches, and working in factories were physically demanding jobs. Lumberjack contests and square dances were vigorous leisure pursuits. Being a wife and taking care of home and family required long hours at arduous tasks. In the early years of this century, much of the energy for operating our factories came from muscle power. By 1970, this figure dropped to less than 1 percent and is reflective of the declining energy demand of our jobs.

The turn of the century found 70 percent of the population working long, hard hours in the production of food. Children of this era walked several miles to school and did chores when they returned home. Today, only 5 percent of the population, using highly mechanized equipment, are involved in the production of food, and their children ride to school. Adults drive to the store, circle the parking lot to get as close as possible to the entrance, and ride elevators and escalators while there. We mow the lawn with a riding mower, play golf in a cart, wash dishes and clothes in appropriate appliances, change television channels with a remote control, open garage doors in the same manner, and so on.

These are simply observations of life in America and are not intended to imply that the fruits of science and technology be repudiated, but rather that their results along with their impact on us be viewed in perspective and acted on accordingly. Mechanization has reached our leisure time and it is in this sphere that we must commit some time to vigorous activity because it has been effectively removed from other areas of life.

John Dryden (1631–1700) recognized the seeds of change two centuries ago and wrote the following:[35]

> *By chase, our long lived fathers earned their food,*
> *Toil strung the nerves and purfied the blood.*
> *But we, their sons, a pampered race of men,*
> *Are dwindled down the three score years and ten,*
> *Better to use your muscles, for health unbought,*
> *Than fee the doctors for a nauseaous draught.*
> *The wise, for cure, on exercise depend,*
> *God never made his work for man to mend.*

Man has inhabited the earth for many centuries but only the last 75 years have generated such drastic changes in lifestyle. Our basic need for physical activity has not changed. Our bodies were constructed for, and thrive, on physical work but we find ourselves thrust into the automobile, television, and sofa age and we simply have not had enough time to adapt to this new sedentary way of living. Perhaps 100,000 years from now the sedentary life will be the healthy life. However, at this stage of our development, the law of use and disuse continues to work, and that which is used becomes stronger and that which is not becomes weaker. For simple verification of this physiological principle, just witness the results of a leg in a cast for eight weeks and note the atrophy that has occurred to the limb during that time.

It is the belief of many people, this author included, that our new ways of living are precipitating or at least significantly contributing to the diseases that are affecting modern affluent man. These diseases are unique to the highly industrialized nations. By contrast, the underdeveloped nations, with their different lifestyles, do not experience this phenomenon to the same extent.

The fitness boom had its roots in this background. The fitness movement that is occurring today started and sputtered several times during this century. World War I draft statistics indicated that many young American males were unfit for military service.[36] This prompted many states to mandate compulsory physical education, emphasizing physical development in the public schools. When the war ended, the emphasis in these programs shifted from physical fitness to sports and games. This scenario was repeated during and after World War II.

During the mid 1950s, a fitness test that was developed for use with clinical patients was administered to normal European and American youngsters. European youngsters scored better on the test (Kraus-Webber test) than American youngsters. This was brought to the attention of President Eisenhower who directed Vice-president Richard Nixon to investigate the problem and upgrade the fitness of American youth. Nixon's representatives contacted the American Association for Health, Physical Education, and Recreation (AAHPER) and together they established the President's Council on Youth Fitness (PCYF).

AAHPER subsequently developed the Youth Fitness Test which has been administered to American youth and national norms have been established from these data. Meanwhile, in an effort to encourage youngsters to pursue vigorous exercise, both organizations established merit awards for fitness. The AAHPER test has been revised in the last few years, and there has been one national administration of the revised test, and two of the original test. According to the results of these tests, the level of fitness of American youngsters has remained stable in the last decade and that level is considered to be sub-par. The President's Council has changed its name and focus since its inception and now encourages exercise for all Americans regardless of age.

The greatest stimulus for an active life, particularly for adults, however, occurred with the publication of Kenneth Cooper's first book entitled *Aerobics.* This text literally started millions of people exercising and Cooper became—and remains—one of this country's leading spokesmen for the benefits of regular physical activity.

Although Cooper did not invent the word "aerobics," he has certainly popularized it. Aerobic exercises include walking, jogging, swimming, cycling, and rope jumping, to name but a few. These activities are performed at a comfortable pace so the participant can meet the energy demand of the exercise on a minute by minute basis for a sustained period of time. These exercises, which employ many large muscles, benefit the cardiorespiratory and muscular systems and significantly impact body composition.

Fitness—Boom or Bust?

The American College of Sports Medicine (ACSM) has established criteria which should be satisfied if exercise is to meet desirable physiological and health related goals.[37] These include the following: the intensity, or vigorousness, of exercise should correspond to 65–90 percent of the maximal heart rate, this heart rate should be maintained for 15 to 60 minutes, and exercise should be pursued three to five days per week. Additionally, the ACSM suggests that beginners select from activities in which the pace can be controlled by the participant, such as walking, jogging, swimming, cycling, skating, and so on. The exerciser can control the pace so as to elicit the training heart rate.

After a period of conditioning, these activities can be supplemented by games and sports for variety. Games and sports are not self-paced. Their intensity is dependent upon the skill level and motivation of the competitors.

When gauged by these criteria, we find first, the results of the various surveys regarding the fitness level of the American public are far from satisfying. The fitness movement has not pervaded all segments of our society. Most of the participants in the movement are young, affluent, and well educated. Second, the activities selected by many proclaimed exercisers, and older respondents in particular, are questionable with respect to meeting the criteria of intensity. Third, the frequency of participation was well below that suggested by the ACSM. However, more Americans are exercising today than at any time during the last 50 years and more are becoming aware of the importance of regular exercise. We have a long way to go, but things are looking up.

SELF-ASSESSMENT
Health/Wellness Inventory[38]

Directions

For each question in the Personal Inventory Table (Table 1.3), circle the number which most closely applies to your behavior according to the following:

  5   if the statement is ALWAYS true
  4   if the statement is FREQUENTLY true
  3   if the statement is OCCASIONALLY true
  2   if the statement is SELDOM true
  1   if the statement is NEVER true

After completing the inventory, enter the numbers you have circled next to the question number in Table 1.4, and total your score for each category. Finally, refer to the section entitled "Wellness Status" to determine your degree of wellness.

Wellness Status

To assess your status in each of the six categories, compare your total score in each to the following key:

  0–34   In need of substantial improvement
  35–44   Good, but some improvement is desirable
  45–50   Excellent. You are doing very well.

Those who are in need of improvement should carefully examine their scores in each category and target one or two areas for improvement and work on those. Do not become overly ambitious and try to change everything at once because this strategy will not work.

TABLE 1.3   Personal Inventory

Situation		Score			
1. I am able to identify the situations and factors that overstress me.	5	④	3	2	1
2. I eat only when I am hungry.	5	④	3	2	1
3. I don't take tranquilizers or other drugs to relax.	⑤	4	3	2	1
4. I support efforts in my community to reduce environmental pollution.	5	④	3	2	1
5. I avoid buying foods with artificial colorings.	5	4	3	②	1
6. I rarely have problems concentrating on what I'm doing because of worrying about other things.	5	4	③	2	1
7. My employer (school) takes measures to ensure that my work (study) place is safe.	5	4	③	2	1
8. I try not to use medications when I feel unwell.	5	④	3	2	1
9. I am able to identify certain bodily responses and illnesses as my reactions to stress.	5	④	3	2	1
10. I question the use of diagnostic x-rays.	5	4	③	2	1
11. I try to alter personal living habits that are risk factors for heart disease, cancer, and other lifestyle diseases.	5	④	3	2	1
12. I avoid taking sleeping pills to help me sleep.	⑤	4	3	2	1
13. I try not to eat foods with refined sugar or corn sugar ingredients.	5	④	3	2	1
14. I accomplish goals I set for myself.	5	4	③	2	1
15. I stretch or bend for several minutes each day to keep my body flexible.	⑤	4	3	2	1
16. I support immunization of all children for common childhood diseases.	⑤	4	3	2	1
17. I try to prevent friends from driving after they drink alcohol.	⑤	4	3	2	1
18. I minimize extra salt intake.	⑤	4	3	2	1
19. I don't mind when other people and situations make me wait or lose time.	5	4	3	2	①
20. I walk four or fewer flights of stairs rather than take the elevator.	5	4	3	②	1
21. I eat fresh fruit and vegetables.	5	④	3	2	1
22. I use dental floss at least once a day.	5	4	③	2	1
23. I read product labels on foods to determine their ingredients.	5	④	3	2	1
24. I try to maintain a normal body weight.	⑤	4	3	2	1
25. I record my feelings and thoughts in a journal or diary.	5	4	③	2	1
26. I have no difficulty falling asleep.	5	4	③	2	1
27. I engage in some form of vigorous physical activity at least three times a week.	⑤	4	3	2	1
28. I take time each day to quiet my mind and relax.	5	④	3	2	1
29. I am willing to make and sustain close friendships and intimate relationships.	5	4	③	2	1
30. I obtain an adequate daily supply of vitamins from my food or vitamin supplements.	5	④	3	2	1
31. I rarely have tension or migraine headaches, or pain in the neck or shoulders.	5	4	3	②	1
32. I wear a safety belt when driving.	⑤	4	3	2	1
33. I am aware of the emotional and situational factors that lead me to overeat.	5	④	3	2	1
34. I avoid driving my car after drinking any alcohol.	5	4	③	2	1
35. I am aware of the side effects of the medicines I take.	5	④	3	2	1
36. I am able to accept feelings of sadness, depression, and anxiety, knowing that they are almost always transient.	5	④	3	2	1
37. I would seek several additional professional opinions if my doctor recommended surgery for me.	5	4	③	2	1
38. I agree that nonsmokers should not have to breathe the smoke from cigarettes in public places.	⑤	4	3	2	1
39. I agree that pregnant women who smoke harm their babies.	⑤	4	3	2	1
40. I feel I get enough sleep.	5	4	③	2	1
41. I ask my doctor why a certain medication is being prescribed and inquire about alternatives.	5	4	③	2	1
42. I am aware of the calories expended in my activities.	5	④	3	2	1

Situation	Score
43. I am willing to give priority to my own needs for time and psychological space by saying "no" to others' request of me.	5 4 3 2 1
44. I walk instead of drive whenever feasible.	5 4 3 2 1
45. I eat a breakfast that contains about one-third of my daily need for calories, proteins, and vitamins.	5 4 3 2 1
46. I prohibit smoking in my home.	5 4 3 2 1
47. I remember and think about my dreams.	5 4 3 2 1
48. I seek medical attention only when I have symptoms or feel that some (potential) condition needs checking, rather than have routine yearly checkups.	5 4 3 2 1
49. I endeavor to make my home accident free.	5 4 3 2 1
50. I ask my doctor to explain the diagnosis of my problem until I understand all that I care to.	5 4 3 2 1
51. I try to include fiber or roughage (whole grains, fresh fruits and vegetables, or bran) in my diet.	5 4 3 2 1
52. I can deal with my emotional problems without alcohol or other mood-altering drugs.	5 4 3 2 1
53. I am satisfied with my school/work.	5 4 3 2 1
54. I require children riding in my car to be in infant seats or in shoulder harnesses.	5 4 3 2 1
55. I try to associate with people who have a positive attitude about life.	5 4 3 2 1
56. I try not to eat snacks of candy, pastries, and other "junk" food.	5 4 3 2 1
57. I avoid people who are "down" all the time and bring down those around them.	5 4 3 2 1
58. I am aware of the calorie content of the foods I eat.	5 4 3 2 1
59. I brush my teeth after meals.	5 4 3 2 1
60. (for women only) I routinely examine my breasts.	5 4 3 2 1
(for men only) I am aware of the signs of testicular cancer.	5 4 3 2 1

TABLE 1.4 Wellness Category Scores

Emotional Health	Fitness and Body Care	Environmental Health	Stress	Nutrition	Medical Self-responsibility
6. ____	15. ____	4. ____	1. ____	2. ____	8. ____
12. ____	20. ____	7. ____	3. ____	5. ____	10. ____
25. ____	22. ____	17. ____	9. ____	13. ____	11. ____
26. ____	24. ____	32. ____	14. ____	18. ____	16. ____
36. ____	27. ____	34. ____	19. ____	21. ____	35. ____
40. ____	33. ____	38. ____	28. ____	23. ____	37. ____
47. ____	42. ____	39. ____	29. ____	30. ____	41. ____
52. ____	44. ____	46. ____	31. ____	45. ____	48. ____
55. ____	58. ____	49. ____	43. ____	51. ____	50. ____
57. ____	59. ____	54. ____	53. ____	56. ____	60. ____
Total ____	____	____	____	____	____

POINTS TO PONDER

1. *What are the components of performance-related fitness? Health-related fitness?*
2. *Are the two types of fitness mutually exclusive? Explain.*
3. *Trace the history of the current fitness movement and identify some of the major contributing forces.*

Chapter Highlights

Wellness is a positive approach to health that emphasizes self-responsibility. It is a continuous process of striving for personal well-being—a concept that is increasingly important because today's leading causes of death are lifestyle induced. The adherence to simple health practices results in a healthier body and a longer life.

Physical fitness has been a topic of interest for centuries, but its systematic study did not begin in earnest until the twentieth century. Physical fitness consists of a number of components which are categorized as either health related or performance related.

Physical fitness is an integral part of a wellness lifestyle and fit people present physical profiles that are synonymous with robust health. In general, active people are leaner, have lower levels of blood fats, lower blood pressure, handle stress more effectively, and smoke less than inactive people.

The fitness movement was spurred by developments in science and technology and their relationship to the changing disease and death patterns of the nation.

Additionally, significant impetus came from organizations who have an interest in the fitness, health, and wellness of the American people. Data from both global wars as well as comparisons between the fitness level of American and European youth produced results that were less than desirable.

The current fitness movement has been dynamic and evolving. It appears to have a strong base of support in the United States and will probably continue for many years. From all indications, it appears as though the fitness movement will endure to embarrass and confound the predictors of its demise. Fitness is in! The trend is toward good health, and the attainment of fitness is an integral part of it. People from all walks of life, from the known to the unknown, have joined (and a few have led) the movement. Physical fitness is perceived not only as necessary for good health, but it is also good business. People in highly visible occupations pursue fitness for its health-related benefits as well as for the positive image it projects. Trim and fit people are looked upon more favorably than fat and unfit people. Celebrities are eager to discuss their exercise programs on talk shows and they write books on fitness, diet, and the ramifications of both for health. Unfortunately, most of them do not have formal training at an accredited institution of higher learning in exercise science or nutrition and have promoted some misinformation as a result.

References

1. G. Edlin and E. Golanty, *Health and Wellness—A Holistic Approach*, Boston: Jones and Bartlett Publishers, 1988, p. 6.

2. J. Grossman, "Inside the Wellness Movement," *Annual Editions Health 83/84*, Guilford, Ct: The Dushkin Publishing Group, Inc., 1983.

3. *Healthy People: The Surgeon General's Report on Health Promotion and Disease Prevention*, Washington, D.C.: U.S. Government Printing Office, 1979.

4. *Orthopedics Today* 1, no. 4 (Reprint,) July-August, 1981.

5. *Healthy People: The Surgeon General's Report On Health Promotion and Disease Prevention*, Washington, D.C.: U.S. Government Printing Office, 1979.

6. "U.S. Health Care Bill $943 Per Person in 1979," *President's Council on Physical Fitness and Sports Newsletter*, Dec. 1980, p. 8.

7. "The Slow Costly Death of Mrs. K," *Harper's Magazine*, 268, 160B (March, 1984): 84.

8. U.S. Department of Commerce. *Statistical Abstracts of the U.S.*, Washington, D.C.: U.S. Government Printing Office, 1988.

9. G. Sheehan, "Living With Style," *The Physician and Sportsmedicine 11, (1983): 65.*

10. L. Breslow, "A Quantitative Approach to the World Health Organization Definition of Health: Physical, Mental, and Social Well-Being," *International Journal of Epidemiology* 1, (1972): 347; L. Breslow, "A Policy Assessment of Preventive Health Practice," *Preventive Medicine* 6 (1977): 242; N.B. Belloc, and L. Breslow, "Relationship of Physical Health Status and Health Practices," *Preventive Medicine* 1 (1972): 409.

11. D. L. Wingard et al., "A Multivariate Analysis of Health-Related Practices: A Nine-Year Mortality Follow-Up of the Alameda County Study," *American Journal of Epidemiology* 116, (1982): 765.

12. G. Sheehan, "Living With Style," 65.

13. C. A. Lambert et al., "Risk Factors and Lifestyle: A Statewide Health-Interview Survey," *New England Journal of Medicine* 306 (1982): 1048.

14. D. B. Ardell, and M. Tager, Planning for Wellness, Dubuque, Iowa: Kendall/Hunt Publishing Co., 1982.

15. "Definition of Physical Fitness," *Journal of Physical Education and Recreation* 50, (Oct., 1979): 28.

16. H. B. Falls et al., *Essentials of Fitness*, Philadelphia: Saunders College, 1980, p. 20.

17. D. E. Cundiff and P. Brynteson, *Health Fitness—Guide to a Life-Style*, Dubuque, Iowa: Kendall/Hunt Publishing Co., 1979.

18. Falls et al., *Essentials of Fitness;* Cundiff and Brynteson, *Health Fitness;* B. Getchell, *Physical Fitness: A Way of Life*, New York: John Wiley and Sons, 1983; R.V. Hockey, *Physical Fitness*, St. Louis, Mo.: The C.V. Mosley Co., 1981; W.P. Marley, *Health and Physical Fitness*, Philadelphia: Saunders College Publishing, 1982; B. J. Sharkey, *Physiology of Fitness*, Champaign, Ill.: Human Kinetics Publishers, 1979.

19. "Perrier Study: Fitness In America," New York: Perrier Great Water of France, Inc., 1979.

20. W. L. Haskell, H.J. Montoye, and D. Orenstein, "Physical Activity and Exercise to Achieve Health-Related Physical Fitness Benefits," *Public Health Reports*, 100 (1985): 202.

21. C. A. Schoenborn, "Health Habits of U.S. Adults 1985: The "Alameda 7" Revisited," *Public Health Reports*, 101 (1986): 571.

22. *Sports Illustrated*, "Sports Poll '86," Time, Inc., 1986.

23. S. N. Blair, R. T. Mulder and H. W. Kohl, "Reaction to 'Secular Trends In Adult Physical Activity: Exercise Boom or Bust?'," *Research Quarterly for Exercise and Sport*, 58, (1987): 106.

24. K. Simmons, "The Federal Government: Keeping Tabs on the Nation's Fitness," *The Physician and Sportsmedicine*, 15, (January, 1987): 190.

25. C. Cinque, "Are Americans Fit? Survey Data Conflict," *The Physician and Sportsmedicine*, 14, (November, 1986).

26. J. Feld, "NSGA Sports Survey," *Club Industry*, 4, (Aug., 1988): 20.

27. C. M. Brooks, "Adult Participation in Physical Activities Requiring Moderate to High Levels of Energy Expenditure," *The Physician and Sportsmedicine*, 15, (1987): 118.

28. J. P. Koplan et al., "An Epidemiological Study of the Benefits and Risks of Running," *Journal of the American Medical Association*, 248 (1982): 3118.

29. S. N. Blair, "Risk Factors and Running Injuries," *Medicine and Science in Sports and Exercise*, 17, (1985): XII.

30. C. Schaefer, ''The Price You'll Pay to Sweat,'' *Changing Times*, 41, (Aug., 1987): 38.

31. P. Gambaccini, ''The Bottom Line on Fitness,'' *Runner's World*, 66 (July, 1987).

32. AFB, ''American Business Gets Fit,'' *Business Week*, 1, (Oct. 7, 1985).

33. American Heart Association, *Heart Facts*, Dallas, Texas: 1988.

34. W.B. Kannell, and others, ''Epidemiology of Acute Myocardial Infarction: The Framingham Study,'' *Medicine Today*, 2, (1968): 50.

35. L.J. Frankel and B.B. Richard, *Be Alive As Long As You Live*, Charleston, W. Va.: Preventicare Publications, 1977.

36. G.F. Anderson, ''A Period of Projects 1955–1980,'' *Journal of Physical Education, Recreation and Dance*, 56, (1985): 72.

37. American College of Sports Medicine. *Guidelines For Exercise Testing and Prescription*, (3rd Edition), Philadelphia: Lea and Fabiger, 1986.

38. Adapted from G. Edlin and E. Golanty, *Health and Wellness*, p. 6.

2

Cardiovascular Disease

Mini Glossary

Aorta: largest artery in the body.

a-vO₂ difference: the amount of oxygen in the venous blood subtracted from the oxygen in arterial blood. This represents the extraction rate of oxygen by the tissues of the body.

Atherosclerosis: a progressive disease which results in the narrowing of arterial channels caused by the build-up of plaque.

Blood platelets: blood cells that are involved in preventing blood loss. They are important components in clot formation.

Cardiovascular diseases: diseases of the heart and blood vessels.

Cerebrovascular accidents: diseases of the blood vessels to the brain or in the brain which result in a stroke.

Congenital heart disease: heart defects which exist at birth and occur when the heart or its structures or the blood vessels near the heart fail to develop normally before birth.

Erythrocytes: the red blood cells that transport oxygen from the lungs to the various tissues of the body and carbon dioxide from the tissues to the lungs.

Hemoglobin: the protein molecule to which oxygen and carbon dioxide attach for transport by the erythrocytes.

Hypertension: medical term for high blood pressure.

Leukocytes: white blood cells that protect the body against invading microorganisms and remove dead cells and debris from the body.

Myocardial infarction: a heart attack. The term literally means "death of heart muscle."

Myocardium: heart muscle.

Introduction

In this chapter you will be introduced to how and why the death and disease patterns in the United States have changed. Infectious diseases have given way to the chronic diseases. **Cardiovascular disease,** the foremost of the chronic diseases, is the number one killer of Americans. This chapter will focus upon (1) the basics of circulation, (2) pediatric origins of cardiovascular disease, and (3) the signs and symptoms of heart disease. The following chapter will concentrate upon the risk factors associated with cardiovascular disease and how some of those factors can be modified through appropriate behavior with special emphasis placed upon the role of exercise.

Changing Patterns of Disease and Death

Infectious diseases such as smallpox, influenza, diphtheria, polio, whooping cough, tuberculosis, and tetanus have been either eradicated or effectively controlled through advances in medical science, improved nutritional practices, better sanitation, and a higher standard of living. Today the leading causes of death and disability are lifestyle in nature: heart disease, cancer, stroke, cirrhosis of the liver, and diabetes. Among the young, accidents, suicide, and homicide are among the leading causes of death. When considering these leading causes of death, it becomes apparent that some can be reduced by a physically active way of life while others can not.

There is an abundance of research, both ongoing and completed, regarding the effects of exercise upon the risk factors and incidence of heart disease. This is particularly appropriate since heart disease is the leading cause of death in the United States and other industrialized countries. Exercise, as part of a multifaceted program, can make a significant contribution to the prevention of heart disease. In addition, it has been shown to be an important tool in after-the-fact rehabilitation.

Cardiovascular disease is the leading cause of death in the United States accounting for 47 percent of all deaths.[1] One in four Americans, or 66 million people, have one or more forms of heart or blood vessel disease. It is estimated that 1,500,000 heart attacks, more than 500,000 of them fatal, will occur in 1989. Five percent of these will occur to people under the age of 40, and 45 percent will occur to people under the age of 65. Strokes, another form of cardiovascular disease, will kill approximately 150,000 Americans during the same year.

While these data are ominous and there is much that remains to be done in the battle against cardiovascular disease, some headway has been made. The death rate from all cardiovascular diseases declined approximately 23 percent from 1976 to 1986.[1] During this same period, deaths from coronary heart disease, which is responsible for the majority of deaths from heart attacks, declined by 28 percent. Deaths from strokes declined by about 40 percent during the same time period. Most authorities attribute the decline in the death rate from cardiovascular disease to lifestyle changes and more sophisticated medical diagnosis and treatment. Lifestyle behaviors, those factors that are under our control, which have contributed to improving the cardiovascular status of the nation include (1) more people exercising, (2) healthy changes in nutritional habits, (3) reduction in cigarette smoking, (4) awareness of the importance of blood pressure screening and control, (5) attempts to manage stress in positive ways, and (6) weight management.

The Basics of Circulation

The Heart and Blood Vessels

The basic anatomy and function of the heart must be grasped, at least in an elementary way, in order to understand circulation and the consequences if the natural order is interrupted. The circulatory system consists of the heart and blood vessels. The heart, a muscular organ made up of specialized cardiac muscle, weighs between eight and ten ounces. About the size of a fist, it lies slightly to the left of center in the chest. The heart is a four-chambered hollow organ whose muscular wall or **myocardium** (*myo*: muscle; *cardium*: heart) is surrounded by a fiberlike bag, the pericardium (*peri*: around) and lined by a strong thin membrane, the endocardium (*endo*: inner). Figure 2.1 shows the various structures of the heart.

The heart is divided into two halves by a wall (the septum) and each half is divided into an upper chamber (the atrium) and a lower chamber (the ventricle). The flow of blood entering and exiting the heart is regulated by valves located between the chambers, the aorta, and the pulmonary artery.

The heart is a double pump. The right heart or "pulmonary pump" (*pulmonary*: lungs) has the singular task of transporting deoxygenated blood to the

FIGURE 2.1

**Gross Anatomy of the
Interior of the Heart**

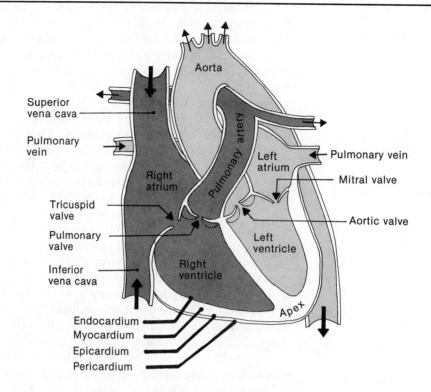

lungs where it can exchange carbon dioxide for a fresh supply of oxygen. From the lungs, the oxygen-rich blood is circulated to the left heart or "systemic pump" (*systemic*: system or body) so that it can be sent to all of the tissues of the body (see Figure 2.2).

The tissues extract their oxygen requirements and in exchange, give up their waste products (principally carbon dioxide) to the blood. The blood, now carrying a reduced oxygen load and an increased amount of carbon dioxide, returns to the right heart where the cycle begins again. Both pumps work simultaneously and continuously. The left pump, which circulates blood throughout the entire body and therefore carries the heavier workload, has a thicker and stronger ventricular wall.

Blood leaves the left heart via the **aorta,** the largest artery in the body. From here it travels through conduits of muscular vessels called arteries. The arteries subdivide into arterioles (the smallest arteries), which eventually empty into the smallest of blood vessels, the capillaries. In the capillaries, oxygen, nutrients, and hormones in the blood are exchanged for waste products from the tissues. The capillaries are so tiny that blood cells pass through them in single file. The arterial and venous systems are joined together by the capillary network. The venules (smallest veins) emanate from these tiny vessels and empty into the veins, allowing the removal of metabolic wastes from the tissues. Providing a constant supply of fuel to the cells while removing their wastes is the principal job of the circulatory system. When red oxygenated blood leaves the left ventricle and courses down the arterial network, it contains 19 milliliters of oxygen (ml O_2) in each 100 ml of blood. The tissues at rest extract about 5 ml O_2 so that the bluish venous

FIGURE 2.2

Circulation of the Pulmonary and Systemic Pumps

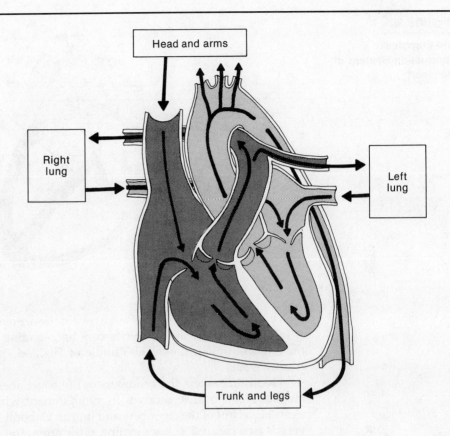

Head and arms

Right lung

Left lung

Trunk and legs

blood that returns to the right atrium contains 14 ml of O_2 per 100 ml of blood. This is called the **arterio-venous oxygen difference (a-vO_2 diff.)** and represents the tissue extraction rate. The oxygen extraction rate increases significantly during vigorous exercise.

The heart's failure to pump blood for a few minutes can be catastrophic. Under usual circumstances, oxygen deprivation for as little as four minutes can destroy the ability of the brain to function normally and it may lead to death. The heart is so vitally important that nature has attempted to protect it by locating it behind the breastbone, encircling it with the ribs and surrounding it with a tough multiple membrane, the pericardium. Fluid between the membranes cushions the heart from trauma and reduces friction as the heart beats against the breastbone and the diaphragm.

At rest, the heart's pumping rate averages between 70 and 80 beats per minute. There is some variance from the average, as endurance athletes often have resting rates in the 30s and 40s while some overweight, sedentary smokers have resting rates in the 90s. Fifty to 100 beats per minute is considered normal by physicians but they have recognized in the last few years that the low heart rates of endurance athletes are adaptations to training and represent normal values for this group.

The heart's beating rate is established by its pacemaker, the sinoatrial node (SA Node), shown in Figure 2.3. The electrical stimulus that causes the heart to contract originates in the SA Node. The atria contract and force blood into

**The Electrical
Conduction System of
the Heart**

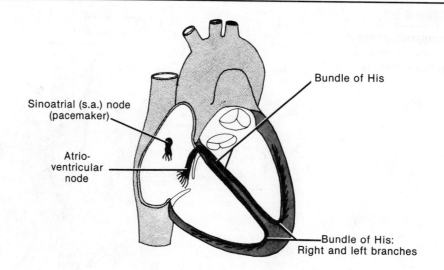

Sinoatrial (s.a.) node
(pacemaker)

Atrio-
ventricular
node

Bundle of His

Bundle of His:
Right and left branches

the ventricles while the impulse travels to the atrioventricular node (AV Node). A split second later the ventricles contract, sending blood through the body as the impulse travels down the Bundle of His and spreads throughout the ventricular walls.

Blood that enters the chambers of the heart does not directly nourish heart muscle. Heart muscle receives its nourishment when the heart contracts and ejects blood out of the chambers and into an elaborate network of coronary blood vessels (see Figure 2.4). Originating at the aorta, the coronary arteries lie around the surface of the heart like a crown and supply the heart muscle with its nutrient needs. The left coronary artery carries the larger volume of blood supplying the cells of the left atrium and ventricle as well as a portion of the right ventricle. The right coronary artery supplies the right atrium and the remainder of the right ventricle. These major vessels divide downstream and eventually culminate in a very dense network of capillaries that is structured precisely so that at least one capillary services each of the heart's muscle fibers. The coronary veins return deoxygenated blood to the right atrium.

The Blood

Plasma, a clear yellowish fluid which carries approximately 100 chemicals, constitutes about 55 percent of the blood. The other 45 percent is made up of several types of cells that are suspended in the plasma. These include the **red cells (erythrocytes), white cells (leukocytes),** and **blood platelets.** The red cells, which represent the majority of blood cells, carry oxygen and carbon dioxide to and from the tissues of the body. **Hemoglobin,** which is the iron-containing protein of the red cells, combines with and transports oxygen to the tissues. The white cells are the body's defense mechanism against invading microorganisms and are actively engaged in combating bacterial infections and other foreign substances that invade the body. The blood platelets are involved in the process of clotting and repair of damaged blood vessels.

FIGURE 2.4

Coronary Circulation

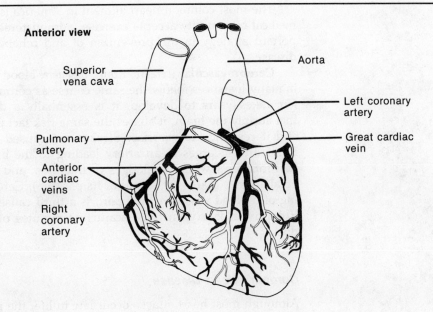

Anterior view

Superior vena cava

Aorta

Left coronary artery

Pulmonary artery

Great cardiac vein

Anterior cardiac veins

Right coronary artery

Cardiovascular Disease: The Twentieth Century Epidemic

Cardiovascular disease is a phenomenon of this century. The reasons advanced for this unfortunate occurrence relate to the living habits discussed in Chapter 1. There are several types of cardiovascular disease.

Congenital heart diseases, which are more accurately labeled as congenital heart defects, exist at birth and result when the heart and its structures or the blood vessels near the heart fail to develop normally before birth. Approximately 25,000 infants are affected annually and 6000 of these die from their defects. Medical scientists are not sure of the causes but it appears that maternal drug and alcohol abuse are implicated. Viral infections may also interfere with the normal development of the heart during uterine life. Many congenital defects can be identified and corrected as a result of new diagnostic methods and sophisticated surgical techniques.

Rheumatic heart disease affects youngsters between the ages of 5 and 15. This form of heart disease is virtually 100 percent preventable because it progresses through a series of stages initiated by a streptococcal infection. The first phase is usually a strep throat and sometimes a strep ear. Antibiotic treatment at this stage will arrest the infection and prevent the possibility of developing rheumatic heart disease.

Congestive heart failure occurs when the heart muscle is unable to contract with sufficient force to effectively pump blood throughout the body. The major causes are high blood pressure, atherosclerosis, heart attack, rheumatic fever, and birth defects. Treatment centers upon drug therapy, including diuretics to remove excess fluid and medication to increase the heart's contractile power.

Exercise makes no contribution to the prevention of congenital or rheumatic heart disease, but it exerts a preventive or delaying effect upon some of the processes that produce congestive heart failure.

The most common heart ailment in America is coronary heart disease. The medical community accepts exercise, administered in proper doses, as an important strategy in the prevention of and rehabilitation from coronary heart disease.

Cerebrovascular (*cerebro*: brain; *vascular*: blood vessels) accidents or strokes in many instances follow the same course as coronary heart disease. The problem takes years to develop, it is essentially a disease of the blood vessels that supply the brain, it shares the same risk factors as coronary heart disease, and it responds to exercise. Strokes are caused by a thrombus (a clot that forms and enlarges in an artery leading to the brain), or an embolus (a clot that forms elsewhere, dislodges or fractures, and circulates to one of the cerebral arteries that is too small for its passage). Cerebral hemorrhage, the bursting of a blood vessel in the brain, is a third cause of stroke. Brain tissue dies if deprived of oxygen for a scant few minutes of time, just as heart muscle does.

Coronary Heart Disease

Although most heart attacks occur late in life, the processes which cause them begin quite early—often prior to adolescence. These processes are insidious and often undetected until, without warning, a heart attack occurs. The attack is sudden but the processes are long-standing.

Coronary heart disease is actually a disease of the coronary blood vessels which supply the heart with oxygen and nutrients. A heart attack or **myocardial infarction** (death of heart muscle tissue) occurs when obstructions or spasms disrupt the flow of blood to a portion of the heart muscle. The loca- of the obstruction or spasm determines the extent of muscle damage. Heart attacks of any magnitude result in irreversible injury and myocardial tissue death. The necrosed tissue forms a scar, contributes no further to the function of the heart and results in a less efficient pump. If the heart attack causes extensive muscle damage, the heart will die and of course, so too will its host.

Heart Attacks in the A.M.

Is there a time of day when heart attacks are more likely to occur? One study has found that people who have coronary heart disease or those who exhibit the risk factors for coronary heart disease have a greater likelihood of suffering sudden cardiac death between 6:00 A.M. and noon. The hour where the greatest incidence of fatal heart attacks occurs is ten to eleven in the morning. The reasons given for this phenomenon include morning increases in hormone levels, blood pressure, and artery tone (persistent contraction of the arterial muscles). Arteries are more constricted in the morning and arterial spasms are more likely to occur in constricted arteries. What about morning exercise? The researchers stated that the risk of sudden death during exercise is very slight and the long-term benefits of regular exercise far outweigh the risk. But they caution that people who suffer from cardiovascular disease might want to give some consideration to the time of day that they exercise.

Adapted from J. E. Muller et al., "Circadian Variation in the Frequency of Sudden Cardiac Death," *Circulation* 75 (January, 1987): 131.

Pediatric Origins: The Silent Phase

The risk factors connected with heart disease were identified in the Framingham Study which began in 1949.[2] This landmark study included more than 5000 residents of Framingham, Massachusetts who were essentially free of coronary disease at the study's inception. Researchers carefully monitored these people for many years as Framingham literally became a "town in a test tube." Gradually the pieces of the puzzle—the risk factors for coronary heart disease—were identified and there evolved the realization that heart disease was not the inevitable consequence of aging but an acquired disease that was potentially preventable. Cigarette smoking, high blood pressure, elevated level of cholesterol, diabetes, overweight, stress, lack of exercise, and a family history of heart disease were found to be highly related to heart attack and stroke.

Investigators have recently turned their attention to the prevalence of the risk factors among children and adolescents and have discovered some alarming facts. Abnormal changes in the coronary arteries, noncongenital in origin, have been identified by autopsy in newborn children through adolescents.[3,4] A survey of 1500 fourth- and fifth-grade students in California indicated that 25 percent had high levels of cholesterol (a harmful substance circulating in the blood), 24 percent had high blood pressure, 32 percent were obese, and 27 percent had a fair or poor heart rate recovery after exercise. The average level of blood cholesterol for the entire group was 200 mg/100 ml (read as 200 milligrams of cholesterol per 100 milliliters of blood), which is significantly higher than the recommended 140 mg/100 ml for this age.

An autopsy study of 18 year olds showed a positive correlation between blood cholesterol levels and the presence of fatty streaks in the coronary arteries and aorta.[5] Some authorities have suggested that a cholesterol level of 110 mg/100 dL of blood is optimal during childhood. The evidence indicates that in overfed, underexercised societies as our own, the average child cholesterol level is 160 mg/100 dL. Children, age 5 to 12, whose percentage of body fat increased over a five-year period developed higher total cholesterol levels than their leaner cohorts during the same period.[6] Cholesterol and triglyceride (another blood fat) testing should begin at 2 to 5 years of age and dietary fat modification is indicated when a child's cholesterol value exceeds 170 mg/100 dL on two successive tests.[7]

A recent poll by the Gallup Organization of youngsters ages 12 to 17 indicated that the majority of these respondents were aware of the importance of eating a healthy diet but they actually practiced poor eating behavior.[8] Ninety-four percent of this group indicated that they were aware of the importance of diet in cholesterol control, but fewer than half of them stated that they tried to avoid high-cholesterol foods.

High blood pressure or **hypertension** (medical term for high blood pressure) has been reported in children as young as three years of age although the tendency for elevated blood pressure may be established earlier. Approximately 2 percent of the nation's elementary school children have persistently high blood pressures. The National Heart, Lung, and Blood Institute has proposed blood pressure guidelines for youngsters which are illustrated in Table 2.1. These are based on nine studies which have a combined total of 70,000 child and adolescent subjects.[9] Authorities are in general agreement that blood pressure levels tend to "track" into adulthood, that is, adolescents whose blood pressures are high are more likley to become hypertensive adults.

On the average, about a fourth of teenager's total daily energy intake comes from snacks.
—M. A. Boyle
E. N. Whitney

TABLE 2.1   Guidelines for Hypertension in Children

Age Group	Significant Hypertension (mmHg)	Severe Hypertension (mmHg)
1 month–2 years	112/74	118/82
3–5 years	116/76	124/84
6–9 years	122/78	130/86
10–12 years	126/82	134/90
13–15 years	136/86	144/92
16–18 years	142/92	150/98

The pharmacologic and behavioral processes that determine tobacco addiction (nicotine addiction) are similar to those that determine addiction to drugs such as heroin and cocaine.
—Surgeon General's report on Nicotine Addiction, 1988

The daily use of cigarettes by high school seniors declined by 35 percent between 1976 and 1985.[10] However, 18.7 percent of high school seniors continue to smoke cigarettes on a daily basis. During that time period, cigarette smoking among teen-age females was slightly higher than that of same age males. Smokeless tobacco usage increased substantially, 8.2 percent, among 17- to 19-year-old men in 1986.

It is estimated that one in five children between the ages of 5 and 17 are substantially overweight, that is, they are a minimum of 20 percent above their desirable weight.[11] Twenty years ago the incidence of child and adolescent obesity was 40 percent less than it is today. More than half of hypertensive children are obese. High levels of blood cholesterol and the predisposition to diabetes mellitus co- exist with childhood obesity. Obese children grow at an accelerated rate maturing faster than lean children and enter puberty sooner. Puberty signals an end to the growth of the long bones of the legs therefore early puberty means that fat children are often shorter as adults. Children who are hypertensive, and/or hypercholesterolemic, and/or cigarette smokers, and/or obese are more likely to carry these risks into adulthood.

These data demonstrate rather convincingly that the risk factors for coronary heart disease appear at a very young age. This suggests that programs of prevention and/or intervention should be started early in life to initiate a reduction in the incidence of premature disease and death. In the last 15 years, lifestyle changes made primarily by middle-aged males have contributed to reducing the death rate from heart attack. If similar changes can be instituted at an earlier age the disease and death rate from heart attack would be reduced further. Autopsy studies of U.S. combat troops who fought in Korea and Vietnam magnify the early development of coronary disease and at the same time show a decline in its incidence during the intervening years between the two encounters. Seventy-seven percent of the U.S. combat casualties in Korea had detectable coronary artery disease and a small percentage of them displayed complete occlusion (blockage) of one of the major arteries.[12] The average age of these soldiers was 22. By comparison, autopsies performed on same-age native Korean combat troops revealed no similar coronary damage. Approximately 18 years later, an autopsy study was completed on U.S. combat troops who died in the Vietnamese War.[13] The incidence of coronary artery disease in these troops (average age of 22) was substantially lower when compared to the U.S. casualties in the Korean conflict. Less than 50 percent of these casualties showed signs of coronary artery disease. The reductions observed during the Vietnamese campaign were paralleled in the general population in the U.S. While the trend of these data is encouraging, the facts indicate that the processes leading to coronary heart disease and death remain appallingly high. Both of these studies depict the insidious time course of a silent disease that begins early in life and usually takes many years to produce overt symptoms.

Atherosclerosis

Atherosclerosis is a slow progressive disease of the arteries that often has its origins in childhood. The atherosclerotic process begins when the arterial lining becomes roughened and acts as an anchoring point for the deposit of fat, fibrin, calcium and cellular debris. These deposits, referred to as plaque, continue to enlarge over many years, progressively narrowing the arterial channel through which blood must flow, causing the affected heart muscle to become ischemic (suffering from a shortage of blood). (See Figure 2.5.) Eventually, the vessel becomes narrowed to the extent that a clot (coronary thrombus) forms, closing the channel completely. The affected heart muscle, deprived of blood, dies. This is a classical heart attack or myocardial infarction (death of heart muscle). At least 80 percent of all cardiovascular deaths are a result of atherosclerosis.[14]

Some heart attacks are silent and imperceptible to the victim. These incidents, which are quite common, involve small areas of heart muscle and may go unnoticed or undetected unless discovered by an electrocardiogram (ECG or EKG). But if a clot occurs in a large vessel supplying a substantial amount of heart muscle, the individual will experience some or all of the various symptoms of a heart attack (see Figure 2.6) and a larger portion of the heart will die. If the attack is of massive proportions, the victim will die.

Atherosclerotic lesions tend to form where single arteries branch into two. The arteries narrow at these points, increasing blood turbulence and wear and tear at these sites and making them prime candidates for plaque build-up. This may occur in the arteries leading to the brain, kidneys, lungs, and legs, as well as the heart. Atherosclerosis is a specific form of arteriosclerosis (hardening of the arteries). Arteriosclerosis causes arterial walls to thicken and lose their elasticity, forcing the heart to pump with greater force to move blood through the circulatory system.

FIGURE 2.5

Schematic of an Artery Undergoing Atherosclerotic Degeneration.

a. Normal artery
b. Early plaque deposits
c. Moderate atherosclerosis
d. Almost complete occlusion

a.　　　　b.　　　　c.　　　　d.

FIGURE 2.6

Signs of a Heart Attack.

1. Uncomfortable pressure, fullness, squeezing, or pain in the center of the chest which lasts longer than 2 minutes.
2. Pain which spreads to the shoulders, arms, or neck.
3. Severe pain, dizziness, fainting, sweating, nausea or shortness of breath may occur.

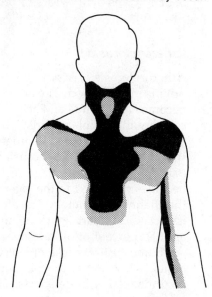

From the American Heart Association.

POINTS TO PONDER

1. *The causes of death in the United States have changed since 1900. How have they changed and why have they changed?*
2. *Discuss the function of the heart as a double pump. What are the functions of the pulmonary and systemic pump?*
3. *What is coronary heart disease?*
4. *Explain what is meant by "the pediatric origins" of atherosclerosis and heart disease.*
5. *What are the signs and symptoms of a heart attack?*

Chapter Highlights

The heart is a double pump whose sole responsibility is to circulate blood throughout the body. The systemic pump sends oxygenated blood to all tissues of the body while the pulmonary pump sends deoxygenated blood to the lungs where a fresh load of oxygen is obtained and carbon dioxide is removed.

The heart is autoregulatory, that is, it contains the mechanisms to produce and deliver its electrical impulses. The sinoatrial node (SA Node), under normal conditions, is the heart's pacemaker and regulates the rhythm of its contractions.

Cardiovascular disease, the leading cause of death in America, is a phenomenon of this century. There are various types of heart disease, some of which are congenital or present at birth. The most prevalent form of heart disease in this country is coronary heart disease. The majority of these are the result of atherosclerosis, which is an insidious process affecting the large and medium sized arteries. The origins of atherosclerosis may be traced to childhood.

It is important to become familiar with the signs and symptoms of a heart attack. When the symptoms appear, it is imperative to seek medical help quickly, preferably at a hospital emergency room. When appropriate medical care is applied within the first few minutes of the initiation of symptoms, a life may be saved and/or the extent of muscle damage may be minimized. Needless to say, either outcome is desirable!

References

1. American Heart Association, *1989 Heart Facts*, American Heart Association, 1988.
2. W.B. Kannell et al., "Epidemiology of Acute Myocardial Infarction: The Framingham Study," *Medicine Today*, 2, (1968): 50.
3. P.D. White, "Preventive Cardiology," *Cardiovascular and Metabolic Diseases*, 1, (1972): 3; H.O. Wolff, "The Pediatrician's Responsibility for Prevention of Coronary Heart Disease," *Postgraduate Medical Journal, 54: 228, 1978.*
4. "Parents Your Children Are Dying," *American Medical Joggers Assoc. Newsletter*, 10 (March, 1984).
5. B. Kirk, "Child Cholesterol Levels, a Medical Controversy," *Medical Journal*, 45, (Sept., 1986): 5.
6. L. Lamb, "Which Child Is At Risk?" *The Health Letter*, 27, (April, 1986): 3.
7. P.N. Herbert and A.H.M. Terpstra, "Diet and Exercise in the Treatment of Hyperlipoproteinemia," *Drug Therapy*, 42, (May 1984).
8. "Teens Aren't Cholesterol Savvy," *Cholesterol Update*, 1 no. 4, (Oct. 1988): 1.
9. Task Force on Blood Pressure Control in Children, "Report of the Second Task Force On Blood Pressure Control in Children— 1987," *Pediatrics*, 79, (1987): 1.
10. U.S. Department of Health and Human Services, *The Health Consequences of Smoking*, Washington, D.C.: U.S. Government Printing Office, 1988.
11. P. Long, "Kids with a Lot to Lose," *Hippocrates*, 2, no. 6, (Nov./Dec. 1988): 72.
12. W.F. Enos et al., "Coronary Disease Among United States Soldiers Killed in Action in Korea: Preliminary Report," *Journal of the American Medical Association*, 152, (1953): 190.
13. J.J. McNamara, et al and others, "Coronary Artery Disease in Combat Casualties in Vietnam," *Journal of the American Medical Association*, 216, (1971): 1185.
14. R. Reed-Flora and T.A. Lang, *Health Behaviors*, St. Paul, MN: West Publishing Co., 1982; Bassler, T.J. "Now the Treadmill," *American Heart Journal*, 94, (1977): 673.

3

Risk Factors for Cardiovascular Disease

Chapter Outline

Mini Glossary

Blood pressure: the force that the blood exerts against the walls of the blood vessels.

Carbon monoxide: a colorless, odorless gas formed by the incomplete oxidation of carbon and highly poisonous when inhaled.

Cholesterol: an organic substance, it is the most abundant steroid in animal tissues, especially in bile and gallstones. Elevated blood cholesterol is a primary risk factor for heart disease.

Chylomicrons: large, buoyant particles which are the primary transporters of triglycerides in the fasting state.

Diabetes mellitus: a metabolic disorder in which the ability to oxidize carbohydrates is more or less completely lost because of faulty pancreatic activity and consequent disturbance of normal insulin mechanisms. This is often accompanied by resistance of receptor cells to insulin.

Diastolic blood pressure: the lowest pressure of arterial blood against the walls of the vessels or heart during diastole.

Distress: normal stress that has become chronic.

Endogenous cholesterol: cholesterol that is manufactured within the body.

Endorphins: one of a family of opioid-like polypeptides originally isolated in the brain but now found in many parts of the body. In the brain they bind to the same receptors that bind exogenous opiates.

Exogenous cholesterol: cholesterol which is received through the diet.

Eustress: good stress; occurs when one accepts and successfully handles a challenge.

HDL-cholesterol: a lipoprotein which transports cholesterol from the blood to the liver for degradation and removal (good cholesterol)

Hypokineses: lack of physical activity

LDL- cholesterol: a lipoprotein which transports cholesterol to the tissues; it is involved in the atherosclerotic process (bad cholesterol).

Mean arterial blood pressure (MAP): the average pressure in the large arteries of the body.

Morbidity: the sick rate or ratio of sick to well in a population.

Nicotine: a stimulant and poisonous drug found in tobacco products.

Obesity: excessive body fat—23 to 24 percent or greater for males; 30 percent or greater for females.

Overweight: excess body weight irrespective of body composition.

Placebo effect: healing that results from a person's belief in the efficacy of a pill, treatment, or other measures when there is no known medicinal value in the substances taken or treatments given.

Systolic Blood Pressure: The greatest pressure in the blood vessels or heart during a cardiac cycle as the result of systole.

Triglycerides: glycerol with three attached fatty acids.

VLDL-cholesterol: Lipoproteins which are the primary transporters of endogenous triglycerides in the fasting state.

Introduction

The risk factors for heart attack and stroke have been identified by several statistical and clinical studies. Several years ago, The American Heart Association (AHA) categorized the risk factors into those that are primary and those that are secondary. Cigarette smoking, elevated cholesterol, and hypertension were the primary factors and all others were secondary. In the AHA publication, *1989 Heart Facts*, the risk factors are categorized as

1. "Major risk factors that can't be changed" (increasing age, male gender, heredity),

2. "Major risk factors that can be changed"' (elevated blood cholesterol, high blood pressure, cigarette smoking), and other contributing factors (obesity, diabetes, stress, and physical inactivity).[1]

Major Risk Factors that Can't be Changed _____

Increasing Age

You begin to realize you're aging when
- *your back goes out more often than you do*
- *after painting the town red you have to take a long rest before applying a second coat*
- *You go all out and end up all in*
- *The little grey haired person you help across the street is your spouse*
- *Your knees buckle—your belt won't.*

The changes associated with aging usually begin after the age of 30. These include decreases in work capacity, muscle tissue, skeletal mass, metabolic rate, nerve cells, and cardiorespiratory function. Blood pressure and the amount of body fat usually increase. These changes are not inevitable, and some need not occur while others may be delayed. The trainability of older people has been documented in many studies. Physically active older people are physiologically the equivalent of younger sedentary people.

The Euro-American Curve (Figure 3.1) illustrates the difference in loss of physiological function between sedentary and active people. This curve was developed from data collected from a cross-section of people in different age

FIGURE 3.1

The Euro-American Curve

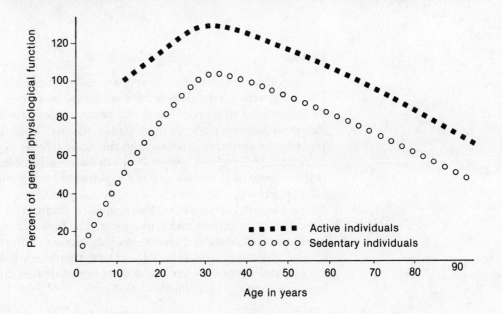

groups. Cross-sectional studies do not represent the best approach in determining the magnitude and type of functional changes which occur during the aging process. However, longitudinal studies, where measurements are made on the same group of people over many years, yield a more accurate profile of the functional age-related changes. The scant longitudinal data indicate that the physical decline depicted in the cross-sectional studies may overestimate the actual decline. Kasch's ongoing study of 15 middle-aged males who exercised consistently for 20 years showed functional declines which were less than half of that observed in the Euro-American Curve.[2] One of the major problems associated with the study of aging concerns the separation of indices of true aging from those changes which are caused by disuse atrophy. Many authorities are convinced that 50 percent of the changes attributed to aging are actually because of physical inactivity.

Since the body thrives upon proper kinds and amounts of physical activity, and since active people are usually more energetic, slimmer, and younger in appearance than inactive people, we might conclude that they are aging according to the way nature intended. Conversely, the sedentary life may accelerate aging.

Age is a risk factor for cardiovascular disease. Fifty-five percent of all cardiovascular deaths occur after the age of 65.[1] No one knows for sure what a lifetime of moderate or vigorous exercise would do to prevent or delay cardiovascular disease because such a study has not yet occurred. However, the evidence for exercise as a modifying agent of the risk factors associated with heart disease is impressive. One study showed that the heart attack rate among sedentary 70- to 79-year-olds was 3.5 times the rate of age-matched people who exercised regularly.[3] There is one irrefutable fact regardless of what we do: unless we die, each of us will age! Ashley Montague advised that it is highly desirable to die young—as late as possible. The quality of the experience and our enjoyment of life during our short stay on this planet may very well depend upon our state of fitness.

Gender

Females have less heart disease than males, particularly prior to menopause. The heart attack rate rises after menopause but does not quite approach the level observed in men. Among the reasons given for the differences between men and women prior to menopause are that the female hormone estrogen protects the coronary arteries from the same degree of devastation that is seen in males, and women generally have more favorable blood fat profiles. Together, these two factors are not conducive to the onset and progression of atherosclerosis.

In the last two decades, the results of changes in female roles and other lifestyle factors are beginning to appear. The heart attack rates in young women have increased because cigarette smoking among young women has risen sharply; oral contraceptives, especially among cigarette smokers, is related to heart disease; and women are assuming more stressful occupational roles—those which have traditionally been filled by males.

Heredity

According to the American Heart Association, "A tendency toward heart disease or atherosclerosis appears to be hereditary, so children of parents with cardiovascular disease are more likely to develop it themselves."[1] The problem of separating genetic factors from a learned lifestyle is complex. An overweight individual with elevated blood pressure and cholesterol may not be the product of heredity, but rather of an overindulgent and underactive lifestyle. First-degree relatives (parents, grandparents, siblings) who have died of coronary disease prior to the age of 60 would strongly indicate the possibility of familial tendencies toward cardiovascular disease. If your family history reads this way, then it is imperative that you attempt to keep the modifiable risk factors in check.

Race

Black Americans are more susceptible to stroke and cardiovascular disease than white Americans. This is probably because of the pervasive hypertension seen among blacks.[4] One of every three Blacks is hypertensive compared to one of every four adults in the remainder of the population. Additionally, Blacks have moderate hypertension twice as often and severe hypertension three times as often as whites. Possible causes for these differences include genetics, sodium sensitivity, and psychological stress.[5] A fourth possible cause involves a particular type of enlargement of the left ventricle of the heart. This form of ventricular hypertrophy tends to become pathological earlier and occurs more often in Blacks. Black women are particularly susceptible to hypertension probably for the reasons listed above but additionally because of obesity and physical inactivity. Black females are much more likely to become pathologically overweight than white females and they have generally been unaffected by the physical fitness movement.[6] The Blacks of South Africa and Haiti have a very low incidence of heart disease.[7] This raises questions regarding the relationship between cardiovascular disease and race. Is the high prevalence of heart disease because of race or cultural influences? Members of the black race living in disparate areas in the world present substantially different cardiovascular disease profiles.

Japanese who reside in Japan have the lowest saturated fat consumption in the industrialized world. This is accompanied by the lowest mortality from cardiovascular disease.[8] Japanese who migrate to the U.S. and adopt typical American dietary habits seem to lose their apparent immunity.[9]

These data demonstrate that environmental elements and lifestyle are influential regarding risk factors for cardiovascular disease. The different races might indulge in divergent lifestyles that may or may not be healthy and may contribute heavily to the incidence—both high and low—of cardiovascular morbidity and mortality.

Major Risk Factors that Can be Changed _____

Cholesterol

Chemically, **cholesterol** is an organic substance classified as a crystalline or solid alcohol. It is a steroid required for the manufacture of hormones as well as bile (for the digestion and absorption of fats), serves as one of the structural components of neural tissue and it is used in the construction of cell walls.[10] A certain amount of cholesterol is essential for good health, but high levels in the blood are associated with heart attack and stroke.

Cholesterol is consumed in the diet **(exogenous cholesterol)** and as a constituent of saturated fat. Both are principally found in animal flesh and dairy products. Some examples of foods containing cholesterol and saturated fats appear in Table 3.1.

A number of population studies over the last 20 years have confirmed that the level of circulating cholesterol in blood plasma was highly related to the development of coronary heart disease (CHD).[11-14] The results of these studies are in remarkable agreement. These studies indicated that the rates of CHD are similar for cholesterol levels below 200 mg/dL (milligrams per deciliter of blood), but above this value the risk increases markedly. Many consumers of this literature concluded from these data that there is no risk associated with cholesterol levels below 200 mg/dL, but this is technically incorrect. The correlation between cholesterol and CHD at low blood concentrations is still positive, so the risk exists but it is well below average. While the risk is significantly reduced at the low end of the cholesterol continuum, it is clear that there is no point below which the risk approaches zero. For example, if a cholesterol level of 200 mg/dL is assigned a ratio of 1.0, then 150 mg/dL carries a lower ratio of 0.7 and a decidedly lower risk. The risk is doubled for 250 mg/dL and doubled again for 300 mg/dL. Another way to examine cholesterol as a risk for CHD is to project from the amount of circulating cholesterol the age at which atherosclerosis reaches a critical stage.[15] The critical stage is that point when 60 percent of coronary vessel surfaces are covered with lesions and this degree of atherosclerosis represents the onset of CHD. The average person with a cholesterol level of 200 mg/dL and no other risk factors will reach a critical degree of atherosclerosis by 70 years of age. A cholesterol level of 250 mg/dL results in a critical degree of atherosclerosis by age 60, and those whose cholesterol is 300 mg/dL will reach that stage by the age of 50. If cholesterol is accompanied by other risk factors, the critical stage occurs sooner.

Ideally, plasma cholesterol levels should be below 200 mg/dL.[16] Table 3.2 illustrates and quantifies the risk. Actually, the ideal cholesterol level for adults is found between 130 and 190 mg/dL.[15]

Some observational studies have demonstrated an inverse relationship between cholesterol and certain types of cancer, that is, people with very low cholesterol levels had a higher than normal death rate from cancer, particularly that of the colon.[17-19] Of course this was very unsettling news considering that low cholesterol levels which decrease the risk of cardiovascular disease seemed to increase the risk of cancer. However, later studies indicated that the decrease in cholesterol occurred secondarily to the onset of cancer or other disease processes associated with an increased risk of cancer.[20-24] In other words, the cancer was in its incipient or preclinical stage and had not yet been detected. Cancerous cells consume more cholesterol than healthy cells and this gives credence to the concept that cancer significantly reduces the level of cholesterol rather than low cholesterol causing cancer. If a substantial drop in cholesterol occurs in the absence of a reason (diet modification, exercise, etc.) you should schedule a medical check-up.

TABLE 3.1 Dietary Cholesterol and Saturated Fat

Item	Cholesterol (in milligrams)*	Saturated Fat (in milligrams)*
Meats (3 oz)		
Beef liver	372	2500
Veal	86	4000
Pork	80	3200
Lean beef	56	2400
Chicken (dark meat)	82	2700
Chicken (white meat)	76	1300
One egg	274	1700
Dairy Products (1 cup; cheese 1 oz)		
Ice cream	59	8900
Whole milk	33	5100
Butter (1 Tbsp)	31	7100
Yogurt (low fat)	11	1800
Cheddar	30	6000
American	27	5600
Camembert	20	4300
Parmesan	8	2000
Oils (1 Tbsp)		
Coconut	0	11,800
Palm	0	6700
Olive	0	1800
Corn	0	1700
Safflower	0	1200
Fish (3 oz)		
Squid	153	400
Oily fish	59	1200
Lean fish	59	300
Shrimp (6 large)	48	200
Clams (6 large)	36	300
Lobster	46.5	75
Other Items of Interest		
Pork brains	2169	1800
Beef kidney	683	3800
Beef hot dog	75	9900
Prime ribs of beef	66.5	5300
Doughnut	36	4000
Milk chocolate	18	16,300
Green or yellow vegetable or fruit	0	trace
Peanut butter (1 Tbsp)	0	1500
Angel food cake	0	1960
Skim milk (1 cup)	4	300
Cheese pizza (3 oz)	6	800
Buttermilk (1 cup)	9	1300
Ice milk, soft (1 cup)	13	2900
Turkey, white meat (3 oz)	59	900

*1000 mg = 1 gram; 454 grams = 1 lb.

TABLE 3.2 Cholesterol Level and Cardiac Risk

Cholesterol(mg/dL)	Risk
Less than 200	Desirable level
200–239	Borderline
240 or greater	High level

Adapted from "Report of the National Cholesterol Education Program Expert Panel on Detection, Evaluation, and Treatment of High Blood Cholesterol in Adults," *Archives of Internal Medicine*, 148, (January, 1988): 36.

Forty percent of the calories consumed by the typical American come from fat, half of which is saturated. In addition, we consume 500 to 600 mg of cholesterol daily. The American Heart Association has suggested recently that we lower our intake of fat to 30 percent of total calories and limit cholesterol intake to 300 mg per day.

Many authorities suggest that it may be more important to limit saturated fat in the diet than to be overly restrictive of cholesterol. A number of years ago, several investigators estimated that increasing cholesterol intake from 250 to 500 mg/day would increase plasma cholesterol by an average of 10 mg/dL.[15] A complicating factor in this estimation comes from the variability of response to dietary cholesterol. Some individuals respond with a substantial increase in plasma cholesterol while others experience little or no increase. On the other hand, the ingestion of saturated fat produces a definite increase in plasma cholesterol. Although the relationship between dietary saturated fat intake and cholesterol level in the blood was quantified two decades ago, it remains valid today.[25] Plasma cholesterol increases by 2.7 mg/dL for every 1 percent increase in dietary saturated fat so that an increase of 5 percent in dietary saturated fat will increase the plasma concentration of cholesterol by 13.5 mg/dL. Most of this increase occurs in the fraction of cholesterol (LDL) which is highly related to the development of atherosclerosis and coronary heart disease. The body manages to manufacture 1000 to 2000 milligrams of cholesterol (**endogenous cholesterol**) each day and saturated fat is the substance that is involved in the process.[26] The evidence is quite clear: the amount of saturated fat and cholesterol in the diet is positively related to blood levels of cholesterol.

An important collaborative study which ended in 1984 provided solid clinical evidence implicating cholesterol as a culprit in coronary artery disease.[27–28] This monumental $150 million study, the Lipid Research Clinics Coronary Primary Prevention Trial (LRC- CPPT), indicated that lowering cholesterol in the blood indeed lowered the risk of having heart disease.

This study began in 1973 and continued for ten years. From 1973 to 1976, 12 cooperating research centers screened 480,000 volunteers and eventually selected 3806 men between the ages of 35 and 59 for participation in the study. All subjects had cholesterol levels in excess of 265 mg/100 dL (the average level for men in this age group is 210–220 mg/100 dL. The subjects were randomly assigned to two groups: one group received a daily dose of cholestyramine, a cholesterol-lowering drug, and the second group was given a daily placebo. Both were administered in a double-blind fashion, that is, each subject was told he was receiving the cholesterol-lowering drug while the experimenter who

We are persuaded that the blood cholesterol levels of most Americans are undesirably high, in large part because of our high dietary intake of calories, saturated fat, and cholesterol.
–National Heart, Lung, and Blood Institute

dispensed the drugs did not know who was getting which. In addition, both groups were given a diet to follow that was designed to lower cholesterol by 4 percent.

This was basically a drug study rather than a diet study because it would have been virtually impossible to control, administer, and measure the daily diet of that many subjects over the 7.4 years of followup. At the completion of the study, the cholestyramine group had reduced their cholesterol level 8.5 percent more than the placebo group, suffered 19 percent fewer heart attacks, and had 24 percent fewer fatal heart attacks.[28] There was also a significant reduction in coronary bypass surgery and angina (chest pain of a temporary nature) in the drug group.

This long-term trial provided the first concrete evidence that decreasing blood cholesterol decreases the incidence of coronary heart disease deaths in human subjects. The researchers estimated that each 1 percent reduction in cholesterol would result in a 2 percent reduction in the risk of coronary heart disease. A 25 percent reduction in cholesterol would translate to a very significant 50 percent reduction in the risk of coronary heart disease. Dr. Antonio M. Gotto, whose primary research interests involve the pathophysiology of atherosclerosis and coronary heart disease, stated that "the implications of this trial extend far beyond the group of middle-aged men with hypercholesterolemia (elevated blood cholesterol) who were studied."[29] The study's principal investigators asserted that "these findings taken in conjunction with the large volume of evidence relating to diet, plasma cholesterol levels, and coronary heart disease, support the view that cholesterol lowering by diet also would be beneficial."[28]

Four years later, the results of another significant study—the Helsinki Heart Study—were reported in the medical literature.[30] Subjects in this five-year study (23,531 middle-aged males) were similar to those in the LRC-CCPT study. The subjects were given a diet that was low in saturated fat and cholesterol and they were advised to stop smoking. lose weight, and exercise. In addition, half of the group was given a cholesterol-lowering drug while the other half received a placebo. During the last three years of the study, the incidence of coronary heart disease decreased by more than 50 percent in the drug versus the placebo group. Total cholesterol and LDL decreased by eight percent while the triglyceride level (another fat to be discussed later) decreased by 35 percent during the five years of the study. Another cholesterol fraction, HDL (protects against coronary heart disease), increased over the study period. This combination of events decreased the incidence of fatal and nonfatal coronary episodes. The Helsinki Heart Study has independently corroborated the findings of the LRC-CCPT and earlier studies that reducing total and LDL cholesterol decreases the risk of coronary artery disease.

Strategies for lowering total cholesterol include (1) reduction in dietary cholesterol and saturated fat, (2) increase in the consumption of soluble fiber (found in oats, beans, fruits and vegetables), (3) weight loss, and (4) cessation of cigarette smoking.

The amount of circulating cholesterol in the blood accounts for only a part of the story. To gain greater insight into cholesterol as a risk factor one must understand how it is packaged and transported in the circulatory system. To begin, the mechanisms of cholesterol distribution are very complex and not completely known at this time but researchers are continuing to unravel the mystery. The following is a brief synopsis of the synthesis, transport, and function of cholesterol. Cholesterol does not dissolve in the blood in a manner similar to sugar and salt. It is transported through the circulatory system attached to protein packages which facilitate its solubility. These transporters, the lipoproteins (fats bound to a protein) include (1) the chylomicrons, (2) very low density lipoprotein (VLDL), (3) intermediate density lipoprotein (IDL), (4) low density lipoprotein (LDL), and high density lipoprotein (HDL). Each of the lipoproteins carries different concentrations of fats (lipids) and protein. See Figure 3.2 for the concentrations and note the size relationship between the lipoproteins. Note also that each of the lipoproteins carries triglycerides, phospholipids, and cholesterol. The greater the concentration of lipids, the less dense the lipoprotein.

The **chylomicrons** are large buoyant particles which are the primary transporters of triglycerides in the fasting state. They originate in the intestine and transport their lipid load to the body's cells which in turn remove the fat that they need. The chylomicrons have essentially been stripped of their contents approximately 12 to 14 hours after eating. The remainder consists of protein remnants and some fat. The liver has receptor sites which recognize, remove and dismantle the chylomicron remnants. From these, **very low density lipoproteins (VLDL)** are manufactured. The VLDL particles are the primary transporters of endogenous triglycerides (those which are made by the body) in the

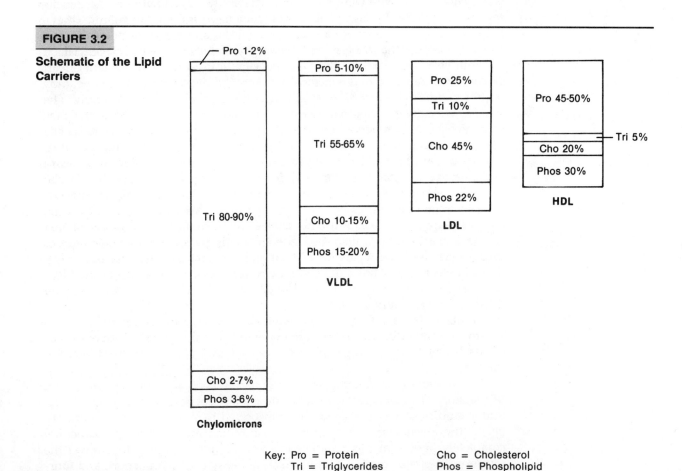

FIGURE 3.2

Schematic of the Lipid Carriers

Key: Pro = Protein   Cho = Cholesterol
     Tri = Triglycerides   Phos = Phospholipid

fasting state. VLDLs circulate through the system releasing their cargo to the muscles and adipose tissue for energy and/or storage. What remains are VLDL remnants from which intermediate density lipoproteins (IDL) are made. IDLs consist of 40 percent triglyceride and 30 percent cholesterol. Some of the IDL particles are quickly captured by the liver but some are catabolized (broken down) and converted to low density lipoproteins (LDL).

Low density lipoproteins are the primary transporters of cholesterol. Cholesterol comprises approximately 45 percent of the elements that LDLs carry. The evidence linking LDL to coronary heart disease has been accumulating rapidly in the last decade. It appears that LDL is the most atherogenic (capable of producing atherosclerosis) of the lipoproteins. Our understanding of the role of LDL transport was substantially increased by the Nobel Prize winning research of Brown and Goldstein.[31] They discovered that the cells have receptor sites that bind LDLs thus removing them from the blood stream. Binding allows cholesterol to enter the cell where it can be stored or used to synthesize plasma membranes, bile acids, and steroid hormones. By removing LDL from the blood for cellular use, the receptors contribute to the prevention of atherosclerosis. However, when the diet is high in animal fat (the American diet), the receptors become saturated and removal of LDL from the blood is significantly reduced. This results in a rise of plasma LDL which leads to the development and/or the exacerbation of atherosclerosis. Animal species who typically do not develop atherosclerosis have plasma LDL levels which are less than 80 mg/dL. Human infants have LDL levels which are approximately 30 mg/dL but this value increases with age. If a low fat diet is maintained during growth and adulthood, LDL will generally remain below 80 mg/dL. The typical American diet usually results in an LDL value which exceeds 100 mg/dL. Heart attacks are rare when the LDL level is below 100 mg/dL. A national panel of experts has developed guidelines for LDL levels and these are presented in Table 3.3. While the panel stated that an LDL level below 130 mg/dL is desirable, they acknowledge that the lower the better. An LDL of 160 mg/dL is roughly equivalent to a total cholesterol (TC) of 240 mg/dL and an LDL of 130 mg/dL is equivalent to a total cholesterol (TC) of 200 mg/dL.

Low density lipoprotein cholesterol may be lowered by reducing saturated fat and cholesterol in the diet.[15] Schaefer concluded after a literature review that the optimal diet for the prevention of coronary artery disease consists of 12 to 15 percent of the total calories coming from protein, 65 percent from carbohydrate (mainly the complex type), 20 to 25 percent from fat (less than 10 percent saturated) and no more than 200 mg of cholesterol per day.[32] The results of at least

> We now have strong evidence that lowering LDL concentrations will reduce the risk of coronary heart disease.
> —Scott M. Grundy

TABLE 3.3 Guidelines for LDL Levels

LDL Cholesterol(mg/dL)	Risk
Less than 130	Desirable level
130–159	Borderline—high risk
160 or greater	High risk

Adapted from "Report of the National Cholesterol Education Program Expert Panel on Detection, Evaluation and Treatment of High Blood Cholesterol in Adults," *Archives of Internal Medicine,* 148, (1988): 36.

two studies have shown that LDL levels respond to exercise and those whose fitness has improved the most experience the greatest reduction.[33,34] Conversely, excessive caloric intake produces an overproduction of VLDL.[35,36] You will recall that LDLs are made from VLDL remnants therefore an increase in the latter will result in an accompanying increase in the former.

Several medications have been shown to be effective in lowering total cholesterol and LDL.[27,28] A relatively new drug, Lovastatin, increases the HDL cholesterol concentration.[37] Taking medication to control cholesterol does not and should not preclude dietary and exercise modalities. In other words, affected individuals should continue taking the prescribed medication but they should not discontinue exercise and dietary approaches. Placing reliance on the medication which requires little effort by the individual, in the absence of lifestyle changes, which requires considerable effort, would be a mistake in the control of cholesterol.

High density lipoproteins are produced in the liver and intestine. It appears that HDLs are involved in "reverse transport," that is, they remove cholesterol from the blood and return it to the liver for degradation, recycling and/or disposal. Through this protective function HDL appears to be antiatherogenic and therefore has been labeled as "good" cholesterol. Obviously, the object is to increase HDL while lowering LDL (labeled as "bad" cholesterol) and TC. Actually a person with a desirable total cholesterol may be at substantial risk for coronary artery disease if the HDL level is low.[13,38] Men whose HDL is below 25 mg/dL and women whose HDL is below 40 mg/dL are at three times the risk for heart disease.[39] The average HDL values for men are 45 mg/dL and for women 55 mg/dL. This biological difference in the HDL values partly explains the lower incidence of heart disease in women compared to men.

Testosterone and HDL

Women live approximately eight years longer than men and one of the primary reasons for this phenomenon is the higher incidence of heart attack deaths among men prior to 55 years of age. There are many reasons why men are more likely than women to have a heart attack at an early age, but a major factor is the male sex hormone testosterone.

Testosterone has a supressant effect on the production of HDL cholesterol. A study by researchers at Baylor University College of Medicine of 57 boys who were at different stages of puberty indicated that increases in testosterone production affected the level of circulating HDL. The subjects were grouped according to their position on the puberty continuum. Those who were prepubertal had an average HDL of 66.6 mg/dL and were producing one-tenth the testosterone of subjects who were at or nearing post-puberty. This latter group had an average HDL level of 54.4 mg/dL. As the stages of puberty advanced toward completion the level of HDL decreased. Some of the prepubertal subjects were given injections of testosterone and the HDL level was significantly reduced in two weeks. The larger the dose of testosterone the greater the decrease of HDL. Adult males produce 10 to 20 times more testosterone than adult females and have HDL levels that are typically below that of females of the same age. Testosterone which is positively associated with virility seems to be negatively associated with longevity.

Many studies have shown an inverse relationship between HDL and coronary heart disease.[13,40–42] In fact, most authorities consider a low HDL level to be a very powerful independent indicator of coronary heart disease. Factors which lower HDL are cigarette smoking,[13,41,42] diabetes,[43] elevated triglycerides,[15,16,32] and the use of anabolic steroids.[44,45] Factors which increase HDL are moderate alcohol consumption,[46,47] weight loss,[48] and physical exercise.[13,48,49]

The effect of alcohol on HDL might prompt few people to substitute a couple of drinks for exercise to produce the same effect. But HDL consists of subfractions, two of which are HDL2 and HDL3. HDL3 appears to be neutral in that it is not involved in the processes of arterial protection or disease. However, HDL2 is established as a protective element which is actively involved in the removal of cholesterol from the arteries.[47,49] Male runners had twice as much HDL2 when compared to male nonrunners.[50] Researchers compared women runners to women nonrunners and found HDL values to be significantly higher in the runners.[49] These researchers had their subjects drink 12 ounces of wine daily during the course of the study. Half of the group also jogged a minimum of 20 miles weekly. The results of this study indicated the exercise level in this group of women, age 18 to 49, was more important than alcohol consumption in elevating plasma HDL2.

Wood and his group found that subjects who lost weight either through exercise or diet experienced an increase in plasma HDL.[48] This effect has also been observed in other studies.[16,51]

The most potent factor for stimulating the production of HDL is aerobic exercise.[13,15,16,33,34,41,42,49] People who regularly participate in endurance-type exercises are leaner, more physically fit, have higher HDL, lower total cholesterol, and lower LDL than sedentary people. This profile is associated with a relatively lower risk for coronary heart disease and conversely reflects high-level wellness. How much, how often, and what kind of exercise is needed to change the pattern of cholesterol into a healthier one? In 1982, a study completed by investigators working in the Stanford Heart Disease Prevention Program provided some of the answers.[52] The researchers concluded that "HDL did not begin to change with (jogging) mileage until nine months of training. The correlation for miles run with HDL is much stronger at one year than at three, six, or nine months." Their analysis indicated that "HDL did not increase unless an average exercise training level of 10 miles/week or more was achieved during a period of one year." This study established a threshold level of training needed to increase HDL. Another significant finding was the the greatest increase in HDL levels was achieved by subjects who ran the most miles per week (20 to 25). This suggests that HDL is responsive to the amount of exercise: the more we do, the more we get.

Evidence is emerging however, which indicates that low intensity exercise and leisure time physical activity may also increase HDL.[53,54] In one study total cholesterol and HDL and its subfractions were evaluated in 35 middle-aged postal mail carriers.[53] The researchers found a significant relationship between consistent, low level intensity exercise (such as the walking that mail carriers do) and increased HDL and HDL2. The implications of this study are enormous from the standpoint of public health. It suggests that one need not be a marathon runner to receive similar health-related benefits. Other researchers are also investigating the relationship between intensity of exercise and several parameters including health-related benefits, longevity, and risk of heart disease. These studies are in general agreement regarding the health-related benefits of low and moderate intensity exercise. These will be discussed later in this chapter under the heading of "Physical Inactivity."

Runners and other exercise participants differ from sedentary people in many ways. It was only natural that questions have been raised regarding the lifestyles of runners. Is their advantageous lipoprotein profile the result of being nonsmokers and lean rather than because they are runners? Blair and coworkers compared the nutritional habits of men and women runners to a same-sex, same-age sample of sedentary people.[55] Compared to the sedentary controls, the runners in this study were significantly leaner, on a weight-adjusted basis they consumed 40 to 60 percent more calories, were more likely to have a few alcoholic drinks, and consumed a lesser percentage of their total calories in the form of protein. This study showed that runners eat a typical American diet so this could not account for their higher HDL, lower LDL and lower total cholesterol. The researchers concluded that the observed differences in plasma lipoproteins between the runners and the controls were probably caused by some factor other than diet, such as their exercise program. The results achieved from consistent participation in aerobic exercise (decreased body weight, increase in HDL, decrease in blood pressure, increase in energy reserve, greater ability to relax, etc.) are consistent with wellness.

Researchers have examined the ratio between total cholesterol (TC) and HDL as a predictor of heart disease. Dividing TC by HDL yields a number which can be interpreted in terms of the risk for heart disease. Ratios of 5 and 4.5 represent the average risk for males and females respectively. Table 3.4 elucidates the risk for values above and below the average.

There have been comparatively fewer studies that have addressed the association between strength and wellness. A logical question is: How much strength is needed for good health? The obvious answer might be enough to function as a human being, to pursue an occupation, and to carry out family and recreational interests. Many people meet these criteria but function at the lower end of the strength continuum so that moving furniture, gardening, changing a flat tire, and the like become burdensome chores. By the same token, a 245-pound male carrying 30 percent of his weight in the form of fat tissue may also have considerable muscle tissue and be very strong. He is clearly obese, a risk for chronic diseases, and not in a state of high-level wellness. So a more appropriate question is not how much strength is needed for good health, but how does *strength training* contribute to good health? Weight training—using moderate weights with 10 to 15 repetitions—rather than weight lifting in which very heavy weights are used in power or Olympic-style lifting can contribute to the objectives of wellness. Weight training and other progressive resistance exercises featuring moderate loads may contribute to health in the following ways: They change

TABLE 3.4   Ratio of Total Cholesterol to HDL Cholesterol

Risk	Male	Female
Very low (½ average)	Under 3.4	Under 3.3
Low risk	4.0	3.8
Average risk	5.0	4.5
Moderate risk (2 × average)	9.5	7.0
High risk (3 × average)	Over 23	Over 11

Adapted from "National Institutes of Health Consensus Development Conference Statement: Lowering Blood Cholesterol." *Journal of the American Medical Association*, 253 (1985): 2080.

body composition by reducing fat and increasing muscle tissue, leading to a more desirable physical appearance; the increase in muscle tissue maintains or increases the resting metabolic rate, which has important implications for weight control; they may help to reduce the incidence of low back problems by developing the abdominal and back muscles; and they may increase HDL while decreasing LDL and total cholesterol. The contributions of resistance exercises will be explained in greater detail in Chapter 8.

Blood Pressure

Blood pressure, which is recorded in millimeters of mercury (mm Hg), is the force exerted against the walls of the arteries as blood courses through the circulatory system. A certain level of pressure, created by contractions of the heart muscle, is needed to circulate blood throughout the body. Blood pressures that exceed normal limits are referred to as *hypertension*.

Blood pressure is routinely measured by an indirect method when you have a medical exam. An inflatable rubber cuff connected to a pressure gauge or tube of mercury is placed around your upper arm. The cuff is inflated with enough pressure to cut off circulation. The air is slowly released from the cuff while a Health professional, using a stethoscope placed on the brachial artery below the cuff, listens for the first sound of blood rushing through the artery. This first sound represents the contraction of the heart and the reading on the pressure gauge at that point is the **systolic** value. The physician or other health professional continues to release the air and listens for the last fading sound that represents the interim, or rest period between contractions. This value, also read from the pressure gauge, is the **diastolic** reading. An average blood pressure for young adults is 120/80. Resting blood pressure which is consistently above 140/90 is considered to be hypertension.

High blood pressure is a silent disease because there are no characteristic or typical symptoms which indicate its presence. In 90 percent of the cases, the cause is unknown. This is referred to as essential hypertension. There is no cure for this type of hypertension but most cases can be managed and controlled through medication and/or other efforts. Hypertension which is not controlled or poorly controlled can lead to serious cardiovascular complications. The remaining 10 percent of the cases of hypertension are secondary to an underlying problem which often can be diagnosed and treated. The cause of this type of hypertension can be identified. When the underlying cause is treated successfully, blood pressure returns to normal.

Approximately one in four Americans has hypertension.[1] This is a serious disease which significantly contributes to the incidence and mortality associated with heart disease and stroke. Recently, mass educational campaigns have produced an encouraging trend: a greater number of hypertensives are seeking and receiving treatment and a growing number of people are becoming aware that they have a blood pressure problem. Even moderate elevations of blood pressure increase the risk. For example, the risk of heart attack doubles and the risk of stroke quadruples for a male whose systolic pressure is in excess of 150 mm Hg compared to a male whose systolic pressure is below 120 mm Hg.

The mean arterial pressure (MAP) is another way to express and evaluate blood pressure. **Mean arterial pressure** represents the average pressure that exists in the major branches of the arterial system. Every 10 mmHg rise in MAP

60,130,000 American adults and children have high blood pressure.
–American Heart Association

increases the risk of cardiovascular disease by 30 percent. The MAP can be calculated for any blood pressure reading. It should be calculated each time blood pressure readings increase so that a trend may be discernible over a period of years. The MAP calculations for a blood pressure of 120/80 is as follows:

$$
\begin{aligned}
\text{MAP} &= \text{DBP} + \tfrac{1}{3}(\text{SBP} - \text{DBP}) \\
&= 80 + \tfrac{1}{3}(120 - 80) \\
&= 80 + \tfrac{1}{3}(40) \\
&= 80 + 13.3 \\
&= 93.3 \\
\text{DBP} &= \text{diastolic blood pressure} \\
\text{SBP} &= \text{systolic blood pressure}
\end{aligned}
$$

The heart is adversely affected by long-standing hypertension. Pumping blood against high resistance in the arteries increases the workload of the heart. As a result it enlarges much as any other muscle which is stimulated over a period of time. The problem for the heart is that the resistance is consistently high therefore it receives inadequate rest. Years of pumping against such a resistance produces muscle fibers that become overly distended or stretched. They progressively lose their ability to snap back, and the end result being a less forceful contraction. The heart becomes and inefficient and weak. Hypertension is one of the leading causes of congestive heart failure. High blood pressure damages the arteries and accelerates atherosclerosis.

Hypertension can usually be controlled with medication, salt restriction, weight loss, and exercise. Since medications for controlling blood pressure may produce undesirable side effects, a better strategy might concentrate upon salt restriction, weight control, and exercise supplemented with such stress reduction techniques as progressive muscle relaxation, Benson's relaxation response, Transcendental Meditation, Yoga, biofeedback, hypnotherapy, and progressive relaxation. Explaining, defining, and demonstrating these techniques is beyond the scope of this text and the interested reader is encouraged to learn from instructors of these methods or possibly from self-help books. However, the following guidelines might provide some insight for budding practitioners of these techniques. One, find a quiet place that is free of interruptions. Sit in a comfortable position, close your eyes and repeat a phrase, such as "I am relaxed" with each exhalation. Do this daily for five minutes for about two weeks and you should be able to determine if this exercise is appropriate for you. Two, select one of the relaxation techniques discussed above. You may need to experiment with more than one of these to find the most effective for you. Three, you must practice the technique every day; most require that you participate twice-a-day. Practice will improve your ability to relax. There is no guarantee that blood pressure can be normalized without medication, but many people have experienced success utilizing these approaches. Control without drugs is highly desirable.

Salt restriction is an important step in the control of blood pressure. A daily intake of 500 milligrams (½ gram) is needed by the body, but Americans consume 20 or more (10–12 grams/daily times this amount). Table salt consists of 40 percent sodium (the real culprit) and 60 percent chloride. Sodium exists naturally in many foods and is added to processed foods by design because it is a cheap flavor-enhancer and preservative.

Sodium increases the blood pressure because it is water-retentive. Excessive salt stimulates the body to hoard fluids that accumulate in all fluid compartments, including the blood stream. An increased amount of blood requires more force to circulate through the vessels. Diuretics are used to rid the body of excess fluid and to lower the blood pressure.

About one-third to one-half of all hypertensives are "salt sensitive" probably because of some genetic anomaly in their ability to process salt. Such people should limit their salt intake because even small amounts may elevate the blood pressure.[56] Most people do not respond to salt in the same manner. Clearly, some hypertension is caused by factors other than salt in the diet. However, it is a good idea to be on the safe side even if your blood pressure is normal by limiting salt intake to less than three grams per day.[57]

There is some evidence that potassium may either neutralize the effects of sodium or that it may have some intrinsic protective influence independent of other factors. When subjects with normal blood pressure consume large amounts of sodium over a period of years, their blood pressures tend to rise.[58] During this time, potassium excretion is accelerated. However, those whose potassium consumption is high during this period of excessive salt ingestion do not experience a rise in blood pressure. Other investigators have shown that people who consume diets low in potassium suffer 4.8 times as many deaths from strokes compared to those whose potassium is average or above.[59] High blood pressure is the leading cause of stroke. The data from studies such as these may possibly shed some light on the effectiveness of the "rice diet" in lowering blood pressure. Undoubtedly, the low sodium content of the diet is a significant contributor to the desirable results attained by users of this diet. However, considerable amounts of fresh fruit (excellent sources of potassium) were an integral part of the "rice diet" and probably added to the success attributed to this regimen. More study is needed to determine the role and amount of dietary potassium needed to aid in the control of blood pressure.

There is evidence that a low calcium intake is related to high blood pressure in some people. See the boxed insert below for further information regarding the relationship between calcium and blood pressure. A number of factors are involved in the development of high blood pressure, and it is becoming increasingly clear that a calcium deficiency is probably one of them.

Hypertension: the Calcium Connection

Recent evidence indicates that there may be a "calcium-sensitive" form of hypertension in addition to the "sodium-sensitive" type with which we are already familiar. This notion was advanced by Dr. David McCarron, who found that high blood pressure, in some people, was accompanied by a calcium deficiency. Other researchers at Cornell University found that 16 of 26 calcium-deficient, hypertensive patients normalized their blood pressures in three months by taking 2000 mg of calcium daily (800 mg is the recommended daily allowance). The other 10 patients required other forms of therapy to lower their blood pressures. The Cornell researchers asserted that one-third to one-half of their patients responded to calcium supplementation. Other researchers think that the Cornell esttimate is much too optimistic and that the true value is closer to 15 percent.

There is considerable disagreement among authorities regarding the role of calcium in the control of high blood pressure. At this point it is probably prudent to conclude that some calcium-deficient patients may normalize their blood pressure by increasing their intake of calcium. It must be noted, however, that all hypertensives are not calcium deficient and that only a fraction of those who are respond well to treatment. Meanwhile, the accepted course of action continues to emphasize salt restriction, weight loss, exercise and medication, if it is prescribed. Calcium supplementation for those hypertensives who are deficient should be used in addition to and not instead of the above approaches. A word of caution: do not begin to take calcium supplements in order to avert high blood pressure. At this juncture there is no evidence to support this practice. If you have high blood pressure, seek medical advice and treatment. But it is important, regardless of the level of blood pressure, to ingest at least the minimum amount of calcium daily.

A diet low in fat, particularly saturated fat, appears to be a viable constituent in a program designed to reduce blood pressure. There appears to be a link between the amount and kind of fat consumed and blood pressure, as studies reported in the *UTCHS Medical Journal* have indicated.[60] Middle-aged subjects in these studies lowered their blood pressure when they reduced their fat intake and consumed more polyunsaturated fat (found in vegetable oils) than saturated fat (found primarily in animal sources).

Weight loss is another component in the management of blood pressure. Excess fat places a strain or greater workload upon the heart which must meet the circulatory demands of the extra tissue. Weight loss usually results in a lowered blood pressure.

Daily drinking of alcoholic beverages will raise the blood pressure of some people. More than two ounces a day seems to be a threshold for raising blood pressure. Two ounces of alcohol can be obtained by drinking two four ounce glasses of wine, two eight ounce glasses of beer or two shots or jiggers of hard liquor. Alcohol should be elminiated from the diet or at worse consumed in moderation.

Exercise is another contributor to blood pressure control. A number of investigators have found that aerobic exercise can lower the blood pressure of hypertensive and borderline hypertensive people. However, many of these studies have been flawed by poor research designs, lack of control groups, too few subjects and exercise programs of varying intensity, frequency and duration. The following examples are a sampling of some of the better recent studies.

Researchers from Duke University Medical Center presented data from an eight and one-half year study at the scientific session of the American Heart Association in 1986 regarding the effect of level of fitness and the risk of heart attack.[61] One of their many conclusions was that physically fit subjects had lower blood pressures than less fit subjects. Montoye was one of the first investigators to consider the occupational and leisure time energy expenditure of a large number of subjects.[62] He found that the least active men had the highest blood pressures. Similar results were obtained in an examination of ten years of data at the Georgia Baptist Medical Center.[63]

Researchers at the Institute for Aerobic Research in Dallas studied the effects of walking and jogging on 56 sedentary men, ages 21 to 37, whose blood pressures were between 140/90 to 160/103 mmHg.[64] None of the subjects showed evidence of heart disease nor were any of them on blood pressure medication. For 16 weeks, half of the group walked and jogged for one hour three days per week while the other half did no exercise. The exercise group gradually diminished their walking time and increased their jogging time over the course of the study. At the end of the 16 weeks, the exercising men reduced their systolic and diastolic pressures by 12.4 and 7 mmHg respectively while the sedentary group reduced their systolic pressure by 6.2 mmHg but increased their diastolic pressure by 2.9 mmHg.

The physical fitness status of 4820 men and 1219 women ages 20 to 65 was assessed at the same Dallas Center.[65] All subjects had normal resting blood pressures at the beginning of this epidemiological study. They were followed for an average of four years—some for only one year and others for as long as 12 years. After adjusting for age, sex, initial body mass index (a gross measure of body composition), and initial blood pressure, the researchers found that those subjects who were in the low fitness category had a 52 percent greater risk of developing hypertension compared to those who were highly fit.

The Harvard Alumni study was another major epidemiological investigation which followed thousands of subjects for many years.[66] The results indicated that those who did not engage in vigorous sports or physical activities had a 35 percent greater risk of developing hypertension than those who were regularly active and this relationship held for all ages from 35 to 74.

A well controlled study by Duncan and coworkers provided some insight into the mechanisms through which blood pressure is lowered through exercise.[67] Adrenaline and noradrenaline are hormones that are important in the regulation of blood pressure. Both are vasoconstrictors, that is, they decrease the diameters of the arterioles which are the smallest arteries. Duncan measured the level of these circulating hormones before and after 16 weeks of exercise. At the end of the study all exercisers had lower resting diastolic blood pressure and lower levels of noradrenaline. The researchers concluded that exercise produced an effect upon resting blood pressure which was independent of other variables (weight loss, stress reduction, etc.) They further concluded that the reduction in the diastolic pressure following training was partially mediated by the exercise induced decrease in noradrenaline.

Investigators at the Veterans Administration Medical Center in Jackson, Mississippi examined the role of aerobic exercise versus eight calisthenics (mostly stretching exercises) on the blood pressures of 19 mildly hypertensive men.[68] Ten of the subjects were put into an aerobics exercise program for 15 to 30 minutes three days per week. The other nine men participated in the calisthenics program. Within ten weeks, the blood pressures of the aerobic group dropped to normal values. The calisthenics group experienced no change in blood pressure during this time. At that point, they too entered the aerobic program and their pressures normalized within a couple of months as well. There was no change in the subjects weight or sodium/potassium levels as measured by urine analysis.

Thirteen sedentary subjects with mild to moderate hypertension (readings persistently above 150/90 mm Hg) were placed in a three-month graduated exercise program.[69] The average age of the group was 44 years. Blood pressures, plasma noradrenaline, and peripheral resistance to blood flow were measured. Peripheral resistance, or the circulatory resistance to blood flow, is one of the major contributors to blood pressure. Peripheral resistance depends on the diameters of the arterioles. The relationship between the two is inverse, the larger the diameters of the arterioles the less the peripheral resistance. The study design called for measurements to be made during the first month of no exercise, the second month with 35 minutes of stationary cycling three days per week, and a final month with the same exercise every day. Exercise three times per week reduced the standing blood pressure to 135/90 and the seven-day per week program reduced the standing blood pressure further to 133/88. This study indicated that frequency of training had an affect on lowering blood pressure and the result was independent of body weight or sodium content. Further, peripheral resistance decreased by 18 percent with three days of exercise per week and 24 percent with daily exercise. Plasma noradrenaline levels fell as well with increasing frequency of exercise and was probably related to the decreased peripheral resistance. These results are similar to those of the Duncan study.

Two researchers examined the effect of quiet rest and aerobic exercise on state anxiety and blood pressure.[70] Half of the 30 subjects had normal blood pressures and half were hypertensive. State anxiety and blood pressure were measured before and after rest and exercise. Both were significantly reduced in each group with rest and exercise but exercise produced a longer lasting effect.

Fifty-one sedentary males (average age of 40) participated in a 30-week marathon training program.[71] Resting blood pressure was measured before and after 15 and 30 weeks of training. Blood pressures improved significantly and the researchers concluded that the reductions were caused by exercise training rather than to the weight and fat loss which occurred.

Children are also the victims of hypertension. In fact, the roots of much adult hypertension can be traced back to childhood. According to the National Heart, Lung, and Blood Institute, most cases of pediatric hypertension can be treated with exercise and diet.[72] This group has recommended that medication for hypertension in children should be considered only after exercise and diet have failed.

Siscovick and his group reviewed the literature on blood pressure from the earliest studies to 1985.[73] They concluded that "habaitual activity and physical fitness may reduce the risk of developing hypertension," and that "habitual exercise may improve control of high blood pressure." I believe that the studies since 1985 support these conclusions also.

Cigarette Smoking

Many medical authorities consider cigarette smoking to be the most potent preventable risk factor associated with chronic illness and premature death. Although cigarette smoking is on the decline, 26.5 percent of Americans over the age of 20 continue to smoke.[74] From 1976 to 1985, smoking incidence among adult males decreased from 42 percent of the population to 33 percent. The decrease for women was not quite as dramatic but dropped from 32 percent of the population to 28 percent. The gap between the number of male and female smokers has been steadily narrowing. The percentage of daily smokers among high school seniors decreased from 28 to 18.7 percent from 1976 to 1986.

The American Cancer Society has estimated that 40 percent of the male smokers and 28 percent of the female smokers die prematurely. Smoking directly contributes to approximately 320,000 deaths annually. Consider the following:

1. Cigarette smoking is responsible for 83 percent of all lung cancer cases. In 1988 there were 139,000 deaths attributable to lung cancer.[74]

2. Smoking is implicated in cancers of the bladder, pancreas, mouth, pharynx, larynx, and esophagus.[74]
3. Smoking is responsible for 30 percent of all cancer deaths and is associated with the development and/or exacerbation of chronic bronchitis and emphysema.[74]
4. Smokers are at twice the risk of heart attack than nonsmokers and are two to four times as likely to die suddenly from heart attack.[1]
5. Smoking causes peripheral vascular disease (narrowing of the blood vessels in the extremities).[75]

Carbon monoxide, a noxious gas that is a by-product of combustable tobacco products, attaches to hemoglobin much more readily than does oxygen. Carbon monoxide effectively displaces oxygen thereby reducing the oxygen carrying capacity of the blood. This contributes in part to the shortness of breath experienced by smokers during moderate physical exertion such as climbing a couple of flights of stairs or walking uphill, and so on.

Nicotine, a powerful stimulant, has a profound effect on the cardiovascular system. Some of its major consequences as determined by the 1988 Surgeon General's Report are:[75]

1. It contributes to heart disease by increasing VLDL and LDL cholesterol and by lowering HDL cholesterol.
2. Nicotine is probably involved in blood platelet aggregation. When the platelets aggregate or clump together, they release a chemical substance that initiates spasms in the coronary arteries. Spasms constrict the blood vessels producing ischemia (diminished blood flow) which can lead to chest pain or heart attack.
3. Nicotine increases the oxygen needs of the myocardium (heart muscle) by increasing heart rate and blood pressure. If the coronary vessels are atherosclerotic, blood flow may not match the demand resulting in ischemia and angina pectoris.
4. Nicotine is a vasoconstrictor of blood vessels particularly those in the extremities. This phenomenon is probably the result of the activation and increased secretion of the catecholamines (adrenaline and noradrenaline) by nicotine.
5. Nicotine also contributes to the development of cardiac arrhythmias (irregular heart beats) and it is involved in reducing the contractile force of the heart muscle.

Heart Attacks in the A.M.

The blood platelets are involved in the blood clotting processes. This is an absolutely necessary function when an artery ruptures. The clotting elements are mobilized at the site of the rupture to repair the damage and stop the hemorrhage. However, when these processes operate in the absence of a break in the blood vessels the results can be catastrophic.

The blood platelets tend to naturally stick together in the morning and they generally do so at sites of existing disease in the arteries. Cigarette smoking stimulates platelet aggregation. Cigarette smokers reach for a cigarette first thing in the morning thus introducing a clumping agent at a time when the platelets are more inclined to stick together. Cigarette smokers increase their risk of heart attack by smoking in the morning.

On November 17, 1983, the Surgeon General of the U.S., Everett Koop, M.D., released a report that focused on the relationship between cigarette smoking and cardiovascular disease. Two of the salient points were: Cigarette smoking should be considered the most important of the known modifiable risk factors for coronary heart disease in the United States, and up to 30 percent of all coronary heart disease deaths are related to smoking. "While lung cancer is the disease most linked to smoking in the mind of the public, the total number of cigarette related deaths because of heart disease is much larger than the number of cigarette related deaths caused by lung cancer."[76,77]

A study of coronary artery bypass patients under 40 years of age revealed that 92 percent of them were cigarette smokers. The researchers concluded that cigarette smoking seemed to be the most prevalent risk factor associated with the need for coronary bypass surgery.[78]

The decrease in cigarette smoking is a satisfying trend, but 51.1 million Americans continue to smoke and this directly contributes to 1000 deaths every day. The ravages imposed by smoking are insidious and take time to appear. The medical profession measures smoking danger in pack-years. For example, smoking one pack per day for 20 years results in 20 pack-years (20 years × 1 pack per day = 20 pack-years). One and one-half packs per day for 20 years equals 30 pack-years (20 × 1½ = 30). Twenty to twenty-five pack years represents a point beyond which medical problems associated with smoking become evident.

It is obvious that smokers should do all in their power to quit. However, it is difficult to stop because of physical dependence on nicotine, psychological dependence on smoking and the development of the habit (situational ties). Complicating the effort to quit for young adults is the fear of gaining weight. Until a couple of years ago researchers and clinicians believed that the fear of weight gain expressed by smokers was exaggerated or a convenient rationalization for those who truly did not want to stop smoking. Women are more likely than men to continue smoking for this reason. According to Klesges, the scientific community has generally accepted the premise that only one-third of those who smoke gain weight when they quit.[79] However, he stated that recent studies indicate that the number who gain weight is closer to 65 percent, however the amount of gain is insignificant. The physiological mechanisms that are responsible for maintaining a lower body weight while smoking behavior persists are not well understood but are thought to include an increase in metabolism (the number of calories needed by the body to support life while at rest) and the rapid advancement of food through the digestive tract resulting in fewer calories being absorbed.[80] When smoking ceases, metabolism and digestive transit slow down and this results in a three to four pound weight gain. Greater weight gains are caused by altered eating habits rather than to physiology. Food smells and tastes better, it may act as a substitute for a cigarette especially during social activities, it may provide some of the oral gratification once obtained from smoking, and it may promote a feeling of relaxation. Weight gain can be avoided through appropriate exercise coupled with sensible eating.

As a group, smokers are approximately 7 percent lighter than nonsmokers.[75] This apparent benefit is actually specious or illusory—it is not as good as it sounds. A group of researchers examined the pattern of fat distribution between smokers and nonsmokers with some interesting results.[81] Even though the smokers were lighter for the same height, their waist to hip ratio (WHR) was signif-

You would have to gain almost 100 pounds to do the physiological damage that smoking one pack of cigarettes a day does.
–Better Health

icantly higher. The higher the WHR the more fat carried in the abdominal region. The subjects were participants in the Baltimore Longitudinal Study of Aging at the Gerontology Research Center from 1960 to 1986. Changes in smoking habits and WHR were observed during this time. As expected, weight increased when subjects stopped smoking and decreased when they started. The WHR of those who quit increased slightly but it was less than that expected if they had continued to smoke. But unexpectedly, the WHR for those who began smoking actually increased despite their losing weight and reflects the influence of cigarette smoking on the distribution of body fat. Not only is this andronergic or masculine fat distribution pattern aesthetically unappealing, it predisposes to such chronic diseases as coronary heart disease, diabetes, stroke, and gout.[82-84] To continue smoking cigarettes for the control of body weight in light of this evidence seems very unwise indeed.

Males have been much more successful than females in quitting the cigarette habit. The incidence of smoking among males has declined by 21.4 percent since 1964, but has only declined by 5.8 percent among females.[85] Women are not immune to the ravages of cigarette smoking. For instance, one study showed that women aged 30 to 55 who smoked 25 cigarettes per day were five times as likely to have a heart attack than nonsmoking women. Even light daily smoking—1 to 4 cigarettes per day—doubled the risk for heart attack and 5 to 14 cigarettes per day tripled the risk.[86]

Today, there are more young women smoking than young men and this represents a reversal of a long-standing trend.[87] The increasing number of female smokers coupled with the number of years that they have smoked has reversed another trend—breast cancer has been replaced by lung cancer as the leading cause of cancer death among females.[74] Smoking women experience menopause approximately two years earlier than nonsmoking women.[85] Cigarette smoking tends to suppress the production of estrogen. Decreased estrogen leads to brittle bones which break easily and early menopause accelerates the process. The antiestrogen effect of cigarette smoking seems to be responsible in part for premature tooth loss. Women who continue to smoke during pregnancy have more spontaneous abortions, premature births, and infants of low birth weight.[87] Smoking women who take birth control pills increase their likelihood of developing blood clots and fatal heart attacks.

The price tag because of smoking is shared by all Americans, smokers and nonsmokers alike, Premature death, medical treatment for smoking-related illnesses, and lost productivity run approximately $65 billion annually—this translates to $2.17 expended for every pack of cigarettes sold.[74] The financial cost to the smoker just to purchase tobacco products for a lifetime of use is staggering and they lose in other financial ways as well.[68] Nonsmoking men and women collect more of their retirement benefits than do smokers simply because they live longer.[85] Nonsmoking men collect $21,000 and nonsmoking women collect $9,000 more than smokers in Social Security benefits.

As the sale of cigarettes declined, the tobacco industry began to invest heavily in the advertisement of smokeless tobacco to take up the slack in sales. Chewing tobacco and dipping snuff have become very popular in certain segments of American Society. A number of surveys—local, state, and national—have indicated that 8 to 36 percent of male high school and college students are regular users of smokeless tobacco products.[74,88,89] The average starting age among youngsters who become regular users of smokeless tobacco products is 10.4

Hard drugs and chemicals claim far fewer victims than tobacco.
–William Chandler

The number of premature deaths due to smoking in the U.S. is the equivalent of 920 fully loaded 747 jumbo jets crashing every year—350,000 people each year.
–American Lung Association

years.[90] The World Health Organization (WHO) has described the growing use of smokeless tobacco as "a new threat to society."[88] The tobacco industry is beginning to aggressively market these products overseas.

Nicotine is an addictive drug regardless of the method of delivery. The effects are the same whether it is inhaled, as in cigarette smoking or absorbed through the tissues of the oral cavity as in chewing or dipping.[91] When the users of either of these products stop using them, they suffer a similar array of withdrawal symptoms—restlessness, anxiety, irritability, and sleep disturbances.

The American Cancer Society estimates that there were 30,600 new cases of oral cancer in 1989.[92] When tobacco is held in the mouth, nicotine and other substances, many of which are carcinogenic (cancer producing), are absorbed through the oral tissues. The prevalence of oral cancer may be 50 times higher among long-term users of smokeless tobacco than for nonusers.[74] The incidence of tooth decay and gum diseases are also significantly higher in users of these products. The data indicates that smokeless tobacco is addictive and deadly.

The advertising of smokeless tobacco was banned from the electronic media but that has not deterred the inadvertant exposure of these products by users who are some of America's top amateur and professional athletes. One of the televised World Series baseball games in 1986 was monitored to determine the amount of time in which smokeless tobacco use was in evidence.[93] A total of nearly 24 minutes of camera exposure of smokeless tobacco use by players and coaches was recorded in this three hour game. Impressionable youngsters observe their sports heroes indulge in these products. Is it not natural for them to emulate their behavior? Meanwhile, the tobacco industry must be sitting on the sidelines, laughing up their sleeves, and enjoying the fruits of this serendipitous and free advertising.

Involuntary or passive smoking is associated with disease and premature death.[94] Studies in Japan, Greece, West Germany, and the United States have shown that nonsmoking spouses of smokers are two to four times more likely to die of lung cancer than nonsmoking spouses who live with nonsmokers. The number of lung cancer deaths occurring to those who inhale the smoke of others either by living and/or working in a smoking environment may be as high as 5000 per year.[95] The average nonsmoking American passively inhales enough cigarette smoke to be the equivalent of smoking one cigarette per day. Nonsmokers who work in smoke-filled environments, such as bars and night clubs, who also live with heavy smokers may passively smoke the equivalent of 14 cigarettes per day! Is it any wonder that laws need to be enacted and enforced to protect nonsmokers in public places and at the worksite? Consider this—you are about three times more likely to die of a heart attack if your mate is a smoker.[96,97] Passive smoking aggravates angina pectoris and induces small airway dysfunction in adults.[98]

Children of smoking parents are more likely to experience higher ratios of respiratory illness including colds, influenza, bronchitis, asthma, and pneumonia.[94] The lung capacity of young male children was decreased by 7 percent when their mothers were smokers and when teenage boys also smoke their lung capacity was reduced by 25 percent. The impact of passive smoking on children can last a lifetime and it may include delayed physical and intellectual development as well as the hazards associated with prolonged exposure to carcinogenic substances.

Almost one-fifth of all deaths in the United States can be traced to the use of tobacco.
–William Chandler

A review of the literature in 1964 indicated no adequate study showing whether exercise diminished the desire for smoking.[99] As far as we know, the issue remains unresolved. That exercise causes smoking cessation is as yet unproven. However, there is evidence, anecdotal in nature, about the relationship between the development of physical fitness and smoking cessation. In a recent article, noted exercise scientist Jack Wilmore stated that, "Experts have also observed the major risk factors associated with heart disease—hypertension, high blood fat levels, even smoking—change in a positive direction as a result of an aerobic training program. (Few people who seriously engage in aerobic exercise continue to smoke.)"[100]

A random sample of 25,000 runners, most of whom were recreational rather than competitive runners, were surveyed prior to participation in the 1982 Atlanta Peachtree 10k race (6.2 miles).[101] They were surveyed regarding their perception of the effects of running upon their health. Two major health benefits emerged: (1) weight loss was achieved, and (2) 81 percent of the male and 75 percent of the female smokers successfully quit the habit subsequent to the inception of their jogging program.

In two separate studies, Blair and his coworkers found that physical exercise and smoking are negatively related but not very strongly.[102] In the second study they were unable to show that individuals who improve their fitness level through voluntary exercise were more likely to quit smoking.[103]

There are thousands of testimonials indicating that people have successfully quit smoking when they have begun to participate with regularity in an endurance exercise program, often after unsuccessfully trying a variety of other strategies. We have witnessed similar results in our Fitness and Wellness Center. This type of evidence is abundant but it does not establish a cause-and-effect relationship between exercise and smoking cessation. Perhaps the most accurate conclusion at this time is that exercise offers another option for cigarette smokers who have inclinations to become nonsmokers. The bottom line may be that if one is truly committed to quitting, one will succeed in spite of the method, but if the resolve is weak, one will fail regardless of the method. Exercise is a viable and valid option because the benefits received from physical activity cannot be maximized while continuing to smoke. Many smokers who become hooked on the exercise and fitness habit become unhooked from the smoking habit.

POINTS TO PONDER

1. *A total cholesterol level of 195 mg/dL means that you do not have to worry about this risk factor for heart disease. Do you agree or disagree and why?*
2. *Which of the lipoprotein fractions carries the most cholesterol; which carries the least?*
3. *How can total cholesterol and LDL be reduced? How can HDL be increased?*
4. *What strategies can one use to lower blood pressure?*
5. *What is essential hypertension and what are its symptoms?*
6. *How does exercise help to control blood pressure?*
7. *How does nicotine effect the cardiovascular system?*
8. *React to this statement: People gain weight when they quit smoking.*

9. *React to this statement: Smokeless tobacco is not as unhealthy as cigarette smoking.*
10. *What are the risks of breathing passive or second-hand smoke for nonsmokers?*

Other Contributing Risk Factors

Physical Inactivity

Physical inactivity (**hypokinesis**) is considered to be a risk factor for heart disease. If carried to an extreme, it is very debilitating to the human body. For example, the changes brought about by the aging process can be simulated in young healthy adults by a few weeks of bed rest.[104] Muscles atrophy (get smaller and weaker), bones demineralize and weaken, and maximum respiratory capacity and cardiovascular endurance decrease. When active young men are subjected to 10 to 11 days of chair rest, they experience substantial reductions in work capacity as well as dizziness, fainting, nausea, vomiting, and circulatory collapse. The old adage "use it or lose it" was very nicely demonstrated by these studies. In our country, growing old all too often is accompanied by inactivity and its attendant physical deterioration. We grow older and become inactive, inactivity breeds inactivity, and aging is inevitable. Without physical activity, physical decline follows a predictable course.

Aerobic exercise pursued on a regular basis is protective in that it favorably influences most of the modifiable risk factors for heart disease. Additionally, we are witnessing the completion of several recent studies which indicate that active people are not only healthier but they live longer than inactive people. One of the salient issues at this point concerns the amount of exercise necessary to confer protection from chronic disease. A second involves the amount of exercise needed to increase life expectancy. Yet another involves the comparison of leisure time physical activity (walking, climbing stairs, gardening, etc.) with physical fitness activities (jogging, swimming, cycling, etc.) in promoting health and improving longevity. The evidence generated from recent studies indicates that the effectiveness of habitual exercise in producing good health and longevity is no longer moot. What remains to be determined is how much, how hard, how long, and what type of activity is required to achieve these ends. The majority of exercise scientists do agree that one does not need to become a marathon runner to achieve the health benefits of physical activity. Somewhere between couch potato status and marathon running lies a threshold of exercise where the health benefits begin to accumulate.

The often-quoted MR FIT study (Multiple Risk Factor Intervention Trial) provided the data for a research group to investigate the level of exercise or physical activity which conferred protection against coronary heart disease.[105] The subjects were 12,000 middle-aged men whose risk of heart attack was in the upper 15 percent of the population at large. The subjects were categorized by activity level based on their leisure time physical activities. The light activity group expended an average of 74 calories per day in physical activity; the moderate activity group expended an average of 224 calories per day in physical activity; and the heavy activity group expended an average of 638 calories in physical activity. The men in the moderate activity group had only 63 percent as many fatal heart attacks as men in the light activity group and only 70 percent as many deaths from all causes. The death rate in the heavy activity group was about the same as that in the moderate activity group, but when these two groups were compared on the basis of combining fatal and nonfatal heart attacks, the heavy activity group had 20 percent fewer events. These data suggest that moderate activity provides substantial protection from heart attack and that heavy activity provides a little more. The effect of physical activity held after other risk factors were statistically controlled. To put the average energy expenditures in this study in perspective, you may consider that 74 calories expended is roughly equivalent to walking three-quarters of a mile; 224 calories translates into walking about two and one-quarter miles; and 638 calories is equivalent to walking six and one-half miles. An eight and one-half year study of 3000 middle-aged men revealed that the least fit subjects had a 3.4 greater risk of suffering a heart attack or stroke than the most fit subjects.[106] These findings held when the data were adjusted for age, smoking habit, blood pressure, and serum cholesterol. Haskell reviewed the literature and concluded that 150 calories expended (walking one and one-half miles) in daily physical activity represented the threshold above which the risk of coronary heart disease decreased.[107] He also concluded that the protective effect of daily energy expenditure increased up to 400 calories and then leveled off.

Paffenbarger's Harvard Alumni study, where 17,000 men were followed for more than 20 years, agreed with the studies of Leon and Haskell.[108] The age-adjusted incidence of coronary heart disease in Paffenbarger's subjects was inversely related to the amount of weekly energy expended walking, stair climbing, and participating in sports activities. Subjects who expended less than 2000 calories per week in these activities were at a 64 percent greater risk of incurring a heart attack than those whose physical activity equalled or surpassed (within limits) the 2000 calorie threshold. Further analysis of the data showed that weekly energy expenditure was inversely related to all causes of mortality.[109] Other conclusions of note were that a past history of participation in athletics had no carryover value into later life regarding lessening the risk for heart disease. It was more important to be currently active. Also, the alumni who became active in later life, regardless of their past history with physical activity, decreased their risk of all-cause mortality. It was significantly better to be currently active than to be an inactive ex-athlete. A series of studies at the Institute for Aerobic Research involving an eight year follow-up of 13,600 middle-age men and 3120 middle-age women showed that subjects who were in the lowest fitness category, regardless of gender, had the highest mortality rates.[110–113] The difference in all-cause mortality was greatest between the low fit category and the moderately fit category. There was little difference in mortality between subjects in the middle fitness categories and those in the high fitness categories even after the data were adjusted for cholesterol, systolic blood pressure, age, and body mass index. Lack of participation in physical fitness activities and/or leisure time physical activities emerged as significant and independent risks for death from any cause. Here again, we see that moderate levels of physical activity have a similar protective effect against mortality from all causes as high levels of physical activity.

Sallis and his co-workers found that moderate levels of physical exertion in this study did not lead to measurable improvements in cardiorespiratory endurance.[114] However, this level of activity was sufficient to produce healthful

Leisure-time activity can be an effective way of physically and mentally separating oneself from stress-producing situations at home or work.
–William Haskell

changes in the coronary risk factors. The most significant of the changes occurred in body mass index. This finding lends support to the notion that physical activity needs to be an integral part of a weight loss plan.

Researchers at the Centers for Disease Control critiqued 43 epidemiological studies which investigated the relationship between physical inactivity and coronary heart disease.[115] While some of the studies were judged unsatisfactory because of faulty research designs or other reasons, the researchers concluded that there is a causal relationship between physical inactivity and coronary heart disease. The strength of this relationship, as evidenced by more than two-thirds of these studies, was similar in magnitude to the relationship between coronary heart disease and elevated cholesterol, high systolic blood pressure, and cigarette smoking. When the active subjects in each of the 43 studies were used as standardizing or reference groups, the average risk for inactivity was approximately 1.9, or said another way: sedentary people are 1.9 times as likely to develop coronary heart disease than the most active people in each study.[116] The most active people in these studies exercised regularly but only for 20 minutes a day, three times per week. This level of exercise will not produce a highly fit individual, so once again, moderate levels of activity provide substantial health enhancement if not high levels of physical fitness. The risk of inactivity (1.9) compares favorably with the risk of the three major modifiable risk factors. They are as follows: 2.1 for high systolic blood pressure ($\geq$150 mmHg versus $\leq$130 mmHg); 2.4 for high serum cholesterol ($\geq$268 mg/dL versus $\leq$218 mg/dL); and 2.5 for cigarette smoking ($\geq$ 1 pack/day versus no smoking). Casperson suggests that lack of physical activity is as strong a risk factor as the other three. But when consideration is given to which of the four would have the most impact upon decreasing mortality, then involvement in physical activity has the edge. The reason is simple: 36 percent of Americans have blood pressures greater than 140/90 mmHg, 32 percent have cholesterol levels in excess of 200 mg/dL, and 27 percent smoke cigarettes.[117] Compare these percentages to the 59 percent of Americans who are inactive and you can readily see that a significant impact on coronary heart disease can occur if this group can be motivated to participate consistently in moderate levels of physical exertion. Van Camp has stated that, "The question is whether it's healthier to run five miles a day or walk briskly five miles a day. The issues are health and fitness. I believe that better fitness leads to better health, but while good fitness leads to good health, great fitness doesn't necessarily lead to even better health."[118] La Porte states with conviction that "Increased activity is associated with increased life expectancy."[118] Blair and his associates have found that physically fit people with high cholesterol levels ($\geq$ 280 mg/dL) were three times less likely to die prematurely of heart disease than unfit people with desirable levels of cholesterol.[119] In the same study, physically fit hypertensives had less chance of dying from coronary heart disease than physically unfit normotensives (normal blood pressure). In other words, it is better to be fit and hypercholesteremic or hypertensive than to be unfit with normal levels of both. Blair stated that the amount of activity required to obtain this degree of protection could be acquired by walking. He further stated that lack of exercise is a potent risk for coronary heart disease and official agencies such as the American Heart Association need to recognize this fact and reflect it in their guidelines. Casperson, Powel, and a growing segment of the scientific community would certainly agree. However, in the *1989 Heart Facts* publication,

There's no doubt whatever that insufficient activity will shorten your life.
−Robert Hyde

It doesn't take an enormous amount of activity to obtain considerable health benefits.
−Steve N. Blair

the American Heart Association continues to state that, "Physical inactivity hasn't been clearly established as a risk factor for heart disease."[1]

The evidence from a number of studies is beginning to show that the level of exercise and physical activity required for the purpose of health enhancement need not be as high as that needed for the development of physical fitness. This is an important point for Americans to understand. Most sedentary people don't like to exercise. To them, the word exercise conjures up sweating and pain, and neither of these is appealing. The approach to motivating them should focus upon everyday activities as opposed to the fitness activities of jogging, swimming, cycling, and so on. Everyday activities such as walking, climbing stairs, carrying our own packages from the store, mopping floors, vacuuming and doing other household chores with enthusiasm, mowing the lawn (without a riding mower), gardening, substituting some physical activity for coffee and doughnuts at the break, and so on, will minimally contribute to physical fitness but they may have a profound effect upon health status. In addition, the Paffenbarger studies showed that the protective effects of exercise are independent of the other known risk factors; that is, exercise produces changes in the cardiovascular system that tend to lower the risk.

Bassler has proposed that marathon runners, or those who jog six miles per day, six days per week, or those who total 1000 miles per year are virtually immune to heart disease provided they are nonsmokers.[120] More study is needed in this regard because people who jog as much as Bassler recommends may practice lifestyle habits in addition to exercise that reduce the risk of heart disease. The influence of jogging upon immunity to heart disease has to be separated from other positive lifestyle factors in order to determine its effectiveness. The fact is that marathon runners have died of heart attacks and some have had coronary atherosclerosis similar to that in the general population.[121] Superior physical fitness did not guarantee protection against the exercise-induced deaths of eighteen runners who died during or immediately after jogging.[122] Nor was marathon running protective for 18 participants who were over 30 years of age.[123]

Death of a Runner

Jim Fixx, jogging guru and author of the best selling text the Complete Book of Running died while on a training run of a massive heart attack in July, 1984 at the age of 52. Fixx had been jogging 80 miles per week so his abrupt death sent shock waves through the running community. It also raised questions about the protective effect of vigorous exercise against heart disease. Also, many pointed to his death as further evidence that vigorous exercise is a risk for precipitating a heart attack.

An autopsy revealed that Fixx had significant coronary artery disease. That he was able to jog 80 miles per week with severely narrowed coronary arteries attests to the trainability and adaptability of the human body. But, did jogging contribute to his death or prolong his life? Prior to becoming a jogger Fixx was a sedentary two pack a day cigarette smoker who was approximately 60 lbs. overweight, working in a high stress job with a family history of heart disease (his father died of a heart attack at the age of 43). This was definitely not a wellness profile. At 35 years of age he turned his life around by starting a jogging program. He lost 60 lbs. and gave up smoking. Many authorities are convinced that these changes in living habits helped to prolong his life—he outlived his father by 9 years. But Fixx refused, for some unknown reason, to heed the advice he offered millions of others through his writings, that is, to submit to a medical examination which would include an EKG stress test.

Ironically, his last refusal to take such a test came just three weeks before his death. After his death it was learned that he had been suffering from angina (chest pain) for at least six weeks and would probably have had an abnormal stress test. Medical intervention at that point might have substantially delayed his death.

Whether jogging increased Fixx's life or caused an early death cannot be answered but the lifestyle changes that he instituted at age 35 were certainly consistent with longer life. Regardless, the quality of his life improved as a result of those changes.

What can we learn from Fixx's death? One, he had a combination of factors that most runners don't have: he had severe heart disease which probably began prior to his change to a healthier lifestyle, he had the risk factors associated with heart disease, and he had a warning (angina) of its occurrence. Two, heart disease is a killer that not even jogging can cure. Three, making positive lifestyle changes should be accompanied by medical feedback prior to initiating vigorous exercise and should continue periodically during the life of the individual. This is particularly appropriate for those who manifest more than one risk factor.

How many jogging-related deaths are the result of chance rather than exercise? When people die under these circumstances, the immediate inference is that the death was caused by jogging because that is what the person was doing at the time. The hypothesis would seem to be that if middle-aged and older adults would abstain from jogging, these premature deaths could be avoided. If we expand upon this ostensibly logical but naive reasoning, we would also have to abstain from sleeping or driving or watching TV because many more heart attacks occur during these activities than from jogging. Obviously, establishing cause and effect is elusive because the atherosclerotic process takes years to culminate in a heart attack. What the individual was doing at the time, except in certain circumstances, probably had little bearing on the result. The expected level of cardiovascular deaths on the basis of chance alone while runners are running has been investigated.[124] Data from the National Center of Health Statistics indicated that 100 cardiovascular deaths per year in runners in the United States could be expected purely on the basis of time. However, the number of reported jogging-related deaths is considerably below this number. Kaplan's research dispels the general notion that jogging is unsafe.

Actually the occurrence of sudden death during exercise is a relatively rare event.[125] The precise number of these deaths is not known but newspaper reports place the incidence between 10 and 25 per year. This is a small number when one considers the millions of competitive and recreational athletes in the United States. The results of a study of U.S. Air Force recruits who participated in 42 days of basic training over a 20-year period reinforced the low prevalence of sudden death among young people (17 to 28 years of age). There were 21 deaths during this time, 19 of them sudden, caused by heart attack which occurred while engaged in or immediately after exercise.[126] During the twenty year period, 1,606,167 recruits went through basic training accumulating millions of hours of exercise time. There was one death for each three million hours of exercise. Only one of the 21 deaths was caused by the build-up of fatty cholesterol deposits in the coronary arteries. The majority of the deaths were attributed to myocarditis (inflammation of heart muscle) and birth defects. Exercise-related cardiac deaths that occur to young people are usually the result of cardiac anomalies,[125] while cardiac deaths in older participants are usually the result of severe atherosclerotic

Exercise-related sudden death can occur in a person with significant cardiovascular disease.
– Steven Van Camp

coronary artery disease.[110,125] Jim Fixx was an example of severe coronary artery disease. On the other hand, Pete Maravich, former basketball great, died suddenly at the age of 40 while playing a leisurely pick-up basketball game with friends. An autopsy revealed that his left coronary artery (the major blood vessel supplying a large portion of heart muscle) and its branches were missing. This was a congenital defect that had gone undetected. Flo Hyman, U.S. Olympic volleyball star in her mid-thirties, collapsed and died during a match.[127] She had Marfan's Syndrome which is an inherited disorder of the connective tissues that is common in very tall people. Her death was caused by a rupture of the aorta (largest artery in the body) which was a consequence of Marfan's disease. The infrequent deaths that do occur to young people during exercise are usually due to congenital problems.

The results of an important long-awaited community based study by Siscovick and his group that examined the relationship between vigorous exercise and the risk of sudden cardiac death was reported in the New England Journal of Medicine.[128] The researchers' approach was unique because they examined concurrently the potential risk of sudden cardiac death during vigorous exercise and the potential benefits associated with habitual exercise in the same population. According to their data, sedentary men who engage in vigorous exercise less than 20 minutes per week are three times more likely to die suddenly than men who exercise vigorously more than two hours and twenty minutes per week. Although the active men have a slightly elevated risk of sudden death during exercise, the long-term health benefits clearly outweigh the mortality risk when compared to the sedentary men. The risk of sudden death during exercise for sedentary men was 56 times greater than their risk at other times. Active men have a mortality advantage at rest and during exercise when compared to sedentary men.

Obesity

According to de Vries, "There are very few, very fat, very old people around. Your own observations—and the national statistics—clearly show that long life does not mean survival of the fattest."[129] Twenty-four percent of males and 27 percent of females between the ages of 20 and 74 weigh at least 20 percent more than that recommended by nutritionists.[130] These people meet or exceed the definition of clinical obesity which was determined by the National Institutes for Health (NIH). Nearly 90 percent of Americans judge their weight to be excessive; approximately 35 percent want to lose at least 15 pounds; 30 percent of the women and 16 percent of the men are dieting at any given time; 80 percent of fourth grade girls are dieting; 31 percent of the women ages 19 to 39 diet at least once-a-month; and 16 percent consider themselves to be perpetual dieters.[130] Approximately 20 percent of this nation's children and adolescents between the ages of 5 and 17 are obese and this figure is 40 percent higher than 20 years ago.[131] This trend was also observed in the National Children and Youth Fitness Study (NCYFS). Skinfold measures of elementary school children were significantly higher in 1986 than they were two decades ago.[132] The problem of overweight is exacerbated for obese children because they tend to develop more fat cells than children of normal weight. The consequences of this phenomenon include difficulty maintaining normal weight and a proclivity to gain weight.

Obese children have a greater probability of becoming obese adolescents and ultimately obese adults. Finally, obese adults are more likely to become the victims of life-threatening diseases.

We are in the midst of a fitness boom: We are consuming less calories today than we did ten years ago; but ironically, instead of getting thinner, we continue to get fatter. Many authorities point to our declining energy expenditure as the primary reason for this predicament. Overweight is this country's foremost nutritional problem.

In this chapter the main consideration centers on obesity as a health hazard rather than as a cosmetic problem. **Obesity** is gender-linked, that is, it is defined as more than 23 to 24 percent body fat for men and more than 30 percent for women.[133] Obesity and overweight are not synonymous terms. **Overweight** may be defined as excessive weight for one's height with no regard for its composition. In the context of this book, this term is useless for counseling people about weight loss. For example, a very muscular male, who is 6' 1" tall with only 10 percent body fat, may weigh 230 pounds. According to the new height/weight charts he is considerably overweight, but his low percentage of body fat indicates that he is carrying a significant amount of muscle tissue. It would be very difficult for this man to lose weight and remain healthy. On the other hand, a sedentary male of the same height who weighs 190 pounds, 24 percent of which is in the form of fat, is not overweight but definitely overfat. This individual falls in the obese range and should be counseled to lose fat tissue while maintaining or building muscle tissue.

Morbidity (the sick rate or ratio of sick to well in a population) and mortality (the death rate or ratio of actual to expected deaths in a population) are greater among the obese than among those of normal weight. Men who are 30 percent above desirable weight experience 70 percent greater mortality than men of normal weight.[26]

The risk of obesity as an independent factor in heart disease is difficult to evaluate. Under any circumstance, ". . . extreme obesity is clearly detrimental to health and longevity, while lesser degrees of overweight worsen the prevalent conditions—high blood pressure and diabetes—and predispose to gallstones."[134] Uncomplicated mild overfatness (accompanied by no other risk factors) probably represents little risk. But obesity generally coexists with other factors and combines with them to increase and complicate the risk.

In 1985, the NIH Consensus Development Conference formally declared obesity a disease.[135] Obesity is highly correlated with coronary heart disease, stroke, atherosclerosis, and diabetes—four of the top ten killers of Americans.[136] Obesity also contributes to gallstones, respiratory disorders, and degenerative changes in the joints (particularly those of the knees and hips). Excessive body weight predisposes men to cancer of the colon, rectum, and prostate while overweight women have a high incidence of cancer of the ovaries, uterus, and breasts. Researchers at Harvard's School of Public Health reviewed 25 studies regarding the relationship between weight and health.[137] The conclusion from some of the studies were erroneous because the researchers did not control for smoking. In those studies where smoking was controlled statistically or when normal weight nonsmokers were compared to obese nonsmokers the results indicated that excess weight caused premature death. Each pound of excess weight increased the death rate by one percent in men 30 to 49 years of age and 2 percent for ages 50 to 62. Every excess pound does count.

Obesity is a complex disease with multiple causes. Genetics, poor nutritional habits, and lack of physical activity are associated with a high percentage of obesity. The genetic influence on the amount of body weight as well as its distribution in the body is becoming more clearly established. Researchers at the University of Pennsylvania studied the relative fatness and body type of adults who had been adopted.[138] They classified 540 adoptees into thin, median weight, overweight, and obese and found that they resembled their genetic parents rather than their adoptive parents even though they learned the lifestyle of the latter. The same group studied identical and fraternal male twins over a period of 25 years.[139] Height, weight, and body mass index (a measure of relative fatness) were first calculated when they entered military service and then 25 years later. Identical twins with identical genes were very similar for height, weight, and body mass index (BMI) at the time they entered the military and again 25 years later. They gained the same amount of weight and at approximately the same time in life. The similarity in the identical twins was twice that observed in the fraternal twins and provides support for the notion that obesity is under substantial genetic control. Identical twins were fed 1000 calories more than they required for 22 days.[140] Each member of the set gained about the same amount of weight and their weight was distributed in the same places. The amount and distribution of weight gain seems to be significantly controlled by genetics. Poor nutritional habits and an inactive lifestyle are also causative factors but these will be discussed in Chapters 8 and 10.

Weight gain generally occurs imperceptibly, or so it seems, over many years. We tend to tolerate it to a certain point or threshold. Crossing the threshold produces dissatisfaction with our appearance and energizes us to map out a strategy aimed at regaining our once-streamlined silhouette. When motivated into action people generally respond by dieting, which means changing eating habits for a period of time until the target weight or a compromise target has been achieved. Most people can successfully lose weight by dieting but they usually find that the accomplishment is temporary as the lost weight is eventually regained—often with a bit more. The often-neglected factor in a weight loss program is exercise. Exercise and diet are not mutually exclusive; they are complementary, with each having a contribution to make. The role of exercise was addressed at an international meeting on obesity in 1983 and the unanimous consensus of the experts was: "if you are about to start a weight reduction program or if you're trying to maintain your present weight, success or failure can depend on whether or not you exercise."[141] Exercise uniquely contributes both to weight loss and weight maintenance by burning calories, speeding up muscle metabolism, building muscle tissue, and balancing appetite with energy expenditure. These factors will be discussed in some detail in Chapter 11.

POINTS TO PONDER

1. *Discuss the following: one can attain the health-related benefits of exercise without becoming physically fit.*
2. *What evidence can you cite to support the notion that regular physical activity may improve longevity?*
3. *Why should inactivity be considered a risk factor for heart disease?*
4. *What risk factors for heart disease can be modified by exercise and what modifications occur?*

5. *How would you respond to this statement: I don't exercise because it is dangerous, people have died while exercising?*
6. *Why should obesity be considered a disease?*
7. *Define overweight and obesity.*
8. *Discuss the influence of genetics and lifestyle in the development of obesity.*

Diabetes Mellitus

Diabetes mellitus (honey-urine disease) is a metabolic disorder in which the body is unable to regulate the level of glucose (sugar) in the blood. It is one of the ten leading causes of death in the United States affecting as many as 10 million Americans. Normal blood sugar levels range from 70 to 110 mg/100 ml of blood. Serious symptoms occur when glucose levels fall significantly out of this range. Individuals suspected of being diabetic are given a glucose tolerance test. They are given a fixed amount of a sugary solution which they must clear from the blood in a standard amount of time. Failure to accomplish this leads to a diagnosis of hyperglycemia and diabetes is suspected. Follow-up tests are then scheduled in order to confirm or refute the diagnosis.

Diabetes mellitus is a significant risk for cardiovascular disease. It is characterized by a relative lack of insulin, a hormone produced by the pancreas that is needed to accompany blood sugar into the body's cells. It does so by binding to special insulin receptors on the surfaces of "target cells," thus stimulating channels to dilate and providing access for glucose to enter the cells where it can be metabolized.

Type I diabetes, or insulin-dependent diabetes, is the most severe form. Type I diabetes was formerly referred to as "juvenile onset" since most of these cases occurred in children and adolescents. People with this type of diabetes usually have enough insulin receptors but they don't manufacture enough insulin so it must be taken by injection. Without insulin, the cells' receptors are not activated, glucose is barred from entry, and blood glucose levels rise. Unable to use glucose, the body switches to fat as the predominant energy source. Ketones are acid bodies that are harmful by-products of fat metabolism. If glucose metabolism remains inhibited while fat metabolism continues unchecked, the blood concentrations of ketones may rise to the point where a diabetic coma occurs. This is a dangerous state that can result in death. Daily injections of the proper amount of insulin prevent this from occurring, but an inherent problem in the treatment of diabetes is that "an injection of insulin is not the same physiologically as the natural secretion of insulin by the pancreas."[142] For example, the pancreas of a nondiabetic automatically monitors blood sugar levels and secretes insulin when it is needed (after a meal) and reduces its secretion when less is needed (during exercise). Insulin-dependent diabetics do not have the luxury of this exquisitely balanced system but instead they inject insulin all at once. Even if a diabetic is living a well-regulated life, occasional imbalances occur between glucose levels and insulin. This results in a lag time between the need for insulin and its availability and contributes to premature deterioration of the cardiovascular system. Diabetes significantly increases the risk for coronary heart disease. It usually co-exists with high levels of cholesterol and triglycerides in the blood. The insulin-dependent diabetic is involved in a continuous balancing act attempting to regulate energy expenditure (rest, work and exercise metabolism), energy intake (food), and insulin. A change in any one requires an adjustment in the others.

Type II diabetes or noninsulin-dependent diabetes usually occurs after 40 years of age in overweight, sedentary people. Eighty percent of all diabetes is of the Type II variety. This type of diabetes is characterized by the production of more than enough insulin but an inadequate number of insulin receptors. As a result, target cells are unable to receive glucose so its level in the blood rises. As Type II diabetes progresses some people will also produce insufficient quantities of insulin. Treatment includes hypoglycemic (sugar lowering) drugs, a low-fat diet, exercise, and weight control. Management of Type II diabetes without drugs is the preferred strategy and for most diabetics it is an achievable goal. Oral hypoglycemic drugs promote the accumulation of fat, making weight loss a difficult proposition. Excessive weight increases the cell's resistance to insulin, which increases dependence upon the hypoglycemic drugs, which in turn inhibits weight loss, and the proverbial vicious cycle becomes firmly established. Exercise and weight loss, however, combine to increase the number of insulin receptors while simultaneously enhancing their sensitivity to insulin. The net result is that more glucose can enter more cells more quickly.[143]

Diabetes cannot be cured but it can be controlled, which is the key to living a long and productive life. Depending upon the type of diabetes, control involves some combination of injectible insulin, oral hypoglycemic agents, meal planning, exercise, and weight loss.

In 1986, a panel of experts from the National Institute of Health (NIH) drafted a statement regarding the role of exercise in the management of noninsulin-dependent diabetes.[144] They stated the major effect of exercise in the control of diabetes was in reducing body fatness. Exercise was also considered to be an adjunct to diet in regulating the glucose level in the blood. An epidemiological study of male insulin-dependent diabetes mellitus (IDDM) patients showed that those who were active in sports in high school or college were less likely to develop cardiovascular disease and less likely to have died than nonpartici-pants.[145] The researchers also found that physical activity decreased the insulin requirements of these subjects. Similar results were found in another study employing former female athletes as the subjects.[146] They had a significantly lower rate of diabetes after the age of 20 than nonparticipating control subjects even though the family histories of the two groups were alike. Donnell D. Etzwiler, Director of the International Diabetes Center, stated that exercise causes a drop in blood glucose level and promotes more effective use of carbohydrates.[147]

Fourteen adolescent male and female insulin-dependent diabetics participated in a 12 week program of exercise which met for 45 minutes, three days per week.[148] Twenty-five minutes were involved with aerobic exercise and the remaining time was devoted to stretching, warm- up, and cool-down. Aerobic capacity increased and LDL cholesterol decreased but there was no change in glycemic control at the end of 12 weeks. Another group of researchers examined the effects of 8 weeks of structured physical fitness (30 minutes of swimming) versus unstructured recreational activities in IDDM adolescents.[149] They found that blood glucose levels declined in both groups but it declined more with structured exercise. The authors also found that while exercise is generally considered to have a glucose lowering effect, it is less predictable than diet or insulin in this regard. Blackett summarized the benefits of exercise for young children and adolescent diabetics.[150] These include: (1) increased cardiac endurance, (2) a decrease in plasma cholesterol and triglycerides, (3) an increase in HDL cholesterol, and (4) a reduction in body fat and prevention of obesity.

Brooks and Fahey discussed the relationship between exercise and diabetes in this way: (1) "Endurance exercise reduces the need for insulin. The lower the insulin dosage, the closer to normal physiology. Therefore, there is less of a roller coaster effect, allowing for easier control of the disease. (2) Endurance exercise reduces platelet adhesiveness for about 24 hours after exercises such as running, swimming, or cycling. (3) Regular endurance exercise reduces the severity of the risk factors of coronary artery disease such as hypertension, obesity, blood lipids, and serum uric acid."[142]

Stress and Its Management

Rules for Handling Stress

- Don't sweat the small stuff.
- Everything is small stuff.
- If you can't "fight" or "flee," then flow.

Robert Eliot, M.D. *Time*, June 6, 1983.

It is estimated that 50 to 75 percent of all people who visit a physician do so for psychosomatic disorders. These are illnesses that originate in the mind and manifest themselves in physical ailments. Animal experiments have shown that the higher centers of the brain can influence the physical state. Human studies are far from conclusive, but certain mental states such as grief over the loss of a loved one increase the risk of contracting infectious diseases on the one hand to dying of a cardiovascular event on the other. In the near future, researchers will be able to delineate the role of emotions in the genesis of health and disease. Shealy discussed the effects of negative emotions:

> *Anger, frustration, depression, hatred, anxiety, fear, and guilt are real stresses. They create physical disease. They weaken the system of immunity. They stimulate the body to produce excess adrenalin and cortisone, and, in general, they upset the homeostasis—the balance—of the various functions of the body.[151]*

It appears that the mind has a profound effect upon the body. Thoughts and emotions directly influence physiology through the regulatory centers of the brain. Conversely, the **"placebo effect"** has worked in a positive fashion to relieve the symptoms of and/or cure disease, to relieve pain, to promote relaxation, and so on. This effect is exemplified by the administration of inert substances, which have no medicinal value, for the purpose of curing illness. The power of the placebo is in the mind of the receiver. Recipients must truly believe that the substance or substances that they take have curative power. Norman Cousins who cured himself of crippling spinal arthritis has studied the placebo effect and describes it as follows:

The placebo, then, is not so much a pill as a process. The process begins with the patient's confidence in the doctor and extends through to the full functioning of his own immunological and healing system. The process works not because of any magic in the tablet but because the human body is its own apothecary and because the most successful prescriptions are those filled by the body itself.[152]

Edlin writes that

Because of the sick person's belief—whether in the placebo, the physician or the healing process—his or her body and brain chemistry are changed. Symptoms disappear. Illness vanishes. Well-being is restored. Scientists are just beginning to unravel the complex changes in body chemistry that can be initiated in the mind. The placebo effect demonstrates quite convincingly that for many people the belief that they have been administered an effective drug is sufficient to provide relief or even to cure their disease. So all people carry within them a powerful source of healing—the beliefs in their minds.[153]

Mention the word "stress" and it immediately congers up a negative image. The prevailing opinion of the general public is that all stress is bad. Stress can be bad—it has been associated with many severe and chronic diseases—but it can also be good and necessary. People who are essentially in control of their lives recognize stress and utilize and channel its energies into productive activities. The ability to control stress resides in each of us. Seliger states that

It is the perception of and attitude about both self and environment that most influences whether a person will be hurt by stress. What researchers are finding is that bad stress is triggered not by the pressures of decision-making but rather by the feeling that one's decisions are useless, that life is overwhelming and beyond personal control.[154]

Upper echelon executives in America's largest corporations actually have a lower mortality rate than same sex people in the general population. These people operate in a corporate pressure-cooker yet they seem to be quite resistant to and experience no adverse effects from their exposure to stress and pressure. Possible explanations for their hardiness include a belief that they are in control of their lives, they have objectives which allow them to proceed with a sense of purpose, and they regard change as a challenge rather than a threat. People who react negatively to stress are in occupations where they do not have the opportunity to enjoy security, status, and/or control. This includes lower management positions, sales jobs, secretarial positions, assembly line positions, and so on. People in these occupations may feel expendable, replaceable, and often see themselves as victims which, of course, leads to bad stress.

Hans Selye, one of the pioneer researchers in this field, defined stress as the nonspecific response of the human organism to any demand, positive or negative, that it encounters.[155] In other words, the body does not discriminate between stressors, good or bad, but reacts the same way regardless of the type.

There are three kinds of stress: normal stress, **distress** (normal stress that has become chronic—bad stress) and **eustress** (good stress). In its attempt to adapt to stress, the body goes through a complex array of physiological changes.

The model of adaptation first described by Selye involves three stages of responses. First is the "alarm" stage where the body prepares for action. Adrenaline, the fight or flight hormone is released, heart rate accelerates, blood pressure increases, extra blood is sent to the muscles and less to the digestive system, pupils dilate to take in more information, blood coagulates more rapidly as a precaution against injury, blood sugar level rises, and the immune system slows down. These are some of the changes that occur which prepare the body to perform in a crisis. These changes represent a significant strain to the body which take a toll should they become numerous and persistent. Second is the "recuperative" stage where the damage sustained during the alarm stage is repaired. Third, is the return to the body's normal state of "relaxed alertness."

Bad stress is normal or acute stress which has become chronic, that is, it lasts for weeks or months thereby precluding the opportunity for repair and recuperation. Unhealthy physical reactions are the result of chronic stress. The underlying mechanisms are not well understood but there are some theories. We begin with the premise that stress probably does not cause disease but that it predisposes or increases one's vulnerability to illness and it may also hasten the process of latent or subclinical disease. The question is why? In a previous section, we saw how the mind can influence and change the body's physiology either positively or negatively. The body's immune system is somewhat depressed during the alarm stage of stress. It returns to fully functioning status during the recuperative stage but when stress is chronic it may remain suppressed for a long period of time thereby increasing susceptibility to illness. The immune system responds to invading microorganisms and environmental insult through a complex series of reactions designed to rid the body of these potentially harmful elements. This is accomplished through the development of specific antibodies and specialized blood cells (lymphocytes) that recognize and attack foreign substances inactivating and preparing them for removal. The immune response is the body's last but most effective line of defense against disease. Oftentimes the immune response is long-lasting conferring immunity for life from specific diseases such as measles or chicken pox. If the immune system is temporarily impaired, as occurs in chronic stress, the individual becomes more vulnerable to disease. Paul Rosch, President of the American Institute of Stress, began research on this topic as a contemporary of Selye three decades ago. He states that cancer and other diseases invade the body when the immune system weakens. The lymphocytes have receptors in their walls which accept hormones such as ACTH (adrenocorticotropic hormone which may assist in resisting stress), endorphins (reduce the perception of pain), and other brain hormones. This network provides a vehicle through which the brain and the immune system communicate. This is the rationale for supporting the connection between thoughts and feelings that cause changes in hormone levels and concomitantly produces responses from the immune system. Chronic stress changes hormone levels and depresses the immune system.

The question then, is how to combat chronic stress since it is pervasive in contemporary America? What tools and techniques are available for us in this perpetual battle that only ends when life does? How can distress be changed into eustress? Stress coping techniques were discussed earlier in this chapter in the section on hypertension. Since this text approaches wellness through physical fitness, the emphasis will be on this vehicle in alleviating and controlling stress. This field of investigation is in its infancy but the preliminary data are encouraging. There are three conclusions which are inherent in the literature regarding the relationship between physical fitness and stress: (1) it reduces the severity of the stress response, (2) it shortens the recovery time from stress, and (3) it reduces stress-related vulnerability to disease. The data leading to these conclusions was generated primarily from studies which employed aerobic exercise. This kind of exercise features continuous movement for at least 10 minutes at an intensity level that can be sustained without stopping to rest.[156] Thirty-four studies which examined the relationship between aerobic fitness and psychosocial stress were reviewed by Crews and Landers.[157] The subjects in these studies were exposed to laboratory-induced psychosocial stressors which included solving math problems under a time deadline, observing films showing accidents or surgery, performing physical exercise of varying kinds, and immersing an extremity, usually an arm, in ice water. After statistical analysis, the researchers concluded that aerobically fit subjects displayed a reduced response to stress compared to unfit subjects and this held regardless of the type of psychosocial stressor that was used. Fit subjects also recovered from stress sooner than the unfit. Some of these studies suggested that physically fit people have a more effective immune system and are better equipped to ward off disease. This may be possible through mechanisms that include an increase in body temperature during and immediately after exercise (this will be discussed in another chapter), the production of endogenous opiates (discussed later in this chapter), and reduction in the levels of epinephrine and norepinephrine (catecholamines which prepare the individual for fight or flight).

The effect of anaerobic activity (high intensity short burst activities such as weight lifting or sprinting 100 yards) on stress reduction is inconclusive. Researchers who support the notion that anaerobic training is effective in reducing the stress response accentuate the natural rhythm of these activities which includes periods of stress followed by periods of recovery.[158] Practice of this sort may facilitate our ability to handle intermittant acute stress and may transfer to life situations enabling us to handle such stress more effectively. Proponents suggest that anaerobically trained people show greater stress-response reduction than people who have had no physical training. Tucker has shown that any kind of exercise which leads to even minimal amounts of fitness may serve as a buffer against stress.[159] Opponents of anaerobic exercise as a stress-reducer, state that activities in this category do not produce the changes in the nervous system that are associated with stress reduction.[160] They add that anaerobic exercise may be counterproductive in relieving stress since these significantly raise the blood pressure.

Howard's longitudinal study has shown that exercise and fitness are beneficial for both mind and body in that they produce positive physiological and personality changes.[161] Improvements in body image and self-esteem result in satisfied individuals who genuinely like themselves. Exercise is a concrete stressor which is easily identified. During participation it replaces ambiguous or nonspecific psychosocial stress. It is also an avenue for the release of excess energy. The social support that one may receive from family and friends, as well as from fellow participants, also seems to be useful to mind and body.

Eustress, or good stress, occurs when one accepts and successfully meets a challenge. Exercise is a stressor and a challenge but one that can be recognized and quantified by participants. This builds confidence which leads to a sense of control over one's destiny. Sensible exercise graded in difficulty to periodically present a greater challenge provides a sense of accomplishment. Success breeds success so the newer challenges should be attainable in order to increase the likelihood of success. Exercise can cause distress when people have unreasonable expectations or objectives and aspirations that cannot be achieved. The rule for training is "train, don't strain" or "relax and enjoy it." When practiced in this manner, exercise is good stress. If exercise is not enjoyable, it may simply become another stressor.

People under chronic stress are constantly secreting adrenaline into the blood stream. Continual activation of this response in the absence of physical activity results in adrenaline storage in the heart muscle and a probable increase is diastolic blood pressure. Circulating adrenaline contributes to the processes involved in cholesterol build-up in the arteries. The best antidote for stress is physical activity because it metabolizes adrenaline while recharging the psychological and emotional batteries.

Physical activity for the purpose of competition may become another stressor for some and a stress reliever for others. For some people exercise is tolerable only when they are competing—running a road race, playing racquetball or tennis, and so on, and they may not participate without competition. Whether competitiveness in physical activity and sports induces or reduces stress needs to be evaluated by each individual.

Since the mind and body function in unison, can we accomplish the reverse? Can we strengthen the body (heart, circulatory, respiratory, muscular systems, etc.) and produce a positive effect upon the mind? The psychological and emotional benefits of endurance-type exercise—which are difficult to quantify—are just beginning to be understood. This area of research became more promising when several types of opiate-like brain chemicals that were reputed to produce elevations in mood, feelings of tranquility, and increased tolerance to pain were identified in the early 1970s. The enkephalins (Greek for "in the brain") were the first to be identified, but these are not very potent because they are rapidly degraded.[162] Later in that decade, the beta **endorphins** (endogenous, made within the body) were identified and proved to be more powerful and more resistant to degradation than the enkephalins. Cooper claims that when present in similar doses as exogenous (taken into the body, as by injection) morphine, the beta endorphins are 200 times more powerful.[163] More recently, the dynorphins (Greek for "power"), another class of chemicals, were identified but little is known about these as yet.

Most of the available research has focused upon the beta endorphins (from this point on referred to simply as endorphins). At the present time, the conclusions about these chemicals are not firm. These chemicals are difficult to measure and many of the tools and techniques used in their assessment are relatively crude. Secondly, these substances are measured in the blood, rather than the brain where the pharmacological effect occurs. Blood elevations may not necessarily translate into brain elevation because of blood-brain barriers that might not allow blood endorphins to filter through.

Most studies have shown an increase in the level of endorphins in response to exercise.[164] In one study, 45 percent of the subjects increased their endorphin level after an easy run, but 80 percent of the same subjects experienced an increase after a strenuous run of equal distance.[165] This suggests that the intensity of exercise might be an important factor in endorphin production.

These researchers used a large number of subjects who ran in natural outdoor settings where the pacing could not be controlled. They surrendered some degree of control in order to achieve realism. Another group used only six subjects and exercised them in a laboratory setting on a treadmill where the pace could be controlled.[166] They measured the subjects' aerobic capacity and then programmed three different intensities based upon these values. They found no increase in endorphin levels as a result of increasing intensities. In another study, a 20-minute run on the treadmill at 80 percent of predicted maximum heart rate increased plasma endorphin levels in five men and four women aged 24 to 36.[167] Endorphin levels were measured in 15 men after a 46 kilometer mountain race.[168] All contestants had an increase, but older runners (over 40 years of age) had a 15 percent lower increase. This suggests that age may be a factor. Endorphin levels immediately after exercise have been measured at five times the resting level. A number of studies have documented the painkilling, mood elevating and tranquilizing effect of the endorphins, but at this point the issue is far from being resolved.

According to the President's Commission on Mental Health, approximately 25 percent of Americans suffer from depression at any given time and 80 percent of all who commit suicide are depressed.[169] Depression is prolonged sadness which persists beyond a reasonable length of time. It is characterized by withdrawal, inactivity, and feelings of helplessness and loss of control. Exercise is now accepted as one component in a spectrum of possible treatments for depression. Several studies have shown that aerobic exercise eases clinical depression.[170-173] Some patients in these studies were "essentially well" after three weeks of training while others were able to reduce their medication. Patients became less depressed with exercise and those who exercised more frequently (five days per week) improved the most.

Many runners have described feelings of euphoria generally referred to as the "runner's high." In his book, *Positive Addiction*, Glasser asserts that jogging provides the opportunity for the mind to "spin free" and relax.[174] He claims that this phenomenon forms the primary stimulus for getting people hooked on jogging. Many joggers insist that they are addicted to running and when denied the opportunity to run, they react with symptoms similar to those observed in some mental and physical disorders. Morgan has labeled this phenomenon, which is characterized by irritability, anxiety and depression, as negative addiction.[175] Some investigators have implied that this type of addition is indigenous to obsessive-compulsive personalities who generally exhibit this pattern in anything that they attempt. They simply transfer this behavior to jogging. Morgan states that the concept of "runner's high" is not supported by the available evidence.[175]

Rethinking the High in Runner's High

We've heard a lot about runner's high in recent years, and there's even a physiological explanation for it. During times of stress, including the exertion of hard running or strenuous exercise, the level of endorphins, the body's "natural opiates," increases. These chemicals, like real opiates, mask pain and have been credited with causing the high many joggers claim to experience during a good run. It has even been suggested that some runners become addicted to the endorphins released during exercise.

Robert G. McMurray of the University of North Carolina at Chapel Hill questions this explanation. An All-American swimmer during college and now an assistant professor of physical education, McMurray says he has never experienced any form of exercise high, and his experiments suggest that even if some people do get high on running, it is not due to the endorphins.

McMurray and his colleagues, David S. Sheps and Diane M. Guinan, injected volunteers with either a control substance or with naloxone, a drug that blocks the action of endorphins. The subjects then walked on a treadmill that gradually became steeper and made walking more difficult. They were asked to stay on the treadmill as long as they could and to rate how hard they were working at intervals. The researchers report in the Journal of Applied Physiology (Vol. 56, No. 2) that there was no difference between the naloxone and control subjects in terms of perceived exertion, the time it took to reach exhaustion and most other physiological measures. And none of the subjects reported feeling anything other than exhaustion during and directly after the exercise.

"Our research suggests that if there really is such a thing as runner's high, it is not being caused by endorphins. It is more likely," McMurray says, "that this feeling of well-being comes from adrenaline or the release of built-up stress." With regard to the possibility of becoming hooked on endorphins, he explains, "The attraction of prolonged exercise is probably psychological. It is so good at relieving stress that some people who are particularly susceptible to stress may begin feeling like they can't do without it."

"Rethinking the High in Runner's High." *Psychology Today*, p. 8, May, 1984. Reprinted by permission.

The data thus far favors the position that aerobic exercise does produce relaxation, feelings of tranquility, and elevations of mood. The mechanisms for explaining these phenomena are not well understood. De Vries summarized the research and concluded that, "A close examination of the available data suggests substantial agreement among researchers that there is a tranquilizer effect from exercise. Although more corroborative evidence is needed, we should draw a cautious conclusion that appropriate types, intensities, and durations of exercise can bring about a significant tranquilizer effect."[176]

In 1969, cardiologists Myer Friedman and Ray Rosenman introduced the concept of behavior type as a risk factor for coronary heart disease. They identified a coronary prone personality which they labeled Type A. Type A people are characteristically competitive, aggressive, time-conscious, tense, and oftentimes hostile. They also identified a more relaxed Type B personality who is easy-going and less time-oriented. The researchers classified 3000 healthy men by personality type and followed them for eight years. They found that Type A people had twice as many heart attacks as Type B people. Since then, other researchers using the same instruments and techniques to categorize behavior type, have been unable to duplicate the results of Friedman and Rosenman. In fact, since the original study, the majority of the evidence indicates that Type A behavior per se does not increase the risk for heart disease nor does it confirm a protective effect between Type B and coronary heart disease. However, there is some agreement that Type A personality coupled with hostility does increase the risk for coronary heart disease.

Scientists who are presently trying to unravel the mysteries associated with the emotional effects of exercise have more questions than answers. But the people who have been exercising consistently voice their opinions unreservedly. They report feeling more relaxed, sleeping more soundly, having more energy, and feeling better than at any other time in their lives. To them, these are the important benefits; how and why they occur are of little consequence. The average participant is not concerned with whether the effect is elicited from the endorphins, or the feeling of well-being associated with exercise, or the feeling of taking charge of this aspect of their lives, or some other reason that has yet to be identified. The important factor is that these effects occur, and the feelings expressed by faithful exercisers are genuine and, in their perceptions, are tied in a causal way to their exercise program. Too many people report similar experiences for it to be in the realm of coincidence. In time, scientists will resolve the whys and hows, but for now we should place some deserved emphasis upon the subjective feelings connected with physical activity. We can predict that these will occur in an appropriately planned and executed exercise program. Perhaps those of us who are involved in motivating others to exercise have relied too much upon objective data focusing upon physiological responses and have slighted to some degree those subjective perceptions that convey to participants that a physically active life is the preferred way to live.

Triglycerides

Triglycerides are found in food, may be synthesized by the liver and intestines, and constitute the most "space-efficient" form of energy storage in the body. Most of the fat in the body is stored in the form of triglycerides. These are composed of fatty acids of varying lengths that are attached to a molecule of glycerol.

The relationship between hypertriglyceridemia (elevated plasma triglycerides) and coronary heart disease remains controversial. The National Institute of Health (NIH) has reported that elevated plasma triglycerides may be associated with heart disease under certain circumstances.[177] These include co-existence with diabetes, kidney disease, obesity, elevated total cholesterol, low concentrations of HDL cholesterol, high concentrations of LDL cholesterol, hypertension, and cigarette smoking.[178] Elevated triglyceride levels do not seem to be independently predictive of coronary risk. Values up to 250 mg/dL are considered to be normal; values between 250 and 500 mg/dL are borderline; and values above 500 mg/dL are excessive. Values below 250 mg/dL do not increase the risk for heart disease unless accompanied by elevated total cholesterol. People whose values are between 250 and 500 mg/dL may be at higher risk particularly if the elevation is caused by familial or genetic factors. Intervention should be established for these people as well as those whose levels are above 500 mg/dL.

Intervention programs designed to lower plasma triglycerides include smoking cessation, alcohol restriction, low fat low cholesterol diet, exercise, and medication.[178] A single bout of aerobic exercise will decrease the concentration of plasma triglycerides.[107] Aerobic exercise performed on consecutive days lowers the level further and keeps it suppressed for 48 to 72 hours. But if several days are allowed to pass without exercise, triglyceride values return to pre-exercise levels. The optimal intensity and duration of exercise for the purpose of reducing plasma triglycerides is not known at this time. It is probably a safe bet that if one follows the American College of Sports Medicine guidelines for exercise, triglyceride values will drop. These guidelines are discussed in Chapter 6.

Cardiac Risk

Now that you have a better understanding of the risk factors associated with heart disease, you are ready to take and appreciate the "Assessment of Cardiac Risk" test in Table 3.5. Examine each category of risk factors carefully and select the description and accompanying score which applies to you. If you don't know your blood cholesterol level, then examine the fat content of your diet and answer ac-

cordingly. If you still cannot decide then select the box which contains 20 percent animal fat for your answer. Total your score for all 8 categories and then determine your degree of risk by comparing your score with the Risk Key at the bottom of the table. (You will note that "stress" is omitted as one of the risks, not because it is unimportant, but because it is difficult to quantify.)

TABLE 3.5   Cardiac Risk Assessment

Factor	Score	Factor	Score
Age		**Exercise**	
10–20	1	Intensive occupational and recreational exertion.	1
21–30	2	Moderate occupational and recreational exercise.	2
31–40	3	Sedentary work and intense recreational exertion.	3
41–50	4	Sedentary occupational and moderate recreational exertion.	5
51–60	6	Sedentary work and light recreational exertion.	6
61–70	8	Complete lack of all exercise.	8
Weight		**Cholesterol**	
More than 5 lb below standard weight.	0	Below 180 mg. Diet contains no animal or solid fats.	1
Standard weight.	1	181–205 mg. Diet contains 10% animal or solid fats.	2
5–20 lb overweight.	2	206–230 mg. Diet contains 20% animal or solid fats.	3
21–35 lb overweight.	3	231–255 mg. Diet contains 30% animal or solid fats.	4
36–50 lb overweight.	5	256–280 mg. Diet contains 40% animal or solid fats.	5
51–65 lb overweight.	7	281–330 mg. Diet contains 50% animal or solid fats.	7
Blood Pressure		**Heredity**	
100 upper reading.	1	No known history of heart disease	1
120 upper reading.	2	One relative with cardiovascular disease over 60.	2
140 upper reading.	4	Two relatives with cardiovascular disease over 60.	3
160 upper reading.	4	One relative with cardiovascular disease under 60.	4
180 upper reading.	6	Two relatives with cardiovascular disease under 60.	6
200 or over upper reading.	8	Three relatives with cardiovascular disease under 60.	8
Tobacco Usage		**Gender**	
Nonuser	0	Female	1
Cigar and/or pipe.	1	Female over 45.	2
10 cigarettes or less a day.	2	Male	3
20 cigarettes a day.	3	Bald Male	4
30 cigarettes a day.	5	Bald, short male.	6
40 cigarettes a day or more.	8	Bald, short, stocky male.	7

RISK KEY

Very low risk = 6–11	Average risk = 18–25	Dangerous risk = 33–42
Low risk = 12–17	High risk = 26–32	Extremely dangerous risk = 42–60

G. Edlin and E. Golanty, *Health and Wellness* (Boston: Jones & Bartlett, 1988). Adapted from an instrument developed by John Boyer.

POINTS TO PONDER

1. Describe and differentiate between Type I and Type II diabetes.
2. Describe the preferred form of treatment for Type II diabetes.
3. Of what benefit is exercise to a diabetic?
4. Define and describe stress.
5. What is the placebo effect?
6. What are the stages of stress and describe each?
7. What effect does chronic stress have upon the body's immune system?
8. How might aerobic exercise alleviate stress?
9. What are the beta endorphins and how are they affected by exercise?

Chapter Highlights

This chapter focused on the risk factors associated with heart disease. The American Heart Association (AHA) has classified these as "major risk factors that can't be changed (increasing age, male sex, and heredity); major risk factors that can be changed (elevated blood cholesterol, high blood pressure, and cigarette smoking); and other contributing risk factors (obesity, diabetes, stress, and physical inactivity)." The AHA devotes little attention to elevated triglyceride level as a risk, but it is included in this text because under certain circumstances it seems to contribute to heart disease.

It is true that several risks are unmodifiable but that should not imply that those who are exposed are destined to die prematurely of heart disease. However, having one or more of these risks does imply that one needs to live a heart-healthy type of lifestyle paying attention to the need for regular exercise, sound nutritional practices, maintenance of ideal body weight, abstinence from tobacco usage, and periodic medical evaluations with particular attention devoted to the cardiac risk profile. While this lifestyle cannot negate these risks, it may ameliorate their effects.

Since this text approaches wellness through physical fitness or physical activity, an attempt was made to delineate the effects of these upon reducing the severity of each of the cardiac risk factors.

References

1. American Heart Association, *1989 Heart Facts,* American Heart Association, 1988.
2. F. W. Kasch et al., "A Longitudinal Study of Cardiovascular Stability in Active Men Aged 45 to 65 Years," *The Physician and Sportsmedicine,* 16 (1988): 117.
3. "Special Report: Risk Factors in Heart Disease," *Medical World News,* 18, (1979): 41.
4. A. Lubell, "Can Exercise Help Treat Hypertension in Black Americans?" *The Physician and Sportsmedicine,* 16, no. 9 (September, 1988): 165.
5. A. Lubell, "Prescribing Exercise to Black Americans," *The Physician and Sportsmedicine,* 16 (1988): 169.
6. P. S. Gartside et al., "Determinants of High Density Lipoprotein Cholesterol in Blacks and Whites: The Second National Health and Nutrition Examination Survey," *American Heart Journal,* 108, (1984): 641.
7. E. Chesler et al., "Myocardial Infarction in the Black Population of South Africa: Coronary Angiographic Findings," *American Heart Journal,* 95 (1978): 691.
8. K. Yano et al., "Dietary Intake and the Risk of Coronary Heart Disease in Japanese Men Living in Hawaii," *American Journal of Clinical Nutrition,* 31 (1978): 1270.

9. T. L. Robertson and others, "Epidemiologic Studies of Coronary Heart Disease and Stroke in Japanese Men Living in Japan, Hawaii, and California," *American Journal of Cardiology,* 39, (1977): 239.

10. The Institute for Aerobics Research, "A Cholesterol Primer," *The Aerobics News,* 1, no. 1 (May, 1986): 1.

11. W. B. Kannel et al., "Serum Cholesterol, Lipoproteins, and Risk of Coronary Heart Disease: The Framingham Study," *Annals of Internal,* Medicine 74 (1971): 1.

12. "Relationship of Blood Pressure, Serum Cholesterol, Smoking Habit, Relative Weight, and ECG Abnormalities to Incidence of Major Coronary Events: Final Report of The Pooling Project Research Group," *Journal of Chronic Disease,* 31, (1978): 201.

13. V. Goldbourt et al., "Total and High Density Lipoprotein Cholesterol in the Serum and Risk of Mortality: Evidence of a Threshold Effect," *British Medical Journal,* 290 (1985): 1239.

14. J. Stamler et al., "Is the Relationship Between Serum Cholesterol and Risk of Death from Coronary Heart Disease Continuous and Graded?" *Journal of the American Medical Association,* 256, (1986): 2823.

15. S. M. Grundy, "Cholesterol and Coronary Heart Disease," *Journal of the American Medical Association,* 256, no. 20 (November, 1986): 2849.

16. "Report of the National Cholesterol Education Program Expert Panel on Detection, Evaluation, and Treatment of High Blood Cholesterol in Adults," *Archives of Internal Medicine,* 148, (January, 1988): 36.

17. A. Kagan et al., "Serum Cholesterol and Mortality in a Japanese-American Population: The Honolulu Heart Program," *American Journal of Epidemiology,* 114, (1981): 11.

18. B. Peterson et al., "Low Cholesterol Level as a Risk Factor for Noncoronary Death in Middle-Aged Men," *Journal of the American Medical Association,* 245, (1981): 2056.

19. R. R. Williams et al., "Cancer Incidence by Levels of Cholesterol," *Journal of the American Medical Association,* 245, (1981): 247.

20. A. J. McMichael et al., "Dietary and Endogenous Cholesterol and Human Cancer," *Epidemiology Reviews,* 6, (1984): 192.

21. A. Keys et al., "Serum Cholesterol and Cancer Mortality in the Seven Countries Study," *American Journal of Epidemiology,* 121, (1985): 870.

22. R. A. Hiatt and B.H. Fireman, "Serum Cholesterol and the Incidence of Cancer in a Large Cohort," *Journal of Chronic Disease,* 39, (1986): 861.

23. R. W. Sherwin et al., "Serum Cholesterol Levels and Cancer Mortality in 361,662 Men Screened for Multiple Risk Factor Intervention Trial," *Journal of the American Medical Association,* 257, (1987): 943.

24. P. Knekt et al., "Serum Cholesterol and Risk of Cancer in a Cohort of 39,000 Men and Women," *Journal of Clinical Epidemiology,* 41, (1988): 519.

25. A. Keys et al., "Cholesterol Response to Changes in the Diet," *Metabolism,* 14, (1965): 776.

26. F. I. Katch and W.D. McArdle, *Nutrition, Weight Control, and Exercise,* Philadelphia: Lea and Febiger, 1988.

27. "The Lipid Research Clinics Coronary Primary Prevention Trial Results: I. Reduction in the Incidence of Coronary Heart Disease," *Journal of the American Medical Association,* 251, (1984): 351.

28. "The Lipid Research Clinics Coronary Primary Prevention Trial Results: II. The Relationship of Reduction in Incidence of Coronary Heart Disease to Cholesterol Lowering," *Journal of the American Medical Association,* 251, (1984): 365.

29. A. M. Gotto, "Can the Progression of Atherosclerosis be Halted? *Drug Therapy,* 37, (1984): 39.

30. V. Manninen et al., "Lipid Alterations and Decline in the Incidence of Coronary Heart Disease in the Helsinki Heart Study," *Journal of the American Medical Association,* 260 (1988): 641.

31. M. S. Brown and J.L. Goldstein, "A Receptor-Mediated Pathway for Cholesterol Homeostasis," *Science,* 232, (1986): 34.

32. E. J. Schaefer et al., "Nutrition, Lipoproteins, and Atherosclerosis," *Clinical Nutrition,* 5, (1986): 99.

33. P. D. Wood et al., "Increased Exercise Level and Plasma Lipoprotein Concentrations: A One-Year Randomized, Controlled Study in Sedentary Middle-Aged Men," *Metabolism,* 32, (1983): 31.

34. P. Hespel et al., "Changes in Plasma Lipids and Apoproteins Associated With Physical Training in Middle-Aged Sedentary Men," *American Heart Journal,* 115, (1988): 786.

35. G. Egusa et al., "Influence of Obesity on the Metabolism of Apolipoprotein B in Humans," *Journal of Clinical Investigation,* 76, (1985): 596.

36. Y. A. Kesaniemi and S.M. Grundy, "Increased Low Density Lipoprotein Production Associated with Obesity," *Arteriosclerosis,* 3, (1983): 170.

37. The Lovastatin Study Group II, "Therapeutic Response to Lovastatin (Mevinolin) in Nonfamilial Hypercholesterolemia," *Journal of the American Medical Association,* 256, (1986): 2829.

38. W. P. Castelli et al., "Incidence of Coronary Heart Disease and Lipoprotein Cholesterol Levels," *Journal of the American Medical Association,* 256, (1986): 2835.

39. D. D. Adams, "Lowering Cholesterol and the Incidence of Coronary Heart Disease" (letter), *Journal of the American Medical Association,* 253, (1985): 3090.

40. A. Keys et al., "HDL Serum Cholesterol and 24-Year Mortality of Men in Finland," *International Journal of Epidemiology,* 13, (1984): 428.

41. D. J. Gordon, "Plasma High-Density Lipoprotein Cholesterol and Coronary Heart Disease in Hypercholesterolemic Men," *Circulation,* 72, (1985): III.

42. L.O. Watkins et al., "High-Density Lipoprotein Cholesterol and Coronary Heart Disease Incidence in Black and White M.R.F.I.T. Usual Care Men," *Circulation,* 71, (1985): 417A.

41. J. A. Cauley et al., "The Relationship of Physical Activity to High-Density Lipoprotein Cholesterol in Postmenopausal Women," *Journal of Chronic Disease,* 39, (1986): 687.

42. R. P. Donahue et al., "Lipids and Lipoproteins in a Young Adult Population: The Beaver County Lipid Study," *American Journal of Epidemiology,* 122, (1985): 485.

43. E. Prader and A. M. Leiken, "High-Density Lipoprotein Cholesterol Determination in the Preventive Health Examination: Effects of Weight and Cigarette Smoking," *Journal of Cardiac Rehabilitation,* 3, (1983): 763.

44. J. C. Cohen et al., "Hypercholesterolemia in Male Power Lifters Using Anabolic-Androgenic Steroids," *The Physician and Sportsmedicine,* 16, (1988): 49.

45. R. M. Mochizuki and K. J. Richter, "Cardiomyopathy and Cerebrovascular Accident Associated With Anabolic-Androgenic Steroid Use," *The Physician and Sportsmedicine,* 16, (1988): 108.

46. W. P. Castelli et al., "Alcohol and Blood Lipids," *Lancet,* 2, (1977): 153.

47. W. L. Haskell et al., "The Effect of Cessation and Resumption of Moderate Alcohol Intake on Serum High-Density Lipoprotein Subfractions," *The New England Journal of Medicine,* 310, (1984).

48. P. D. Wood et al., "Changes in Plasma Lipids and Lipoproteins in Overweight Men During Weight Loss Through Dieting as Compared with Exercise," *The New England Journal of Medicine,* 319, (1988): 1173.

49. G. H. Hartung et al., "Effect of Alcohol Intake and Exercise on Plasma High-Density Lipoprotein Cholesterol Subfractions and Apolipoprotein A-1 in Women," *American Journal of Cardiology,* 58, (1986): 148.

50. P. D. Wood et al., "The Distribution of Plasma Lipoproteins in Middle-Aged Male Runners," *Metabolism,* 25, (1976): 1249.

51. R. Sorbris et al., "Effect of Weight Reduction on Plasma Lipoproteins and Adipose Tissue Metabolism in Obese Subjects," *European Journal of Clinical Investigation,* 11, (1981): 491.

52. P. T. Williams et al., "The Effect of Running Mileage and Duration on Plasma Lipoprotein Levels," *Journal of the American Medical Association,* 247, (1982): 2674.

53. T. C. Cook et al., "Chronic Low Level Physical Activity As a Determinant of High Density Lipoprotein Cholesterol and Subfractions," *Medicine and Science in Sport and Exercise,* 18, (1986): 653.

54. G. H. Hartung et al., "Relation of Diet to High-Density Lipoprotein Cholesterol in Middle-Aged Marathon Runners, Joggers, and Inactive Men," *New England Journal of Medicine,* 302, (1980): 357.

55. S. N. Blair et al., "Comparison of Nutrient Intake In Middle-Aged Men and Women Runners and Controls," *Medicine and Science in Sports and Exercise,* 13, (1981): 310.

56. T. R. Ratto, "The Great Salt Controversy," *Medical Self-Care Magazine,* 69, (1986): 35.

57. E. N. Whitney et al., *Understanding Normal and Clinical Nutrition,* St. Paul: West Publishing Co., 1987.

58. G. Kolata, "Value of Low Sodium Diets Questioned," *Science,* 216, (1982): 38.

59. K. T. Khaw et al., "Dieting Potassium and Stroke Associated Mortality. A 12 Year Prospective Population Study," *New England Journal of Medicine,* 316, (1987): 235.

60. B. Kirk, *University of Tennessee Center for the Health Sciences Medical Journal,* July 8, 1983.

61. L. Lamb (ed.), "Exercise Prevents Deaths From Heart Attacks," *The Health Letter,* 29, (February, 1987): 3.

62. H. J. Montoye et al., "Habitual Physical Activity and Blood Pressure," *Medicine and Science in Sports,* 4, (Winter 1972): 175.

63. G. F. Fletcher, "Exercise for High Blood Pressure," *Medical Journal,* 45, (1986): 9.

63. G. F. Fletcher, *Exercise In the Practice of Medicine,* New York: Futura Publishing Co., 1982.

64. B. Kirk, "Exercise for High Blood Pressure," *Medical Journal,* 45, (1986): 9.

65. S. N. Blair et al., "Physical Fitness and Incidence of Hypertension in Healthy Normotensive Men and Women," *Journal of the American Medical Association,* 252, (1984): 487.

66. R. S. Paffenbarger et al., "Physical Activity and Incidence of Hypertension in College Alumni," *American Journal of Epidemiology,* 117, (1983): 245.

67. J. J. Duncan et al., "The Effects of Aerobic Exercise on Plasma Catecholamines and Blood Pressure in Patients with Mild Essential Hypertension," *Journal of the American Medical Association,* 254, (1985): 2609.

68. L. Lamb (ed.), "Aerobic Exercise Lowers Blood Pressure," *The Health Letter,* 26, (December 13, 1985): 1.

69. L. Nelson et al., "Effect of Changing Levels of Physical Activity on Blood-Pressure and Hemodynamics in Essential Hypertension," *Lancet,* (1986): 473.

70. J. S. Raglin and W. P. Morgan, "Influence of Exercise and Quiet Rest on State Anxiety and Blood Pressure," *Medicine and Science in Sports and Exercise,* 19, (1987): 456.

71. I. N. Findlay et al., "Cardiovascular Effects of Training for a Marathon Run in Unfit Middle-Aged Men," *British Medical Journal,* 295, (1987): 521.

72. "Report of the Second Task Force on Blood Pressure Control in Children—1987," *Pediatrics,* 79, (1987): 1.

73. D. S. Siscovick et al., "The Disease-Specific Benefits and Risks of Physical Activity and Exercise," *Public Health Reports,* 100, (1985).

74. American Cancer Society, *Cancer Facts and Figures—1988,* New York: 1988.

75. *The Health Consequences of Smoking—Nicotine Addiction,* A Report of the Surgeon General (Rockville, Maryland: Department of Health and Human Services, 1988).

76. "1983 Surgeon General's Report Health Consequences of Smoking," *Smoking and Health Reporter,* 1, (January, 1984): 1.

77. "Focus on Smoking Cessation," Smoking and Health Reporter 1, no. 3 (April 1984): 4.

78. E. T. Gelfand et al., "Coronary Artery Bypass in Patients Under Forty Years of Age," *Canadian Journal of Surgery,* 26, (1983): 188.

79. L. Scago, "Weighty Fears," *MSU Magazine,* 6, (1987): 11.

80. "Stop Smoking: Don't Gain Weight," *Better Health IV,* (October, 1987): 2.

81. H. Shimokata et al., "Studies in the Distribution of Body Fat—III. Effects of Cigarette Smoking," *Journal of the American Medical Association,* 261, (1989): 1169.

82. S. M. Haffner et al., "Upper Body and Centralized Adiposity in Mexican Americans and non-Hispanic Whites: Relationship to Body Mass Index and Other Behavioral and Demographic Variables," *International Journal of Obesity,* 10, (1986): 493.

83. P. R. M. Jones et al., "Waist-Hip Circumference Ratio and Its Relation to Age and Overweight in British Men," *Human Nutrition Clinical Nutrition,* 40c, (1986): 239.

84. D. J. Lanska et al., "Factors Influencing Anatomical Location of Fat Tissue in 52,953 Women," *International Journal of Obesity,* 9, (1985): 29.

85. L. Lamb (ed.), "Cigarettes and Women," *The Health Letter,* 31, (March 25, 1988): 4.

86. W. C. Willett et al., "Relative and Absolute Risks of Coronary Heart Disease Among Women Who Smoke Cigarettes," *New England Journal of Medicine,* 317, (1987): 1303.

87. M. Manly, "Smoke Damage—The Health Effects of Tobacco," *Annual Editions—Health 89/90,* Guilford, Conn.: The Dushkin Publishing Group, Inc., 1989.

88. R. Wolfe, "Smokeless Tobacco—The Fatal Pinch," *Annual Editions—Health, 89/90,* Guilford, Conn.: The Dushkin Publishing Group, Inc., 1989.

89. G. N. Connolly et al., "The Reemergence of Smokeless Tobacco," The New England Journal of Medicine, 314, (1986): 1020.

90. Office of Inspector General, *Youth Use of Smokeless Tobacco: More Than a Pinch of Trouble,* (U.S. Dept. of Health and Human Services, 1986).

91. G. N. Connolly and others, "Use of Smokeless Tobacco in Major League Baseball," *New England Journal of Medicine,* 318, (1988): 1281.

92. E. Silverberg and J. A. Lubera, "Cancer Statistics, 1989," *Ca—A Cancer Journal for Clinicians,* 39, (1989): 3.

93. R. B. Jones, "Use of Smokeless Tobacco in the 1986 World Series," *New England Journal of Medicine,* 316, (1987): 952.

94. W. U. Chandler, "Banishing Tobacco," *Annual Editions—Health 89/90,* Guilford, Conn.: The Dushkin Publishing Group, Inc., 1989.

95. *Smoking and Health Reporter,* 2, (January, 1985).

96. L. Lamb (ed.), "Passive Smoking Causes Heart Attacks," *The Health Letter,* 29, (March, 1987): 4.

97. P. Gunby, "Wives Ischemic Heart Disease Linked with Husband's Smoking," *Journal of the American Medical Association,* 253, (1985): 2945.

98. C. Garland, "Effects of Passive Smoking on Ischemic Heart Disease Mortality of Nonsmokers," *American Journal of Epidemiology,* 121, (1985): 645.

99. S. M. Fox and J. S. Skinner, "Physical Activity and Cardiovascular Health," *American Journal of Cardiology,* 14, (1984): 731.

100. J. H. Wilmore, "Exercise: The Aerobic Edge," *Food and Fitness,* The First International Videoconference on Good Eating, Exercise and Health, 47 (March 30, 1984).

101. J. P. Koplan et al., "An Epidemiologic Study of the Benefits and Risks of Running," *Journal of the American Medical Association,* 248, (1982): 3118.

102. S. N. Blair, et al., "Relationships Between Exercise or Physical Activity and Other Health Behaviors," *Public Health Reports,* 100, (1985): 172.

103. S. N. Blair et al., "Comparison of Dietary and Smoking Habit Changes in Physical Fitness Improvers and Nonimprovers," *Preventive Medicine,* 13, (1984): 411.

104. B. Saltin et al., "Response to Exercise After Bed Rest and After Training," *Circulation Supplement,* 7, (1968): 1.

105. A. S. Leon et al., "Leisure-Time Physical Activity Levels and Risk of Coronary Heart Disease and Death," *Journal of the American Medical Association,* 258, (1987): 2388.

106. B. Kirk (ed.), "Fitness Influences Risk of Death," *Medical Journal,* 52, (1987): 3.

107. W. L. Haskell, "Physical Activity and Health: Need to Define the Required Stimulus," *The American Journal of Cardiology,* 55, (1985): 4D.

108. R. S. Paffenbarger et al., "A Natural History of Athleticism and Cardiovascular Health," *The Journal of the American Medical Association,* 252, (1984): 491.

109. R. S. Paffenbarger et al., "Physical Activity, All-Cause Mortality, and Longevity of College Alumni," *New England Journal of Medicine,* 314, (1986): 605.

110. D. G. Clark et al., "Physical Fitness and All-Cause Mortality in Healthy Women," *Medicine and Science in Sports and Exercise,* 20, (1988-supplement): 57.

111. L. W. Gibbons et al., "Physical Fitness and Mortality From Any Cause in Hypertensive Men," *Medicine and Science in Sports and Exercise,* 20, (1988-supplement): 57.

112. H. W. Kohl and S. N. Blair, "Physical Fitness and Mortality From Any Cause in Adult Men With Chronic Disease," *Medicine and Science in Sports and Exercise,* 20, (1988-supplement): 57.

113. S. N. Blair and H. W. Kohl, "Physical Activity or Physical Fitness: Which Is More Important For Health?" *Medicine and Science in Sports and Exercise,* 20, (1988- supplement): 58.

114. J. F. Sallis et al., "Moderate-Intensity Physical Activity and Cardiovascular Risk Factors: The Stanford Five-City Project," *Preventive Medicine,* 15, (1986): 561.

115. K. E. Powell, "Physical Activity and the Incidence of Coronary Heart Disease," *Annual Reviews of Public Health,* 8 (1987): 253.

116. C. J. Casperson, "Physical Inactivity and Coronary Heart Disease," *The Physician and Sportsmedicine,* 15, (1987): 43.

117. "Physical Activity: Prevents Coronary Heart Disease," *Better Health V,* (January, 1988): 4.

118. T. Monahan, "From Activity To Eternity," *The Physician and Sportsmedicine,* 14, (1986): 156.

119. S. N. Blair, "Low Physical Fitness and Increased Risk of Death and Disability," Speech delivered at the SDAAHPERD Convention, Chattanooga, TN, Feb. 24, 1989.

120. T. Bassler, "Marathon Running and Immunity to Heart Disease," *The Physician and Sportsmedicine,* 3, (April 1975): 77.

121. B. F. Waller and W. C. Roberts, "Sudden Death While Running in Conditioned Runners Aged 40 Years or Over," *American Journal of Cardiology,* 45, (1980): 1291.

122. P. D. Thompson et al., "Death During Jogging Or Running," *Journal of the American Medical Association,* 242, (1979): 1265.

123. T. D. Noakes, "Heart Disease in Marathon Runners: A Review," *Medicine and Science in Sports and Exercise,* 19, (1987): 187.

124. J. P. Kaplan, "Cardiovascular Deaths While Running," *Journal of the American Medical Association,* 242, (1979): 2578.

125. S. P. Van Camp, "Exercise-Related Sudden Death: Risks and Causes," *The Physician and Sportsmedicine,* 16 (1988): 96.

126. L. Lamb (ed.), "Sudden Cardiac Deaths in Young Men," *The Health Letter,* 29 (June 12, 1987): 1.

127. S. P. Van Camp and J. H. Choi, "Exercise and Sudden Death," *The Physician and Sportsmedicine,* 16 (1988): 49.

128. D. S. Siscovick et al., "The Incidence of Primary Cardiac Arrest During Vigorous Exercise," *The New England Journal of Medicine,* 311, (1984): 874.

129. H. A. de Vries, *Health Science,* Santa Monica, CA: Goodyear Publishing Co., 1979.

130. "Dieting: The Losing Game," *Time,* (January 20, 1986): 54.

131. S. L. Gortmaker et al., "Increasing Pediatric Obesity in the United States," *American Journal of Disabled Children,* 141, (1987): 535.

132. J. G. Ross and R. R. Pate, "The National Children and Youth Fitness Study II: A Summary of Findings," *Journal of Physical Education, Recreation, and Dance,* 58, (1987): 51.

133. E. T. Howley and B. D. Franks, *Health/Fitness Instructor's Handbook,* Champaign, IL: Human Kinetics Publishers, Inc., 1986.

134. P. D. Wood, "The Science of Successful Weight Loss," *Food and Fitness,* The First International Videoconference on Good Eating, Exercise and Health, 3, March 30, 1984.

135. W. R. Foster and B. T. Burton (eds.), "Health Implications of Obesity: National Institutes of Health Development Conference," *Annals of Internal Medicine,* 103, (1985, Supp. 6 part 2): 977.

136. D. Groves, "Is Childhood Obesity Related to TV Addiction?" *The Physician and Sportsmedicine,* 16, (1988): 117.

137. J. E. Manson et al., "Body Weight and Longevity: A Reassessment," *Journal of the American Medical Association,* 257, (1987): 353.

138. A. Stunkard et al., "An Adoption Study of Human Obesity," *New England Journal of Medicine,* 314, (1986): 193.

139. A. Stunkard et al., "A Twin Study of Human Obesity," *Journal of the American Medical Association,* 256, (1986): 51.

140. E. T. Poehlman et al., "Genotype Controlled Changes in Body Composition and Fat Morphology Following Overfeeding in Twins," *American Journal of Clinical Nutrition,* 43, (1986): 723.

141. J. S. Stern, "Movement Makes the Difference," *Food and Fitness*, The First International Videoconference on Good Eating, Exercise and Health, 49, March 30, 1984, p. 3.

142. G. A. Brooks and T. D. Fahey, *Exercise Physiology*, New York: John Wiley and Sons, 1984.

143. N. R. Day, *Controlling Type II Diabetes*, Daly City, CA: Krames Communications, 1983.

144. National Institutes of Health (NIH) Consensus Development Conference on Diet and Exercise in Noninsulin-Dependent Diabetes Mellitus, Draft Statement," Bethesda, MD: National Institute of Diabetes and Digestive and Kidney Diseases and the NIH Office of Medical Applications of Research, 1986.

145. R. E. LaPorte et al., Pittsburgh Insulin-Dependent Diabetes Mellitus Morbidity and Mortality Study: Physical Activity and Diabetic Complications," *Pediatrics*, 78, (1986): 1027.

146. R. E. Frisch et al., "Lower Prevalence of Diabetes in Female Former College Athletes Compared With Nonathletes," *Diabetes*, 35, (1986): 1101.

147. M. Duda, "The Role of Exercise In Managing Diabetes," *The Physician and Sportsmedicine*, 13, (1985): 164.

148. B. N. Campaigne et al., "The Effects of Physical Training on Blood Lipid Profiles in Adolescents with Insulin-Dependent Diabetes Mellitus," *The Physician and Sportsmedicine*, 13, 1985: 83.

149. R. Stratton et al., "Acute Glycemic Effects of Exercise in Adolescents with Insulin-Dependent Diabetes Mellitus," *The Physician and Sportsmedicine*, 16, (1988): 150.

150. P. Blackett, "Child and Adolescent Athletes with Diabetes," *The Physician and Sportsmedicine*, 16, (1988): 133.

151. C. N. Shealy, *90 Days to Self-Health*, New York: Bantam Books, 1977.

152. N. Cousins, "The Mysterious Placebo: How Mind Helps Medicine Work," *Saturday Review*, (Oct. 1, 1977): 9.

153. G. Edlin and E. Golanty, *Health and Wellness*, Boston: Jones and Bartlett, Publishers, 1988.

154. S. Siliger, "Stress Can Be Good For You," *Annual Editions—89/90*, Guilford, Conn.: The Dushkin Publishing Group, Inc., 1989.

155. H. Selye, *Stress Without Distress*, New York: Signet, 1974.

156. H. Higdon, "12 Minutes Does It," *American Health*, (June, 1988): 41.

157. D. J. Crews and D. M. Landers, "A Meta Analytic Review of Aerobic Fitness and Reactivity to Psychosocial Stressors," *Medicine and Science in Sports and Exercise*, 19, (suppl. 1987): 5114.

158. D. J. Crews et al., "Psychosocial Stress Response Following Training," *Medicine and Science in Sports and Exercise*, 20, (suppl. 1988): 585.

159. L. A. Tucker et al., "Physical Fitness: A Buffer Against Stress," *Perceptual and Motor Skills*, 63, (1986): 955.

160. E. Roskies et al., "The Montreal Type A Intervention Project: Major Findings," *Health Psychology*, 5, (1986): 45.

161. J. H. Howard et al., "Physical Activity As a Moderator of Life Events and Somatic Complaints: A Longitudinal Study," *Canadian Journal of Applied Sports Science*, 9, (1984): 194.

162. V. J. Haber and J. R. Sutton, "Endorphins and Exercise," *Sports Medicine*, 1, (1984): 154.

163. K. H. Cooper, *The Aerobics Program for Total Well-Being*, New York: Bantam Books, 1982.

164. W. M. Bortz et al., "Catecholamines, Dopamine, and Endorphin Levels During Extreme Exercise," *New England Journal of Medicine*, 305, (1981): 305.

165. E. W. D. Colt et al., "The Effect of Running on Plasma Beta Endorphin," *Life Sciences*, 28, (1981): 1673.

166. P. A. Farrell et al., "Increases in Plasma Beta-EP and Beta-LPH Immunoreactivity After Treadmill Running in Humans," *Journal of Applied Physiology: Respiratory, Environmental and Exercise Physiology*, 52, (1982): 1245.

167. "Beta-Endorphin Seen After Treadmill Exercise," *The Physician and Sportsmedicine*, 11, (1983): 16.

168. D. Appenzeller et al., "Neurology of Endurance Training: V. Endorphins," (Abstract), *Neurology*, 30, (1980): 418.

169. T. Monahan, "Exercise and Depression: Swapping Sweat for Serenity?" *The Physician and Sportsmedicine*, 14, (1988): 192.

170. J. H. Greist et al., "Running Out of Depression," *The Physician and Sportsmedicine*, 6, (1978): 49.

171. R. S. Brown et al., "The Prescription of Exercise for Depression," *The Physician and Sportsmedicine*, 6, (1978): 35.

172. R. M. Hayden and G. J. Allen, "Relationship Between Aerobic Exercise, Anxiety and Depression: Convergent Validation by Knowledgeable Informants," *Journal of Sports Medicine*, 24, (1984): 68.

173. R. M. Carney et al., "The Relationship Between Depression and Aerobic Capacity in Hemodialysis Patients," *Psychosomatic Medicine*, 48, (1986): 143.

174. W. Glasser, *Positive Addiction*, New York: Harper & Row, 1976.

175. W. P. Morgan, "Negative Addiction in Runners," *The Physician and Sportsmedicine*, 7, (1979): 57.

176. H. deVries, "Tranquilizer Effect of Exercise: A Critical Review," *The Physician and Sportsmedicine*, 9, (1981): 53.

177. "Treatment of Hypertriglyceridemia. NIH Consensus Development Conference Summary," *Arteriosclerosis*, 4, (1984): 296.

178. E. L. Bierman, "The Treatment of Hypertriglyceridemia: Views From the National Institute of Health Consensus Conference," *Cholesterol and Coronary Disease . . . Reducing the Risk*, 2, (1988): 6.

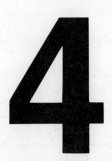

4

Other Chronic Diseases

Chapter Outline

Mini Glossary

Oligomenorrhea: scanty menses

Amenorrhea: absence of menses

Asthma: widespread narrowing of the airways of the lungs because of varying degrees to spasm of smooth muscle, edema of the mucosa, and mucus in the bronchi and bronchioles.

Cancer: a large group of disorders that are characterized by abnormal cellular growth.

Cortical bone: the dense, hard outer layer of bone such as that which appears in the shafts of the long bones of the arms and legs.

Metastasis: the spread of cancer from the original site to other sites in the body.

Neoplasm: growth of new tissue (tumor).

Osteoarthritis: a degenerative joint disease characterized by the deterioration of articular cartilage particularly in the weight bearing joints. Often referred to a "wear and tear" arthritis.

Osteoporosis: reduction in the quantity of bone as a result of demineralization and atrophy of skeletal tissue.

Trabecular bone: spongy bone, not as dense as cortical bone.

Introduction

This chapter focuses upon osteoporosis, low back problems, osteoarthritis, asthma, and cancer. These prevalent chronic diseases are covered because most Americans are affected by one or more, and there is a relationship between them and exercise. For instance, many people do not exercise because they fear that it contributes to the wear and tear of joints thus resulting in osteoarthritis. We will explore that possibility by presenting samples of the available evidence and then we will arrive at some conclusions. Many asthmatics do not exercise because it generally induces an asthma attack. While this certainly does occur, should they deny themselves the health benefits of exercise? Can asthmatics exercise in safety? How do osteoporosis, low back problems, and cancer respond to exercise? These and other questions and concerns will be discussed in this chapter.

Osteoporosis

Osteoporosis (bone-thinning) is a major affliction of the elderly. Postmenopausal women are particularly susceptible. The osteoporotic process, like other degenerative disease processes, follows a long insidious course usually beginning about age 35. Prior to this age there is a net increase in the bulk and strength of bones but afterwards more bone is lost than is deposited. This bone demineralization occurs at a faster rate for females than males and is accelerated in the first few years after menopause. This loss is exacerbated by the fact that women have lighter bones than men of the same weight and age. The result is that compared to men, women have less to lose but they lose it faster.

Osteoporosis is responsible for approximately 1.2 million bone fractures annually, and 530,000 of these involve the vertebral bones in the spinal column and another 227,000 are fractures of the hips.[1] The yearly cost of medical treatment and rehabilitation to the victims of osteoporotic-induced fractures is in excess of $1.6 billion.

Bone is a living tissue which responds to physical stress and compression. It is continuously undergoing remodeling. Skeletal growth and development occurs during the years of growth. Bone deposition or formation occurs more rapidly than bone resorption or removal. In adulthood, the remodeling process is constant, that is, the addition of new bone equals the removal of old bone. However, in osteoporosis, bone is lost at a faster rate than it is replaced leading to weakened and brittle bone.

Cortical bone is the dense, hard outer layer of bone such as the shafts of the long bones of the arms and legs. **Trabecular bone** is spongy and less dense and is surrounded by cortical bone. The vertebrae consist primarily of trabecular bone. The trabecular bone is weaker than cortical bone and breaks more easily because of its spongy consistency. This accounts for the high incidence of fractures of the vertebrae and ball of the femur (thigh bone). Women with advanced osteoporosis will lose 35 percent of their cortical and 50 percent of their trabecular bone.

Researchers have identified several factors which increase the risk of osteoporosis. The primary risk factors include female gender, white or Oriental race, slender body type, and early menopause. The secondary risks include alcohol and tobacco abuse, calcium deficiency, family history, sedentary lifestyle, and use of certain medications (anticonvulsants and thyroid hormone). Osteoporosis is more likely to occur to people who have more than one risk.

Two types of osteoporosis, each caused by different pathogenetic mechanisms, have been identified.[2] Type I affects eight times more women than men, and it occurs after menopause (age 50 to 65).[3] The fracture sites, in their order of prevalence in Type I osteoporosis, are vertebral crush fractures and fractures of the arm above the wrist. These fractures are caused by accelerated bone loss because of estrogen dificiency after menopause. Type II osteoporosis affects twice as many women as men, and usually occurs to both sexes in the 70 years of age group. Hip fractures are the most frequent events and estrogen deficiency is only one of many possible contributing factors in this type of osteoporosis.

Authorities agree that osteoporosis is best prevented than treated because much of the deformity associated with it is irreversible. Prevention and/or treatment includes estrogen replacement, calcium supplementation, fluoride intake, and exercise.

Women who are deficient in estrogen will develop osteoporosis. The incidence and severity of osteoporosis in these women can be reduced with estrogen replacement.[4] Estrogen replacement slows bone loss and seems to be most effective in the prevention of osteoporosis. However, it does not reverse the course of the disease. Today, estrogen is administered with progestin because estrogen alone is associated with cancer of the lining of the uterus.

Two-thirds of the weight of bone consists of minerals and calcium with calcium representing 40 percent of that weight.[5] Adequate calcium intake is necessary to maintain skeletal mass and healthy bones. Inadequate intake or poor absorption of calcium can adversely affect the skeletal system. Adult women are encouraged to take a minimum of 1000 mg. daily, and middle-aged women 1500 mg. daily.[5] Heaney states, "There should no longer be any doubt about the basic relationship of exogenous calcium deficiency and osteoporosis."[5] Calcium intake is positively related to bone mass and negatively related to bone loss.[6] However, calcium replacement is effective only when the primary cause of osteoporosis is calcium deficiency.

Estrogen would prevent at least 90 percent of the vertebral fractures among postmenopausal women.
–Robert Lindsay

Flouride treatment is experimental and has not been approved as therapy for osteoporosis by the Food and Drug Administration. Fluoride increases bone mass and is effective in treating osteoporosis whereas calcium supplementation and estrogen replacement are more effective in prevention.[7] Fluoride treatment produces some unpleasant side effects in some users. Nausea, vomiting, peptic ulcers, hemorrhagic anemia, and ankle, knee and foot pain have been reported in users. These are not life-threatening and abate when usage is discontinued.

Bone responds to the force of gravity and muscle contraction. The stimulus produced by exercise is important in the treatment and prevention of osteoporosis.[8] Enforced bed rest (4 to 36 weeks) occurring to healthy people results in significant bone loss. Inactivity and the absence of gravitational force (weightlessness) produce the same deleterious effect upon the skeletal system. Some degree of stress must be periodically imposed upon the skeletal system for bone to maintain its integrity. Disuse osteoporosis results from prolonged periods of inactivity. Physical activity forces bone to adapt and respond to the stresses imposed upon it and, as with other body tissues, it hypertrophies (grows larger and stronger). When unstressed, bone atrophies. The development of muscle tissue is important to the development and maintenance of bone mass.

Athletes have greater bone density than age-matched sedentary persons (controls) and this is probably because of their greater muscle mass.[9, 10, 11] Strong muscles capable of exerting strong forces upon the bones, result in thicker, stronger bones. In addition, athletes participating in different sports show different skeletal adaptations based upon the load to which bone is subjected. When the thigh bones of athletes competing in different sports were compared, the greatest bone density was found in the weight lifters, followed by the weight throwers, runners, soccer players, and swimmers in that order. "Swimmers were not significantly different than age-matched sedentary controls in bone density. Weight bearing activities are more effective in maintaining skeletal integrity than nonweight-bearing activities such as swiming and cycling."[8] Nonweight-bearing activities seem to be effective for participants who are at a low initial fitness level because they help to build muscle tissue and strength.

Unilateral athletes are excellent candidates for studying the effects of physical activity upon selected sites of the skeletal system. Tennis players and baseball pitchers make extensive use of the dominant arm as they practice and perform in their sports. Their dominant arms are larger caused by muscle and bone hypertrophy compared to their nondominant arm. The bone density of the dominant arms of male tennis players was as much as 35 percent greater than the nondominant arm,[12, 13] and female tennis players showed a 28 percent difference.[14]

Studies employing mild to moderate exercises for the elderly in the 60 to 95 years age group have shown increases in bone mineral content and/or cessation of mineral loss.[15, 16] The subjects in these studies were females whose average ages were 82 and 72 years.

Oligomenorrhea (scanty menses) and **amenorrhea** (absence of menses) are two to four times more prevalent among athletes than nonathletes, and higher among runners than swimmers and cyclists.[17, 18] One of the concerns when the menses is interrupted or stopped is its relationship to the loss of mineral from the bones. Bone losses tend to increase the incidence of fractures for women who are in heavy training.[19] Athletic amenorrhea is characterized by persistent low levels of endogenous estrogen (made in the body), bone mineral loss, loss of body weight, and low body fat.[20] According to Smith, "the etiology (cause of amenorrhea) has not been established conclusively. The factors include low body fat; dietary factors such as low-calcium intake, vegetarianism, low-dietary protein or fat, and high-iron intake; high intensity and length of training; weight loss; delayed menarche; and training at a young age."[8]

Amenorrhea and concomitant bone loss can be avoided or delayed by maintaining body fat above 14 to 15 percent of total weight, sensible exercise, and proper nutrition including adequate calorie intake.

Males seem to be affected by Type II osteoporosis and usually quite late in life. They too can profit from sound nutritional practices and regular exercise. Smith has stated that, "physical activity, as a stimulus, affects human bone in two ways: First, there is an increased stress and strain on the skeletal system because of muscular contraction and gravity; and second, increased metabolic demands of working muscles result in an increased blood flow and blood pressure in the cardiovascular system."[21] Consistent muscular contractions from exercise and/or physical work which leads to the development of muscular strength plays a significant role in development and maintenance of the skelatal system. It follows then, that weight bearing aerobic exercises not only develop the cardiovascular system but they also stimulate the skeletal system. Progressive resistance exercise, such as weight training, has little impact upon the cardiovascular system but great potential for developing all of the major muscle groups and most of the skeletal system. This is a good reason for including both types of exercise in one's fitness program.

One of the critical factors involving one's susceptibility to osteoporosis concerns the initial size and density of bones. This is one of the reasons why small thin women are at great risk, and men, whose skeletal systems are larger and denser, are at less risk. Also, there is a direct relationship between the size of muscles and the size of bones, and men have more muscle tissue than women.[22] The best time to influence the skeletal system is prior to the age of 30. Regular participation in weight bearing aerobic activities together with resistence exercises, and proper nutrition combine to build dense healthy bones which are resistant to osteoporosis.

Care in selecting and participating in exercise is a must for one who is osteoporotic. Forceful contraction of muscles or high impact activities may result in fractures. Exercises and activities should be modified for safety. Swimming, water aerobics, and light weight training are good activities for those with osteoporosis.

The exact cause or causes of osteoporosis is not known. Inadequate amounts of dietary calcium and vitamin D, hormonal changes, sedentary living habits, and reduced exposure to sunlight have been investigated as possible causes.

Fractures are very common as a result of the bone loss that occurs at the rate of 0.75 to 1.0 percent per year in women beginning at age 30 to 35, and for men at age 50 to 55.[21] Most commonly affected are the vertebrae of the spinal column, which tend to collapse in the forward, weight-bearing portion. If enough of the vertebrae are involved, the spinal column will curve abnormally and shorten, resulting in a condition referred to as "hunchback" or "dowager's hump."

The earlier a person starts a regular exercise program, the greater the likelihood of meaningful osteogeneses (bone growth).
—Morris Notelovitz

Low-Back Problems

Basic knowledge of the major anatomical components of the back is important in order to understand the causes and treatment for low-back pain. The vertebral column consisting of 33 bones is the only bony connection between the upper and lower halves of the body (see Figure 4.1). It supports the weight of the torso, surrounds and protects the spinal cord, and its landmarks are sources of attachment for muscles and ligaments. The spinal cord extends downward from the base of the brain through most of the length of the vertebral column. Nerves exit from the spinal cord through openings between each of the vertebra. Discs are located between each of the vertebra where they act as shock absorbers and keep the vertebrae from rubbing against each other. Discs contain a ring of tough fibrous tissue with white sponge-like nucleus in the center.

Eight of every ten Americans, it is estimated, will suffer a back injury sometime during their lives.[23] Low-back pain is the second leading cause of lost work time for people under the age of 45. It costs business and industry $250 million in workers' compensation and approximately one billion dollars in lost output annually. Twenty-five to thirty percent of all disability payments are paid for back injuries.[24] Humans are particularly susceptible to back injury because of our upright posture. We have lost the structural advantage conferred by walking on all fours, so the burden of supporting the weight of the torso falls upon the lower portion of the spine. The spinal column is not

---

FIGURE 4.1

Normal Curvature of the Spine

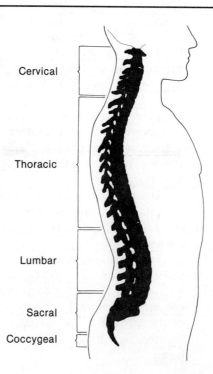

Cervical

Thoracic

Lumbar

Sacral

Coccygeal

straight; it curves inward in the lower region (lumbar area) and when the curvature is accentuated (lordosis, sway back) the likelihood of injury increases markedly.

The problem is concisely stated by Root, who remarks, "a simple law of physics states that when a force or weight is applied to a curved structure, the greatest stress is exerted on the concave or inner side of the curve. Therefore the more pronounced a curve in the spine is, the more uneven is the load of pressure over its surface, with the greatest loads concentrated at the apex of the curve. This in turn will cause excessive wear (a form of chronic trauma) on the intervertebral joints at the curve's apex so that degenerative changes and the wear and tear factor will occur earlier than normal in the spine's life."[25]

Low-back pain can occur from a variety of causes, the majority of which can be classified as resulting from "mechanical factors." These include excessive body weight, poor posture, and lack of physical fitness.[23] The majority of low-back pain involves muscle and ligament strain as well as inflamed joints along the vertebral column. Some injuries involve discs that herniate or tear, and their jell-like exudate exerts pressure on the spinal nerves. Back pain also occurs from injuries sustained from accidents, falls, lifting heavy objects, and athletic injuries. Arthritis and osteoporosis also cause low-back pain.

Strategies for preventing low-back problems include the maintenance of normal body weight; strength development exercises for the back and abdominals; flexibility exercises for the back, hips and legs; and correct lifting techniques. However, if a problem does occur there are avenues of treatment.

Today, exercises may be selected to treat the specific problem. Williams flexion exercises (see Table 4.1) are used for low-back problems caused by extension movements.[26] These involve the posterior elements of the spine, that is, those structures behind the body of the vertebrae. Extending the back in activities such as walking or others which involve arching the back usually increase the pain. Flexion activities such as forward bending, sitting, and driving usually reduce the pain.[27] McKenzie's extension exercises (Table 4.1) are more appropriate for disc problems.[28] In these instances, flexion movements cause pain while extension movements (arching the back and walking) provide some relief. The option of different exercises for low-back problems is a recent change in treatment. This was accompanied by another change. Not many years ago people with discogenic low-back problems were kept in bed for weeks. Today, they remain in bed for only a few days. Roos states that, "movement is the key to life. Immobility affects the tissues of the low back the same way it affects the other joints.[27]

In addition to recommending either the Williams or McKenzie exercises, patients are encouraged, at the appropriate time, to participate in exercises that develop cardiovascular endurance and muscular strength. Cardiovascular endurance is important because it increases one's level of energy which should help with the maintenance of good posture. Fatigue causes people to slouch deviating from the normal spinal curve. The cardiovascular endurance level of firefighters who participated in a large-scale study was the one factor that made a difference in back patients.[29] The cardiovascular activities not only promoted aerobic endurance but they contributed to muscle conditioning and a healthy back.

For beginners, light weight resistance exercises should accompany the cardiovascular conditioning program. There should be a gradual progression of resistance as physical fitness improves. Exercises should work the major muscles of the back, hips, and legs as well as the abdominal muscles. The abdominal muscles may be developed by employing modified sit-ups or variations of trunk curls.[30] The majority of people can benefit from trunk curls where the trunk is flexed no more than 30 degrees which is approximately that point when the shoulder blades clear the floor.

TABLE 4.1   Exercises for Low-Back Pain

Certain exercises can help alleviate low-back pain and help prevent recurrence. The choice of exercises depends on your specific diagnosis; extension exercises generally are best for persons with disk problems, while flexion exercises usually are best for persons with pain from other causes. Your physician can advise you as to which exercises are appropriate for you, and he or she may prescribe additional exercises to build strength and flexibility.

Flexion Exercises

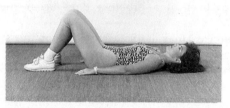

Pelvic Tilt. Lie on your back, feet flat on the floor with knees bent as shown. Press the lower back to the floor by contracting your stomach muscles. Do not push down with your legs. Hold 5 to 10 seconds.

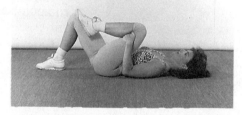

Alternate knee to chest. Lie on your back with knees bent and feet flat on the floor. Place your hands under the right knee and pull your right leg to your chest. Hold 5 to 10 seconds and lower to starting position. Repeat with left leg.

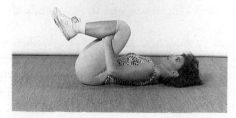

Double knee to chest. Starting position is identical to the pelvic tilt. Pull right knee to chest and then pull left knee to chest. Hold both of these for 5 to 10 seconds and then slowly lower one leg at a time to starting position.

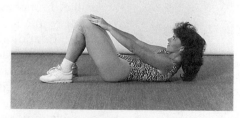

Partial sit-up. Slowly curl your head and shoulders off the floor until your fingers touch your knees, hold 1 to 2 seconds, and return to starting position. **Caution:** make sure your low back stays in contact with the floor.

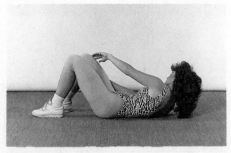

Partial sit-up with a twist. Proceed as in the partial sit-up except that both hands touch the left knee. Return to the starting position and repeat with both hands touching the right knee.

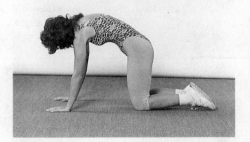 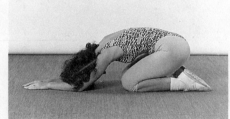

Trunk flexion. Start on your hands and knees, tuck your chin to your chest, slowly sit back on your heels, and simultaneously lower your shoulders to the floor. Hold for 5 to 10 seconds and return to starting position.

Extension Exercises*

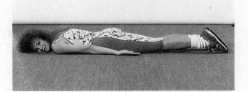 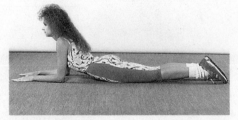

Lying prone. Lie on your stomach, head turned to one side and arms at your sides. Lie in this position for 5 to 10 minutes.

Lying prone propped on elbows. Lie on your stomach with the weight supported on your elbows and forearms. Relax your back and allow hips to sag and contact the floor. Hold 5 to 10 minutes. If pain occurs, repeat the lying prone exercise and try it again.

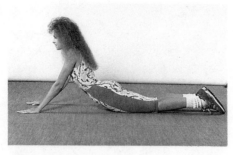

Prone press-ups. Lie on your stomach, palms on the floor near the shoulders. Slowly push your shoulders up but keep your hips in contact with the floor by letting your back and stomach sag. Slowly return to starting position. Repeat 5 to 10 times.

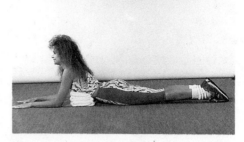

Progressive extension with pillows. Lie on your stomach with one pillow under your chest. Add a pillow every two to three minutes until you are lying on three pillows. Stay in this position for 5 minutes and then remove the pillows one at a time over a period of two to three minutes.

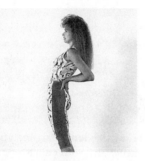

Standing back extension. Stand with your feet approximately shoulder width apart with your hands against the back of the pelvis. Arch your back as far as is comfortable while pushing forward with your hands. Keep your head erect. Repeat 5 to 10 times.

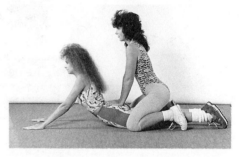

Assisted prone press-ups. Do the same prone press-ups but have a partner press down on your pelvis to stabalize it. This exercise can increase range of motion in the lumbar spine.

*Caution: It is acceptable to have mild back pain associated with these positions. But if a particular position causes pain to develop in a new location or increases existing hip or leg pain, it should be discontinued.

Flexibility of the hip joint, hamstrings, quadriceps, hip flexors, and gluteals is essential to normal maintenance of the spine. Loss of flexibility in the muscles increases the probability of low-back problems.

Excess weight and an enlarged waistline contribute to low back problems. The further out front the weight is carried, the greater the force exerted on the low back. Slimming the waist and losing weight are an important part of a healthy back program.

In essence, a program designed to produce a healthy back includes strengthening the abdominal and back muscles, stretching the lower back, hip flexors and hamstring muscles, postural improvement, weight loss if needed, and lifting and carrying objects correctly.

POINTS TO PONDER

1. *Define and describe osteoporosis.*
2. *Who is most at risk for developing osteoporosis and why?*
3. *What are the most common fracture sites in Type I and Type II osteoporosis?*
4. *Describe the role of exercise in preventing, delaying, and treating osteoporosis.*
5. *What are the causes of low-back problems?*
6. *What strategies might you imploy in preventing low-back problems?*
7. *Describe the role of exercise in the treatment of low-back pain.*

Osteoarthritis

Osteoarthritis is a degenerative joint disease characterized by the deterioration of articular cartilage particularly in the weight bearing joints. It is called the "wear and tear" disease. Since the cartilage wears out, it is believed that the habitual participation in activities which produce trauma would accelerate the course of the disease. Weight bearing activities have been studied to determine their impact upon the development or exacerbation of osteoarthritis. The activity that has received the most attention is jogging.

Weight bearing activities expose the joints to substantial forces. Compared to walking, the forces generated by jogging are twice as great at the hip, six times as great at the knee, and twice that at the ankle, however, forces such as these can be accepted by the body without detriment.[31] The joints are capable of dissipating the forces produced by weight bearing impact-loading activities. This occurs because the joints are supported by the voluntary muscles and movement is buffered by compressible shock-absorbing cartilage whose surfaces articulate in an essentially friction free environment. The development of strong muscles surrounding the joints, particularly that of the knee, is imperative in the prevention of injury.

Osteoarthritis is the most common joint disease in the United States, and its causes are not known but its prevalence is.[32] Osteoarthritis is a progressive disease which worsens with age and ultimately affects most people to some extent. The degeneration of some joints begins prior to age 20 and continues throughout life. Thirty-five percent of the 30-year-olds have clinically identifiable osteoarthritis of the knee. The weight bearing joints of most 40- to 50-year-olds are affected and 85 percent of the 75-year-olds have diagnosable osteoarthritis.

Does jogging aggrevate preexisting osteoarthritis? Moskowitz presents the majority opinion when he states that, "It is my belief that jogging may aggravate osteoarthritis, especially when the hip or knee are already symptomatic."[32] Does jogging cause osteoarthritis in normal joints? The answer is "No" and there is considerable evidence to support this position. In fact, there is evidence which suggests that jogging may slow the functional aspects of musculoskeletal aging. For several years, 498 runners and 365 nonrunners were followed.[33] The runners visited a physician less often and had less physical disability than age-matched nonrunners and osteoarthritis seemed to be developing more slowly.

The same group of researchers compared 41 runners age 50 to 72 with matched controls who exercised one-fourth as much and ran one-tenth as much.[10]

The bones of the hands, knees, and lumbar spine were evaluated by x-ray, but the evaluations were made under anonymous conditions, the evaluators were not told whose x-ray they were examining. This technique maintains objectivity and removes experimentor bias from clouding the results. The results of the evaluations showed that runners had 40 percent more bone mineral content in the vertebrae and secondly, there was no difference between the two groups in the clinical manifestations of osteoarthritis. Thirty-five years of data collected in the Framigham study showed a strong relationship between obesity and development of osteoarthritis of the knee later in life.[34] The researchers concluded that obesity is probably a major cause of osteoarthritis of the knee and that running probably is not. Even high milage running (an average of 28 miles per week for 12 years) was not associated with the premature development of osteoarthritis.[35]

Asthma

Bronchial **asthma** is characterized by widespread narrowing of airways because of contraction or spasm of smooth muscle and/or swelling of the mucus membranes in the pulmonary air passages. Breathing becomes very difficult during an asthmatic attack and such attacks can be frightening experiences.

Nine million Americans are asthmatic and 4000 die of asthma each year. Allergies may trigger the asthma response. Ninety percent of the asthmatics under the age of 30 have allergies. Hay fever caused by allergies to specific substances such as ragweed, tree and grass pollen, cat dander, mold spores, mites, and other allergens may trigger an asthma attack. Allergens are substances which cause allergic reations in some people while producing no abnormal reaction in others. Asthma may be caused by environmental factors (extrinsic) or intrinsic factors where no external factors can be identified. There is no cure for asthma, but there are many effective medications to prevent or reduce the length and severity of an attack.

Exercise may precipitate an asthma attack. Seventy to eighty percent of all asthmatics develop bronchospasms during or following exercise.[36] Bronchial narrowing peaks about 5 to 10 minutes subsequent to physical exertion but recovery is spontaneous and complete within 30 to 90 minutes.[37] Exercise-induced asthma is characterized by moderate airway obstruction and is usually not life-threatening. The severity of an attack depends upon the intensity of the exercise or more specifically on the level of ventilation required to meet the metabolic demands of the task. The environmental conditions in which the task is performed also influences the severity of the attack. Cold dry air produces greater airway obstruction than warm moist air. Cold weather masks or scarves worn over the mouth are useful in preventing cold-induced asthma.

The fear of exercise-induced asthma keeps many people sedentary. However, some asthma sufferers have participated in athletics at the national and international level as amateurs and professionals. The Americal College of Allergy and Immunology and the American Accademy of Allergy and Immunology agree on the necessity of regular exercise for asthmatics.[36] Regular exercise benefits the asthma sufferer in much the same way as it benefits other individuals. Improvements in aerobic endurance, muscular strength and flexibility, and general health status all occur to asthmatics. In addition to these outcomes, participation in fitness activities results in a decrease in the frequency and severity of exercise-induced asthma.[38,39] Thirty weeks of swim training for youngsters 9 to 16 years of age resulted in a significant decrease in the total number of asthma attacks and a significant decrease in the need for medication.[39] Swimming, and probably other water activities, seems to be excellent because of the warm moist environment in which they take place and also because the high ventilation rates required to precipitate bronchospasms are difficult to achieve. Swimming appears to be the least asthmogenic (asthma producing) of the aerobic exercises and running and cycling appear to be the most asthmogenic.

Even severely asthmatic hospitalized patients made significant gains in cardiopulmonary fitness after a conditioning program of stationary cycling. Their pulmonary function tests did not improve significantly, but 92 percent of them improved their endurance and were able to increase their work capacity.[40]

Strange as it may sound, some people are allergic to exercise and experience annoying physiological reactions which include hives, itching, allergic shock (anaphylaxis), hypotension, bronchial spasms, irregular heartbeat, and gastrointestinal problems.[41,42] Affected people may have one or more of these symptoms beginning about five minutes after the onset of exercise. The reactions usually subside spontaneously in 30 minutes to four hours but persistent headaches may occur and last for several days. Some of these reactions are potentially life-threatening but there have been no fatalities reported thus far.

There are several approaches to treating exercise-induced allergy. First, it may be possible to identify co-contributors without which the allergic reaction may not have occurred. For instance, a particular kind of food eaten prior to exercise may produce the allergic response when in fact neither the food nor the exercise alone would have. Avoiding that particular food would allow the individual to exercise safely. Secondly, a host of medications are available from inhalants to injections which can be used to prevent or mitigate an attack. Exercising asthmatics should be following the treatment and advice of an allergist. It is probably a good idea for people who have allergic reactions to exercise with a friend or family member in case they need help.

Cancer

As many as 2,000 industrial chemicals may pose a cancer risk.
–Jeffrey McKenna

Cancer involves a large group of disorders which are characterized by abnormal cellular growth. Any cell may become cancerous if it is exposed to carcinogenic (cancer causing) substances. These substances produce mutant cells that divide and grow uncontrollably. Normal cells follow an orderly pattern of division and growth which in adulthood is restricted to the replacement of lost cells. Mutant cells are recognized as deviations from normal and are attacked and destroyed by specialized cells which form a part of the immune system. Occasionally, mutant cells escape detection by the immune system and grow into tumors (**neoplasms**). Slow growing tumors that remain in their original location and do not invade surrounding tissue are usually benign or noncancerous. Rapidly growing tumors that break away from their original site and infiltrate other tissues are malignant or cancerous. These tumors shed cancerous cells which are transported by the lymph and circulatory systems to all areas of the body where they invade other tissues and rapidly proliferate. **Metastasis** is the term which defines the spread of cancer from its original site to other areas of the body resulting in multiple cancer sites.

Early detection and treatment is essential if cancer is to be cured. Surgery is the prescribed course of action as long as cancer is localized but it is ineffective after metastasis. Cancer which has metastasized is treated with chemotherapy and/or radiation. These modalities destroy cancerous cells or interfere with their division and growth. Unfortunately, normal cells respond to and are affected in the same manner particularly those whose growth rate is rapid. Fast growing blood cells and cells lining the digestive tract are susceptible to radiation and chemotherapy. Side-effects associated with their destruction cause substantial discomfort for patients who must be treated in this manner.

Cancer is a deadly disease. Malignant cells grow wild, competing with normal cells for space and nutrients. They crowd out and destroy normal cells but are unable to perform the functions of those cells. As a result the affected organs cannot operate normally as expected and death will occur eventually.

> In theory, stress could directly cause cancer by setting changes in the neuroendocrine system, causing a biochemical reaction that could transform normal cells into malignant ones.
> –Steven Locke

About 66 million Americans or 30 percent of the population will contact cancer in their lifetimes.[43] Cancer kills more youngsters between the ages of 3 and 14 than any other disease.[44] Approximately 494,000 people died of cancer in 1988 making it the second leading cause of death in the United States.

Many persons in health-related and the medical profession agree that approximately 80 percent of all cancers may be avoided by intelligent lifestyle choices.[45] About 35 percent of the total cancer death toll is associated with diet and another 30 percent is attributed to cigarette smoking.

Some energy is currently being expended by researchers who are examining the role of exercise in the prevention of cancer. Animal studies suggest that exercise and low-fat, low-calorie diets reduce the risk of cancer and improve longevity. One cannot extrapolate the results from animal studies to humans but the possibilities are intriguing enough to have stimulated studies with human subjects.

The Harvard Alumni study showed that cancer mortality was highest in those who exercised least even after age and cigarette smoking were accounted for.[46] Approximately 5400 college alumnae were evaluated on the basis of their participation in physical activities when they were students.[47] The women were categorized as either athletes or nonathletes. Athletes were women who participated as members of a varsity, dormitory, or intramural team for at least one year or who were involved in regular exercise such as running 10 miles per week or its equivalent. The results indicated that nonathletes had twice the risk of breast cancer and two and one-half times the risk of cancer of the reproductive system (uterus, ovaries, cervix, and vagina). Since these cancers account for 40 percent of the total number of cancers occurring to women, the researchers stated that the results of this study need to be interpreted carefully. They further stated that the role of exercise in reducing the incidence of cancer requires further research. The risk of colon cancer in 1.1 million Swedish men was 1.3 times greater for subjects in sedentary versus active occupations.[48] These results were corroborated by an investigation in the United States in 1987.[49] Men in sedentary jobs had twice the risk of colon cancer as those in active jobs and sedentary women tended to have a higher risk for breast and colon cancer than active women. The results of another recent study showed a negative correlation between fitness level and the development of cancer.[50] The most fit of the 19,000 subjects in this study had less cancer than the least fit.

Just as exercise and a low-fat diet help prevent coronary heart disease, they may also help prevent cancer.
—Edward Eichner

The evidence of a relationship between pnysical fitness and cancer is mounting but it falls short of establishing cause and effect. However, the results of the epidemiological studies, which are investigating this relationship, are encouraging as they reveal a role for exercise and physical fitness in preventing cancer. Several hypotheses have been advanced to explain the mechanism through which exercise operates to prevent cancer. The first of these concerns the role of exercise in reducing body fat. The amount of body fat is positively correlated with the incidence of cancer.[51,52] Frisch suggested that the relative leanness of the female athletes in her study protected them from cancer of the breast and uterus.[47] The fat in the adipose tissue stimulates the production of estrogen while slimness reduces the estrogen drive. The risk of cancers of the female reproductive system are positively associated with high estrogen levels. Second, exercise may act as a stimulant to the body's immune system. The immune system usually recognizes and destroys cancerous cells early in their development. There are three types of immune cells which function in an integrated manner to guard against the development of cancer: (1) cytotoxic T cells, (2) natural killer cells, and (3) macrophages. All three of these cells directly attack and destroy cancer cells and all three secrete interferon. Interferon (a family of proteins that defend against viral infection) enhances the killing capacity of the immune cells and inhibits the proliferation of cancer cells. However, the fact that cancer does occur indicates that the immune system is not infallible in recognizing and/or destroying carcinogenic cells.

Several studies have shown that exercise may augment or boost the immune system. Plasma interferon levels doubled when eight untrained men exercised on a stationary cycle for 60 minutes at 70 percent of their aerobic capacity.[53] Plasma levels returned to normal two hours after exercise. Vigorous exercise stimulated the release of Interleukin-1 (IL-1) which in turn promotes the release of Interlukin-2 (IL-2) which enhances the activity of the cytotoxic T cells and natural killer cells.[54,55] Theoretically then, exercise boosts the immune response by provoking the secretion of Interleukin-2 which is an antineoplastic agent (prevents the formation of tumors). Strenuous exercise increases blood levels of natural killer cells,[56] and B and T lymphocytes.[57] The natural killer cells lyse (rupture) and destroy many kinds of virus-infected host and tumor cells. The B lymphocytes produce antibodies which attack substances that are recognized as foreign to their host. These include viruses, bacteria, organ transplants, cancerous cells, and so. The T cells defend the host against most viral and fungal infections and are involved in an important way with the regulatory control of the immune mechanisms. Simon stated that, "Exercise is a known remedy for the weakness and low spirits that cancer patients experience during their recovery. It boosts energy and endurance, and also builds confidence and optimism. But, within the past five years, several medical investigations have revealed a surprising new fact: Exercise may also help prevent cancer."[58] Recognition of the potential of exercise to prevent cancer came in 1985 when the American Cancer Society began recommending exercise to protect against cancer.[59]

POINTS TO PONDER

1. Respond to this statement: Exercise causes and worsens osteoarthritis.
2. Asthma sufferers should not exercise. Do you agree or disagree and why?

3. *What is cancer and why is it a deadly disease?*
4. *How might exercise boost the immune system?*

Chapter Highlights

Osteoporosis, low-back problems, osteoarthritis, asthma, and cancer were briefly reviewed, defined, and described. Particular attention was given to the manner in which they are affected by regular exercise.

Exercise is only one of the strategies which may be employed in preventing, delaying, and treating osteoporosis. Exercise develops strong dense bones that are resistant to fracturing. Other strategies include estrogen therapy, and increased intakes of calcium and fluoride.

Exercise contributes to the development of a strong healthy back and it is also a treatment modality of significant importance.

Osteoarthritis is a progressive disease primarily affecting the weight bearing joints. Normal joints do not become osteoarthritic as a result of exercise and there is considerable evidence in support of this point. The causes of osteoarthritis are not known but it is becoming increasingly clear that exercise is not one of them.

Asthma sufferers benefit from exercise in the same way as anyone else except they must be more careful. There are safe and effective medications available today which allow asthmatics to exercise safely. Asthma patients should be under the care of an allergist who can guide their treatment and their exercise program.

Cancer is the second leading cause of death in the United States. Several recent epidemiological studies have shown that active people have less incidence of cancer. While these studies fail to establish a cause and effect relationship between exercise and the prevention of cancer, they are encouraging particularly in light of the consensus among these investigations in favor of an active lifestyle.

References

1. B. L. Riggs and L. J. Melton III, "Involutional Osteoporosis," *New England Journal of Medicine*, 314, (1986): 1676.
2. B. L. Riggs and L. J. Melton III, "Evidence for Two Distinct Syndromes of Involutional Osteoporosis," *American Journal of Medicine*, 75, (1983): 899.
3. C. C. Johnston and C. Slemeda, "Osteoporsis: An Overview," *The Physician and Sportsmedicine*, 15, (1987): 64.
4. R. Lindsay, "Estrogen and Osteoporosis," *The Physician and Sportsmedicine*, 15, (1987): 105.
5. R. P. Heaney, "The Role of Calcium in Prevention and Treatment of Osteoporosis," *The Physician and Sportsmedicine*, 15, (1987): 83.
6. "NIH Consensus Development Conference on Osteoporosis," *Journal of the American Medical Association*, 252, (1984): 799.
7. L. R. Hedlund and J. C. Gallagher, "The Effect of Fluoride in Osteoporosis," *The Physician and Sportsmedicine*, 15, (1987): 111.
8. E. L. Smith and C. Gilligan, "Effects of Inactivity and Exercise on Bone," *The Physician and Sportsmedicine*, 15, (1987): 91.
9. V. Brewer et al., "Role of Exercise in Prevention of Involutional Bone Loss," *Medicine and Science in Sports and Exercise*, 15, (1983): 445.
10. N. E. Lane et al., "Long Distance Running, Bone Density, and Osteoarthritis," *Journal of the American Medical Association*, 255, (1986): 1147.
11. B. Nilsson and N. Westline, "Bone Density in Athletes," *Clinical Orthopedics*, 77, (1971): 179.
12. E. R. Buskirk et al., "Unilateral Activity and Bone and Muscular Development in the Forearm," *Research Quarterly*, 27, (1956): 127.

13. H. H. Jones et al., "Humeral Hypertrophy in Response to Exercise," *Journal of Bone and Joint Surgery*, 59, (1977): 204.

14. P. C. Jacobson et al., "Bone Density in Women: College Athletes and Older Athletic Women," *Journal of Orthopedic Research*, 2, (1985): 328.

15. E. L. Smith et al., "Physical Activity and Calcium Modalities for Bone Mineral Increase in Aged Women," *Medicine and Science in Sports and Exercise*, 13, (1981): 60.

16. A. Rundgren et al., "Effects of a Training Programme for Elderly People on Mineral Content of the Heel Bone," *Archives of Gerontology and Geriatrics*, 3, (1984): 243.

17. M. M. Shangold, "Athletic Amenorrhea," *Clinical Obstetrics and Gynecology*, 28, (1985): 664.

18. C. F. Sanborn and others, "Is Athletic Amenorrhea Specific to Runners?" *American Journal of Obstetrics and Gynecology*, 143, (1982): 859.

19. R. Marcus et al., "Menstrual Function and Bone Mass in Elite Women Distance Runners: Endocrine and Metabolic Features," *Annals of Internal Medicine*, 102, (1985): 158.

20. B. L. Drinkwater et al., "Bone Mineral Density After Resumption of Menses in Amenorrheic Athletes," *Journal of the American Medical Association*, 256, (1986): 380.

21. E. L. Smith, "Bone Changes in the Exercising Older Adult," *Exercise and Aging: The Scientific Basis*, E. L. Smith and R. C. Serfuss (eds.) Hillside, N.J.: Enslow Publishers, 1981.

22. L. Lamb (ed.), "Osteoporosis in Men" *The Health Letter*, 30, (Oct. 23, 1987): 1.

23. "Low Back Pain" *Mayo Clinic Health Letter*, 7, (Feb. 1989): 4.

24. D. A. Shaw, "Back to Back Fitness," *Corporate Fitness and Recreation*, 2, (1983): 31.

25. L. Root and T. Kiernan, *Oh, My Aching Back*, New York: David McKay Co., 1973.

26. P. C. Williams, *Low Back and Neck Pain: Causes and Conservative Treatment*, Springfield, Ill: Charles C. Thomas, 1974.

27. R. Roos, "Active Treatment for Patients with Low Back Pain," *Your Patient and Fitness*, 1, (1988): 5.

28. R. A. McKenzie, The Lumbar Spine: *Mechanical Diagnosis and Pain*, Waikanae, New Zealand: Spinal Publications, 1981.

29. L. D. Cady et al., "Strength and Fitness and Subsequent Back Injuries in Firefighters," *Journal of Occupational Medicine*, 21, (1979): 269.

30. W. Liemoher et al., "Unresolved Controversies in Back Management—A Review," *The Journal of Orthopedic and Sports Physical Therapy*, 9, (1988): 239.

31. M. Pascale and W. A. Grana, "Does Running Cause Osteoarthritis?" *The Physician and Sportsmedicine*, 17, (1989): 156.

32. R. W. Moskowitz, "Primary Osteoarthritis: Epidemiology, Clinical Aspects, and General Management," *American Journal of Medicine*, 83, (1987): 5.

33. N. E. Lane et al., "Aging, Long-Distance Running and the Development of Musculoskeletal Disability," *American Journal of Medicine*, 82, (1987): 772.

34. D. T. Felson, "Obesity and Knee Osteoarthritis. The Framingham Study," *Annals of Internal Medicine*, 109, (1988): 18.

35. R. S. Panush et al., "Is Running Associated With Degenerative Joint Disease," *Journal of the American Medical Association*, 255, (1986): 1152.

36. S. I. Wolf and K. L. Lampl, "Pulmonary Rehabilitation: The Use of Aerobic Dance as a Therapeutic Exercise for Asthmatic Patients," *Annals of Allergy*, 61, (1988): 357.

37. E. R. McFadden, "Exercise and Asthma," *New England Journal of Medicine*, 317, (1987): 502.

38. K. D. Fitch et al., "The Effect of Running Training on Exercise-Induced Asthma," *Annals of Allergy*, 57, (1986): 90.

39. K. D. Fitch et al., "Effect of Swimming Training on Children With Asthma," *Archives of Disabled Children*, 51, (1976): 190.

40. S. K. Ludwich et al., "Normalization of Cardiopulmonary Endurance in Severly Asthmatic Children After Bicycle Ergometry Therapy," *Journal of Pediatrics*, 109, (1986): 446.

41. W. S. Eisenstadt et al., "Allergic Reactions to Exercise," *The Physician and Sportsmedicine*, 12, (1984): 94.

42. J. Lweis et al., "Exercise-Induced Urticaria, Angiodema, and Anaphylactoid Episodes," *Journal of Allergy and Clinical Immunology*, 68, (1981): 432.

43. S. Locke and D. Colligan, "Is the Cure For Cancer in the Mind?" *Annual Editions—Health 89/90*, Guilford, Conneticut: The Dushkin Publishing Group, 1989.

44. American Cancer Society, *Cancer Facts and Figures—1988*, New York: American Cancer Society, 1988.

45. J. McKenna and J. Shea, "How to Cut the Risk of Cancer," *Annual Editions—Health 89/90*, Guilford, Conneticut: The Dushkin Publishing Group, 1989.

46. R. S. Paffenbarger et al., "A Natural History of Athleticism and Cardiovascular Health," *Journal of the American Medical Association*, 252 (1984): 491.

47. R. E. Frisch "Lower Prevalence of Breast Cancer and Cancers of the Reproductive System Among Former College Athletes Compared to Non-Athletes," *British Journal of Cancer*, 52, (1985): 885.

48. M. Gerhardsson et al., "Sedentary Jobs and Colon Cancer," *American Journal of Epidemiology*, 123, (1986): 775.

49. J. E. Vena et al., "Occupational Exercise and Risk of Cancer," *American Journal of Clinical Nutrition*, 45, (1987): 318.

50. S. N. Blair, "Low Physical Fitness and Increased Risk of Death and Disability," Speech delivered at the SDAAHPERD Convention, Chattanooga, TN, Feb. 24, 1989.

51. A. P. Simopoulous, "Obesity and Carcinogenesis: Historical Perspective," *American Journal of Clinical Nutrition*, 45, (1987): 271.

52. L. N. Kolonel, "Fat and Colon Cancer. How Firm is the Epidemiological Evidence," American Journal of Clinical Nutrition, 45, (1987): 336.

53. A. Viti et al., "Effect of Exercise on Plasma Interferon Levels," *Journal of Applied Physiology*, 59, (1985): 426.

54. J. G. Carmon et al., "Physiological Mechanisms Contributing to Increased Interleukin—1 Secretion," *Journal of Applied Physiology*, 61, (1986): 1869.

55. E. R. Eichner, "The Marathon: Is More Less?" *The Physician and Sportsmedicine*, 14, (1986): 183.

56. A. J. Edwards et al., "Changes in the Populations of Lymphoid Cells in Human Peripheral Blood Following Physical Exercise," *Clinical and Experimental Immunology*, 58, (1984): 420.

57. A. J. Robertson et al., "The Effect of Strenuous Physical Exercise on Circulating Blood Lymphocytes and Serum Cortisol Levels," *Journal of Clinical and Laboratory Immunology*, 5, (1981): 53.

58. H. D. Simon, "Derailing Cancer," *The Walking Magazine*, 4, (March/April 1989): 17.

59. M. M. Gauthur, "Can Exercise Reduce the Risk of Cancer," *The Physician and Sportsmedicine*, 14, (1986): 170.

5

Motivation

Chapter Outline _____

Mini Glossary

Adherence: long-term participation

Blood Lactate: a metabolite that produces fatigue; results from incomplete breakdown of sugar.

Burnout: a loss of energy, creativity, and direction.

Extrinsic Reward (external reward): any positive reinforcement emanating from an outside source, i.e., friends, coaches, etc., that increases the strength of a response.

Goal: something toward which effort or movement is directed; and end or objective to be achieved.

Intrinsic Reward (internal reward): reinforcement coming from within; The degree of satisfaction derived from participation in the absence of some visible reward.

Motivation: the internal mechanisms and external stimuli that arouse and direct behavior.

Positive Reinforcement: a reward; increases the strength of a response or responses.

Self-Concept: the set of people's beliefs about and evaluations of themselves as persons.

Stimulus: any energy impinging upon an organism that results in a response.

Introduction

In Chapter 1 the importance of self-responsibility as the cornerstone of a wellness lifestyle was established. Adherence to a regular program of exercise is one of its vital elements. This chapter addresses the problem of motivating people for involvement in those lifetime activities that facilitate and maintain fitness.

According to Wilmore, initiating and complying with an exercise program is dependent upon education and motivation.[1] Education includes explaining why and how people should exercise. Both are important because many sedentary adults plunge into exercise with unrealistic impressions of what constitutes effective yet safe training practices. The importance of education was attested to by the results achieved with the publication of Kenneth Cooper's first book, *Aerobics.* He provided the whys and hows in that text, which embarked literally millions of people on exercise programs. The timing of this book was right; Americans were ready to do something positive for themselves, but they needed a plan, and Cooper's book seemed to provide that plan. The print and broadcast medias also got into the act and the public soon began to learn about the value of exercise.

Motivation is a second crucial element. There must be sufficient motivation to sustain the program during the first six months because 40 to 50 percent of those who start exercising drop out within six months to one year,[2, 3] with the largest percentage of these occurring during the first three months.[4] Exercise programs lasting a year or longer experience less than 50 percent adherence (continuation in the program) and the situation worsens as time goes by. Dishman labeled the first six months of a beginner's adventure into exercise as the "critical period."

Exercise Drop-Outs and Adherers

Recent research is indicating strongly that exercise and physical activities consist of behaviors which are more complex than other health-related behaviors. Ex-

The acquisition of habits of increased physical activity is viewed as a process with three stages: (a) the decision to start exercising, (b) the early states of behavior change, and (c) maintenance of the new behavior.
–Dorothy Knapp

Although numerous variables affect participant exercise compliance, perhaps the most important is the exercise leader.
–Barry Franklin

Exercise programs should be designed not only to develop optimal fitness but also to enhance long-term adherence to training.
–Michael Pollack

ercise shares some common dimensions with other health behaviors but it has inherent uniqueness (effort, exertion, sweat, etc.) which separates it from these. As a result of its uniqueness, researchers are currently attempting to develop a model of behavior indigenous to exercise which will enable them to predict who will be the potential drop-outs and adherers. The advantages of such a model are obvious. If the potential drop-outs can be identified early, they can be targeted for appropriate interventions by program staff in order to increase the probability of adherence.

Studies of this type are complex and difficult because (1) terminology has not yet been standardized, and (2) participants change their behaviors. For instance, many people who enroll in supervised exercise programs drop out but continue to exercise on their own while others drop out and do not exercise on their own. This confounds the adherence statistics unless viable follow-up of dropouts occurs to determine their exercise status.

The reasons most often offered by exercise dropouts include lack of time, inconvenient or inaccessible exercise site, work conflicts, and poor spouse support.[2] It is difficult to determine whether these are actual barriers or perceived barriers to exercise. Evidence indicates that adherers often live further away from the exercise facility and have no more leisure time than dropouts. Spousal support repeatedly has been shown to be a predictor of adherence but some adherers have indicated that it is less important than other factors. Perhaps one of the differences between those who continue to exercise and those who don't is that impediments to exercise are perceived as real barriers by dropouts. These same barriers are perceived by adherers as mere inconveniences which are easily surmounted. Turning dropouts into adherers may be accomplished by changing their perceptions. This may be affected by providing instruction in time management, by providing flexible exercise hours and developing home exercise programs for them.

Wood has advanced several additional reasons for dropping out.[5] One reason includes a poor attitude toward exercise. Wood states, "Our schools have produced two or three generations of adults who, generally speaking, are philosophically opposed to exercise." A second problem involves poor choice of exercise. Exercise comes in many forms so there is ample opportunity to select activities that are fun, enjoyable, and appropriate for one's needs. Third, people drop out because of injuries. Wood claims that many of these injuries are preexisting, that is, they were sustained early in life primarily through participation in contact sports in the schools. The majority of these involve knee problems resulting from cartilage damage. These are aggravated, rather than developed, by vigorous exercise of the wrong type later in life. The advent of an injury during the program is generalized to all exercises and not merely the one in which it occurred. Actually, people with preexisting injuries should be evaluated and guided into activities that will not exacerbate those injuries. For instance, severe lower limb injuries might not be aggravated by nonweight bearing activities such as swimming and cycling.

Some generalizations regarding exercise adherence may be advanced which tend to endure regardless of subjects, methods, time-frames, and programs.[2] These include the following: (1) blue collar workers, smokers, and the obese are less likely to begin and sustain exercise either in a supervised or individual program; (2) people who are highly self-motivated are more likely to continue nonsupervised exercise; (3) perception of lack of time and inconvenience lead to dropping out, but some exercisers continue despite the same barriers, and (4) health-enhancement encourages adopting an exercise program but reinforcement from health and exercise professionals, support from significant others, and the feelings of well-being and the attainment of one's goals seem to be more important for continuation.

Who Is Exercising?

Although a healthy lifestyle is theoretically within reach of almost anyone, it is the relatively wealthy, educated, white American who is the typical practitioner. A national survey of upper management regarding their attitudes about health and physical fitness are presented in Tables 5.1 and 5.2 Sixty-four percent of these executives exercise regularly, only 10 percent smoke, and their average blood pressure was an excellent 124/79. Even though they devote an average of 54 hours per week to their jobs, they find time to exercise. Some of their tips include:

> Schedule exercise as a regular business appointment, to minimize the likelihood that the day's demands will intrude; park a mile or two away from the office (or commuting point) and "walk-in;" never stay in a hotel that doesn't have a pool, fitness center or exercise path (nearby if not on the premises); and finally, don't treat travel as an excuse to interrupt your routine. Your running or walking shoes can be a reminder and incentive. Never leave home without 'em![6]

While the wealthy were discarding bad health habits, the poor were not.[7] Cardiovascular disease has decreased among those with higher socioeconomic status, but the poor continue to suffer more than their share.[8] Some researchers

TABLE 5.1   Attitudes of 3000 Executives Regarding Health and Exercise*

	Very Important (%)	Important (%)	Not Important (%)
Healthy Habits			
Don't smoke	87	8	5
Exercise regularly	76	19	5
Eat less sugar, salt, fat	73	21	6
Get adequate sleep	56	33	11
Control stress	55	35	10
Limit alcohol intake	51	39	10
Exercise Motivation			
Overall health benefits	87	10	3
Improved sense of well-being	74	20	6
Weight control	71	19	10
Reduced stress	56	26	18
Better productivity	53	31	16

*Figures represent percent of respondents.

Adapted from K. M. Cahill, "The 3-Martini Lunch Is Long Gone," *The Walking Magazine*, (March/April 1989): 33.

TABLE 5.2 Physical Fitness Participation of 3000 Executives*

Favorite Activities	Percent Who Participate	Percent of Participants 3 times a week or more
Jogging/running	35	72
Tennis	35	7
Golf	32	2
Fitness walking	31	66
Stationary cycling	22	64
Weight training	27	56
Calisthenics	18	94
Racquetball	12	26
Outdoor cycling	10	10

*Figures represent percent of respondents.

Adapted from K. M. Cahill, "The 3-Martini Lunch Is Long Gone," *The Walking Magazine*, (March/April 1989): 33.

have concluded that the high prevalence of chronic disease among Blacks and other minorities is evidence that the fitness movement has passed them by.[9] LaPorte has stated, "the exercise boom has been a result of efforts to target the sedentary white-collar executives who have money. But those excluded from the fitness boom are the ones who need it the most. If researchers want to use activity to reduce the prevalence of chronic disease, they have to go where the chronic diseases are—among the lower socioeconomic groups."[10] Efforts aimed at this segment of society are underway in California, Arizona, and Georgia and each program has achieved success in changing health and exercise behaviors. Health professionals administering these programs are convinced that it is fruitless to bring Jane Fonda and Richard Simmons to the ghetto but it is much more productive to develop fitness programs that respect cultural values.[9] A sound fitness program developed for middle-class America will not work in these settings but a sound program adapted for local consumption will.

Motivation: Some Basics

Motivation is a label invented by people to describe a characteristic type of behavior. It cannot be measured directly; therefore it is inferred through observations of behaviors and actions. Such imprecision often results in inaccurate perceptions about presumed levels of motivation. The matter is confused further because motivation, as with other aspects of human behavior, lacks a uniformly acceptable definition. For this text, we will adopt Sage's definition that motivation is "the internal mechanisms and external stimuli that arouse and direct behavior."[11] According to this definition, **motivation** is affected by both internal and external forces. External forces, represented by **extrinsic** (external) **rewards,** often are a necessary stimulus for people to continue in an exercise program during those critical early months. For instance, membership in an exercise group provides a setting where compliments and positive strokes from one's peers furnish the external reinforcement for adherence during this time.

The rewards provided to the novice exerciser can be: (1) symbolic (a badge, pin, T-shirt), (2) material (money, prizes, payment of fitness club dues), or (3) psychological (attention, recognition, encouragement, etc).[12] Rewards such as these are important, particularly during the early stages of exercise, since at this point many facets of the program—cost of exercise apparel, equipment, investment of time, pain, discouragement, failure to realize goals, fatigue, and possible alienation of family—may be perceived as deterrents to continuation. An event of considerable import in exercise motivation occurs when the individual transcends dependence on external rewards and begins to internalize the feelings of well-being as prime motivators of exercise.

Franklin stated, "the benefits derived from extrinsic rewards, while initially important, are also short-lived. Ultimately, the motivation to continue an exercise program must be intrinsic rather than extrinsic in nature. The individual must develop an attitude toward exercise which reinforces adherence."[13] Buffington stated that each individual is his or her own best motivator, as the greatest motivational energy comes from within.[14] When the reward comes from the degree of satisfaction derived from participation, it is referred to as **intrinsic (or internal) reward.**

Motivation: How Important?

There are those who argue that motivation is the most-valued human commodity. It separates the successes from the failures, the winners from the losers, and the spectacular from the mundane. What does motivation look like? Take a good look inside yourself. You'll find it.

Buffington, P. W., "Getting Going." *Sky*, 112, April, 1985.

There is some question regarding the staying power produced solely by external rewards and there is speculation regarding its possible depressant effect upon intrinsic motivation. For instance, two researchers showed that "play could be turned into work,"[15] and two others declared that "token rewards may lead to token learning."[16] The epitome of the adverse effect of external reward upon intrinsic motivation is represented by the fable recounted below.

Pay Prevents Play

Once upon a time, there was an old man who was bothered by the noise made by a group of young boys who would play in an area near his house. As the story is told, the old man, desperately trying to come up with a way to rid himself of the disturbances, decided to pay the boys. He offered them 25 cents apiece to return the next day and play by his house. Naturally, the boys thought they had found a good thing and returned to play the next day, at which time the old man offered them 20 cents if they would repeat their performance on the morrow. When they returned the next day they found that the ante had been reduced to 15 cents and the old man told them that in the next few days he would give them only a nickel for their efforts. At that point, the boys became very agitated and decided that their efforts were worth more than a nickel. They told the old man that they would not return.

Siedentop, D. and G. Ramey, "Extrinsic Rewards and Intrinsic Motivation," *Motor Skills: Theory Into Practice*, 2, No. 1: 49, 1977.

The drive producing long-term **adherence** in any endeavor, exercise included, must be intrinsically motivated. But more recent research indicates that external rewards do not necessarily subvert internal motivation. In fact, prudently selected external rewards that are contingent upon quality of performance do not impair (and may even augment) intrinsic motivation.

Human behavior is purposeful; that is, it is goal-directed. The objective of motivated behavior is the achievement of our goals. **Positive reinforcements** (intrinsic supplemented with extrinsic) motivate us to persist in the attainment of these goals. A workable plan for achieving **goals** involves knowing what we want to accomplish in the long run. In other words, we should be able to identify our long-range goals. Then we should set realistic short-term goals which may be reached within a reasonable time. The achievement of each short-term goal acts as both a reinforcer and a stimulus motivating us to strive for the next goal, while each accomplishment brings us closer to realizing our long-term goal. The key is realism: setting goals that are difficult enough to provide a challenge but that we have a reasonable chance of achieving. This is a functional plan for achieving objectives and physical fitness should be approached in this manner.

Some psychologists have determined that a moderate level of motivation is optimal.[17] Too little is likely to result in early failure and too much may result in injury and burnout. In either case, motivation is adversely affected, adherence wanes, and the program, with all of its good intentions and potential benefits, is terminated. In order to avert this all-too-familiar scenario, we must cultivate the philosophy that our fitness goals should be approaced slowly and patiently, albeit progressively. We must learn to contain our enthusiasm so as not to attempt too much too soon during the early phases of the program. Remember, physical fitness is not achieved with two weeks of training. The development and maintenance of physical fitness should be a life-long affair. This requires a sizeable commitment of time and knowledgeable effort, but the results are eminently worthwhile. You supply the time and the effort and this text will provide you with the necessary knowledge. The appropriate application of these ingredients will increase your likelihood of success.

Why People Exercise

People participate in physical activities for a variety of reasons. Knowledgeable people in the fitness business can list many reasons why people in general are attracted to exercise. A carefully studied approach was presented by Kenyon, who developed a conceptual model regarding why people participate and why they select certain kinds of activities.[18] We know, in general, why people participate. We need to learn more about which stimulus or combination of stimuli will motivate a given individual to exercise.

It is a reasonable assumption, considering the multidimensionality of physical activity (i.e., aerobic dancing, biking, running, swimming, racquetball, etc.), that there are movement experiences that have the potential to provide some degree of satisfaction for everyone. Kenyon's scale (Kenyon Attitude Toward Physical Activity Scale) consists of the following dimensions: (1) social experiences, (2) health and fitness, (3) the pursuit of vertigo which refers to risk taking activities such as rock climbing, white water canoeing, rappelling, etc., (4) aesthetic experiences, (5) catharsis, and (6) ascetic experiences.[18]

Most of the reasons given for joining the physical fitness movement may be found embedded within these six dimensions. The dimension cited most often as the motivation for exercise relates to health.[19, 20] This category includes psychological and emotional as well as physiological reasons for exercise. A 1985 Gallup Survey reconfirmed the desire to improve one's health status as the major motive for initiating an exercise program.[18] More than half of the respondents indicated that exercise was part of a general overhaul of their lives. Seventy-four percent of the women and 59 percent of the men indicated that being "out of shape and/or overweight" stimulated them to begin exercising. The cluster of responses associated with health were cited most often, by most respondents, and the data showed that exercisers were more likely to change living habits to those that are related to good health. They were more willing and more successful in eating more nutritiously and giving up smoking than their nonexercising peers. The survey also indicated that multiple motives were often involved in establishing the exercise habit. Many respondents stated that in addition to health reasons they were motivated to exercise because they did not want to be in as poor physical condition as many of the people with whom they interacted. These negative models helped to convince these respondents of the need for fitness. Twenty percent of the sample began to exercise because their jobs had become more demanding and a sizeable segment of this group exercised to combat on-the-job burnout. **Burnout,** a relatively vague term, implies a loss of energy, creativity, and direction. Forty-three percent of the Gallup respondents, who exercised a minimum of five hours per week, reported more creative energy as well as more total energy devoted to their jobs. Becoming and remaining fit may do as much for occupational health as it does for personal health.

It is important to consider enhancement of body image and self-concept as motivators for exercise. **Self-concept** refers to our perceptions about ourselves and it is molded from how we see ourselves and how we think others see us. It involves the personal self, physical self, moral and ethical self, and family self. Body image, which represents the physical self, is an important constituent of self-concept.

A national panel of experts was convened by the National Institute of Mental Health in order to produce a state-of-the-art summary regarding the effect of exercise on mental health.[21] They concluded that long-term participation in exercise leads to a significant increase in self-esteem and significantly enhances one's estimation of the physical self. Body image improves as fitness level improves.

Loss of excess weight, development of muscle tissue, and desirable changes in body composition all contribute to a better physical appearance and thus to a better body image. The research indeed suggests that the enhancement of physical fitness is pervasive. It leads to an improvement of body image that enhances the entire self-concept. Folkins and Sime stated that, "The personality research with the highest payoff has been that which focuses on self-concept variables."[22] These two authors, in a comprehensive review of the research, concluded that those experiments with the best research designs and that were continued for a long enough period of time for exercise to produce a training effect resulted in improvements in self-concept. In a later study, Callen found that "almost all runners derive important mental and emotional benefits, which include relief of tension, improved mood, and better self-image."[23]

Scientists at the National Center for Health Statistics in Maryland have been studying the relationships between exercise and mental health. After analyzing data from surveys which collectively involved more than 75,000 adults representing a broad spectrum of individuals in the United States and Canada, they concluded that a positive association exists between exercise and mental health.[24] Initially, exercise may seem stressful but those who continue begin to feel better about themselves.[5] The gains in self-esteem, coupled with decreased feelings of tension, become powerful positive reinforcers. These desirable changes, which are subtle at first, do not become evident until the tenth or twelfth week of exercise. Unfortunately, many would-be exercisers drop out prior to this time having never fully experienced these benefits. Psychologist Robert Brown indicated that his files are packed with cases which support the notion that many people exercise primarily to control their moods and because of the way they feel about themselves.[24]

An interesting aspect of the effects of physical fitness upon self-concept relates to one's perceptions of one's level of fitness. Several studies reported that subjects' perceptions of their improved level of fitness, even in the absence of an actual improvement, beneficially affected their self-concept.[25,26,27] This suggests that merely participating in an exercise program has the potential to positively impact the self-concept.

The importance of developing a positive self-concept, or the degree of satisfaction that we derive from who and what we are, was most appropriately advanced by Dr. Norman Vincent Peale, who stated that "you have to spend every minute of your life in your own company. If you don't enjoy it, you're going to be miserable." By comparison, a few minutes spent in fitness activities three to five times per week may help us enjoy living with ourselves. Fitness is not a panacea, but the evidence indicates that it improves the self-concept.

As previously stated, it takes some time and effort—a small price to pay for such a profound payoff. A poor self-concept often leads to feelings of inferiority. Eleanor Roosevelt once said, "no one can make you feel inferior without your consent." We do not have to accept our lot in life: we can make a change. Do something positive for yourself: Make exercise a part of your life.

Psychological Effects of Exercise

Most regular exercisers not only feel healthier, but they also think exercise helps them feel good about themselves. In a recent study most seasoned runners said that their good feelings about running stem from psychological rather than physical satisfaction. For example, vigorous exercise may act as a release for anxiety and tension, and it has been favorably compared with tranquilizing drugs, meditation, and various relaxation techniques as a means of reducing muscle tension.

Good self-esteem is another strong deterrent to psychological problems. Feelings about the body and especially about appearance are intimately related to self-concept, so improved fitness usually results in improved self-esteem.

Weltman, A and B. Stamford, *The Physician and Sportsmedicine*, 11, No. 1: Jan., 1983.

Some people enjoy the social interactions with others while they exercise. They jog with a partner or group, participate in aerobic dance, compete in sporting activities, enjoy backpacking, and so on, partially to satisfy a need to do things with others but also to receive the benefits of exercise. This is carried to the extreme by those individuals who exercise because it is the "in thing" to do. This may not be the best of reasons but, from our perspective, the motive that initiates the program is irrelevant as long as the program endures. If the program is continued, the superficial motives that spurred the individual to exercise will probably yield to more substantial ones.

Some people exercise for "the pursuit of vertigo." According to Kenyon, this dimension is satisfied through activities presenting some degree of physical and/or psychological risk such as hang gliding, skydiving, mountain climbing, and white water canoeing, among others. Participants involved in these activities are often in quest of the ultimate physical and psychological experience and are willing to assume whatever risks are necessary to attain their objectives.

Some people are influenced by the aesthetic appeal or beauty of graceful and proficient physical movement while others are attracted by the potential that movement has to improve physical appearance. Favorable changes in body composition—loss of fat and gain of muscle—enhance physical appearance and, at least by Western standards, create a more pleasing silhouette.

Exercise to eat. Working out offers one of the few remaining excuses to eat more, to indulge occasionally without guilt.
–James Rippe

The evidence is quite clear that the majority of middle-aged and older adults exercise primarily for health enhancement. Several investigations of college students also indicated that health was the major reason for engaging in exercise.[28,29] However, a recent study of this population suggested that previous studies may have misinterpreted student motives by not including questions related to aesthetics. As a result, student interest in exercise and weight control were interpreted as reflective of their desire to enhance their health status. Koslow's study indicated that student interest in exercise and weight control were motivated primarily by their desire to develop aesthetically pleasing physical appearance instead.[30] Exercise for health was rated highly by this group but second to aesthetics. The appeal of exercise for this group should stress both, but greater effort should be devoted to the potential of exercise to effect desirable changes in physical appearance.

Others are drawn to exercise for catharsis, that is, to reduce that twentieth century ubiquity known as chronic stress. We covered this aspect of exercise in some detail in Chapter 3, but to summarize, regular exercise is one of the excellent ways for dealing with chronic stress. A final group participates for ascetic reasons. To this group the discipline associated with the rigors of training holds the most appeal.

Reasons why people exercise may be found within Kenyon's scales. The remaining problem is that we still don't know what motivates a given individual to begin to exercise. Factors that motivate one person may not have the same effect on another because of differences in experience, values, interests, objectives, intelligence, and so on. The selection of the exact factor or factors that might motivate a given individual to participate is conjectural at best. There is general agreement that adherence on a regular basis for a long period of time is greatly enhanced if the activity selected is fun and enjoyable.[2, 5, 13, 19, 31] You can readily see how a given activity (for example, jogging) may be fun for some and drudgery for others. Therefore, we must try to match activities with people on the basis of what provides enjoyment while meeting their physiological needs, interests, and objectives. This is not always easy to do. This task would be much more manageable is we had highly qualified physical education teachers in the elementary schools. During these formative years, children who are exposed to top-notch programs—that teach the need for and the physiology of fitness as well as the motor skills to attain it—may retain the interest, knowledge, and skill bases for later participation. We cannot prove this but it seems to be a logical place to begin establishing lifelong exercise habits.

POINTS TO PONDER

1. *Describe the characteristics of those who are unlikely to exercise.*
2. *Who is more likely to exercise over the long-term and why?*
3. *Name and define the six components of Kenyon's Attitude Toward Physical Activity Scale.*
4. *Identify the primary reasons why middle-aged people and college-age people exercise.*

Motivational Strategies

Approaches to Motivation

Two disparate motivational techniques, the educational/promotional and the individualized/behavioral approaches, have been employed to stimulate greater involvement in fitness enterprises.[32] With regard to exercise, educational/promotional approaches are based on two premises: that individuals are motivated for self-enhancement, and that knowledge of the how and why of exercise is the only stimulus needed for people to become more active. The effectiveness of this technique is questionable for making long-term changes in health practices. In fact, the research indicates that knowledge of appropriate health practices unaccompanied by action is an inadequate basis for sustaining these practices.

The transmittal of information and the accumulation of knowledge is, for most, not enough to change behavior. By now, most cigarette smokers know that smoking is harmful because it predisposes them to serious chronic diseases but they continue to smoke anyway. By now, most sedentary people know that an active lifestyle featuring leisure time exercise is healthful but they continue to remain inactive. For these people, knowledge is not enough to change behavior. Promotional efforts to sell exercise to the general public often rely upon educational information which shows how exercise reduces the risk of cardiovascular disease.[33] Education alone regarding potential health benefits has generally been ineffective. Most individuals think of themselves as relatively invulnerable to major health problems. The mentality that these diseases will happen to the other person still persists.

Educational/promotional techniques have attempted to produce mass changes in behavior through media approaches. The results have often been disappointing probably because of the heavy emphasis upon providing only factual information.[33] Researchers in Sweden attempted to encourage behavioral changes through a one-year newspaper campaign to educate the readership on cigarette smoking, nutrition, and exercise.[34] The follow-up indicated that only 5 percent of the people who began to exercise did so because of the information provided in the newspaper. The researchers concluded that the campaign was not successful in motivating nonexercisers to change their behavior.

The individualized/behavioral approach is very specific, being targeted to a given individual. Exercise prescription, motivational strategies, and reinforcement are built into the package. Case histories indicate that this approach is capable of initiating substantial behavioral changes. The limitations of this method are that it is labor-intensive, cost-inefficient, time-consuming and reaches a limited audience.[35]

Define Your Goals

Because exercise is multifaceted and can be programmed in numerous ways, it can meet many different objectives. The selection of appropriate types of activities and the proper application of exercise principles can help the overweight to lose and the underweight to gain, but first it must be determined what is to be accomplished through the exercise program. The more specific your goals the better. Do you wish to gain or lose weight, increase your energy level, reduce your risk for chronic disease, or improve your physical appearance? Would you like to participate competitively in swimming, cycling, running, court games, and so on? Your reasons for participation will determine which types of activity are best as well as how hard and how often they should be performed. If you have several goals, rank them in order of importance and work on them one at a time. Often, more than one goal may be pursued concurrently. For instance, weight loss and an increase in energy level can be accomplished together and an increase in muscle tissue and strength may also be accomplished at the same time.

Set Realistic Goals

Set goals that are realistic, attainable, and behavioral. The more specific the goal the better. An example of a nonspecific goal is reflected in the commonly heard statement: "I have finally had it; I'm going to lose weight." Contrast that statement with, "I'm going to lose 30 pounds and I'm going to do it by losing two pounds per week." This statement is specific and provides a time-table or a plan of attack. A nonbehavioral goal is, "I'm going to reduce my resting heart rate to 56 beats per minute." It can be made behavioral by adding, "I'm going to reduce my resting heart rate to 56 beats per minute by jogging 30 minutes per day, four days per week." Realistic goals expressed specifically and behaviorally are more helpful because they provide information and guidance for their attainment.

Don't expect too much too soon. Be patient because fitness takes time. At the same time, don't become excessively goal-oriented. Remain flexible and change your goals and activities if and when the need arises. Do not go beyond your exercise capacity by raising the intensity too abruptly. This will lead to discomfort and possibly injury. In either case, you will probably terminate the program. The injury rate rises when you exercise more than five times per week for more than 45 minutes per session.[36] Beginners would do well to exercise every other day and limit the duration of each workout to 20 to 30 minutes exclusive of warm-up and cool-down.

Exercise recommendations for the average participant would do well to decrease the intensity while increasing the frequency and duration. High intensity exercise is inappropriate, it is not enjoyable nor is it well-tolerated by those

The commonly used phrase "do your best" does not result in as great a performance improvement as does a specific goal.
–Richard MaGill

who participate for reasons other than competition.[4] Nor is it appropriate for the overweight, the sedentary, older people, and people who have cardiovascular disease. Studies have shown that increasing the frequency and/or duration of exercise is an effective way to equalize the caloric expenditure of higher intensity exercise. The increase in aerobic capacity is similar for both training schedules. The intensity of exercise should be sufficient to meet the exerciser's objectives but not so high as to be a deterrent.

People differ genetically in their potential for aerobic activity. We cannot all achieve the same level of performance, but we can all improve our level of fitness. Consistency is the key: you must exercise regularly to achieve your objectives. Set short-term goals that can be achieved in a few weeks. This will give you the feeling of success and provide a boost for you to achieve the next goal because success breeds success and motivates you to work harder. If the ultimate goal is to lose 30 pounds, it can be approached in stages with each stage covering a loss of six to eight pounds. If the task is not broken down into a series of small steps it may appear to be insurmountable. Reward yourself upon the successful completion of each stage. The closer you get to the ultimate goal, the more reinforcement you will get from other people who notice the positive changes in your physical appearance.

You may occasionally experience a setback or two on the way to your goals but don't let these deter you. You may not be progressing as rapidly as you would like or a minor injury or illness might keep you out of action temporarily. These and similar delays occur to almost everyone who exercises so expect occasional problems, handle them philosophically, and don't get discouraged. If an injury means that you cannot engage in your favorite physical activity, then find a substitute. A knee injury might prevent you from playing tennis or racquetball or jogging, but swimming or stationary cycling might be acceptable alternatives. They may not be your favorite forms of exercise but concentrate on the results rather than the means of attaining those results. Above all, don't become impatient with temporary setbacks. A classic example of maintaining motivation in spite of a string of setbacks was displayed by a nineteenth century politician. He lost his business, was defeated for the legislature, failed in business once again, suffered an emotional breakdown, lost an election for the U.S. Congress twice, U.S. Senate twice, and vice-president of the United States once, but in 1860 he was elected president. In the face of adversity Abraham Lincoln never lost his motivation to succeed.[15]

Exercise with a Group

Two investigators compared Cooper's individualized aerobics program to the group approach and found that after 28 weeks only 47 percent of those in the individualized program continued to participate compared to 82 percent in the group system.[37] An attractive feature of group participation is the possibility of developing social relationships with other participants. The group provides reinforcement, camaraderie, and an element of competition as well as a spirit of cooperation. In the early days of exercise, allegiance to a group enhances compliance; one's commitment to the group is not as easily dissolved as a commitment to oneself.[33] When the individual becomes committed to regular participation in exercise, the need for group support will probably decrease and the program can be continued without it.

Enlist the Aid of Significant Others

Spouses, family members, friends, and coworkers—those with whom the individual frequently interacts and who are considered to be special by the prospective exerciser—can be a primary source of support. Social support from these people (particularly one's spouse) includes a favorable attitude and encouragement toward the individual's exercise endeavors. Spouse support has been a source of positive motivation in a number of studies.[38, 39] A better scenario exists when spouses and/or other family members are regular exercisers. They can be role models who can draw on their experiences and knowledge to provide information, counsel, and advice. They may act as reinforcers of exercise by working-out with the novice exerciser.

Exercise with a Buddy

The effectiveness of the buddy-support system was examined in two independent investigations.[40, 41] They indicated that this model might provide the necessary support for sustaining an exercise program. Two people with similar training routines and compatible levels of fitness can reinforce each other. Knowing that your training buddy will be waiting for you at a designated time and place makes it difficult to skip the workout even when you would rather do something else.

Associate with Other Exercisers

Associate with people who motivate you in a positive manner and avoid those who are negative and pessimistic. Don't allow them to give you a negative attitude. Seek out others who exercise and, with them, discuss training, nutrition, weight loss, the reasons why they began exercising, what they have already accomplished, what you hope to do and learn from each other. Catch their enthusiasm and give them some of yours. Enthusiasm is prevalent and contagious when people who exercise get together; as a result of this interaction you will eagerly approach your next workout.

Keep a Progress Chart

Maintaining a daily record (self-monitoring) of one's exercise may be motivating particularly if the record sheet is posted where it may be regularly observed.[42] A daily record provides objective data which shows the actual rate and amount of progress that has been achieved. Exercisers who keep records increase their level of exercise substantially.

Looking back at the record and observing the gains that have been made can be a source of motivation when one becomes discouraged. The chart should reflect changes in body weight, type and amount of exercise, duration, and the exercising and resting heart rates. There should also be room for a short accompanying statement on how the participant felt during and after the workout. See Table 5.3 for a workable progress chart.

Weighing oneself prior to and after the workout is important particularly in hot weather when fluid loss can become a major problem. Most of the weight lost during the workout is liquid so the difference between pre- and post-exercise

TABLE 5.3 Progress Chart

Date	Body Weight		Exercise		Intensity**			Comments
	Pre	Post	Type	Duration*	RHR	THR	PE	

*Time, distance, etc.
**RHR = resting heart rate; THR = training heart rate; PE = perceived exertion.

weight is an approximation of the amount of fluid loss. This figure should not exceed 4 to 5 percent of the body's weight. This process of determining and/or approximating fluid loss is one of the functional aspects of the progress chart. Over the long term, a trend for weight loss, type and amount of exercise, distance covered, and heart rates (exercise and resting) will become discernible and you will have a record of improvement.

Exercise to Music

Music provides a sense of rhythm and it tends to take the mind off the effort. A researcher at the Ohio State University tested experienced runners with and without upbeat music.[43] The runners stated that music made the bout of exercise seem easier. They ran both trials, one with and one without music, at the same workload. Measures of working heart rates and **blood lactate** indicated that the runners were working equally hard on both trials, only their perceptions of the difficulty of the workload were changed.

Music can be easily provided indoors and portable radio headsets are gaining in popularity for outdoor exercise.

Set a Definite Time and Place for Exercise

It is best to set a definite time and a convenient place in the initial stages of the program. Resolve to exercise at least three times per week and schedule your workout as you would any other important activity.

Cardiologist James Rippe suggests that the day and time of each work-out should be written on one's daily calendar so that it will be scheduled in the same way as appointments and other important activities.[44] Resist the temptation to replace your workout with some other pursuit that might be more appealing. Skipping workouts becomes habit-forming; the more you do it the easier it becomes. After you become hooked on exercise, the time and/or place may be varied to meet the vagaries of weather, job responsibilities, and aesthetic sensibilities.

Participate in a Variety of Activities

Varying the activities is one of the ways to maintain enthusiasm and combat boredom. Select activities that are enjoyable and randomly rotate participating in them. You may also wish to participate in more than one activity on any given day. If you are not participating competitively in a particular activity, then you have great flexibility of choice.

Dwell on the Positive

We tend to notice the negatives associated with the workout such as the sore muscles, the effort required, and the feelings of fatigue. Instead, concentrate on the positives—as the song states, "accentuate the positive and eliminate the negative." Pay attention to the sense of accomplishment and the feeling of relaxation after exercise. Notice that your mind roams freely during exercise. Let it go where it may. You may work out the solution to a nagging problem while you jog or bike, or you may organize in your mind that paper that is due next week or you may simply daydream. Also, as the weeks pass you will notice a difference in energy level and a feeling of general well-being. Concentrate on these factors and they will keep you in the right frame of mind about exercise.

Don't Become Obsessive About Exercise

You should relax and enjoy exercise—it should be recreative, not obstructive. Don't become so obsessive that you feel and act miserable because you missed a day of exercise. Sometimes unplanned circumstances make it difficult to exercise on a particular day. Develop the mature philosophy that tomorrow is another day and you will get your chance then. If you become ill, don't exercise. Resume your program when you feel better. The major point is that missing an occasional day of exercise will not detract from the fitness benefits that you have achieved. Later on in this text you will find that a couple of days off from exercise in a week's time is important. The second point is that one need not feel guilty because occasionally a day slips by without a workout. If you rest two days per week, you can use one of these to make up the missing workout.

There Are No Failures

Physical fitness may be attained without competing against others or the clock. McGlynn[45] has summarized this concept very nicely in this manner, "There are no complex skills to learn, no condescending instructors, no embarassing situations, no last-place finishes, no critical peers, no intimidation." In other words, just go out and do your thing.

Select Activities that You Enjoy

Enjoyment is one of the cornerstones of adherence. Activities which are not enjoyable, will have a short life span. There are not many of us who fit in the ascetic category and exercise for the sheer discipline regardless of the lack of fun and enjoyment.

SELF-ASSESSMENT
Exercise Adherence Scale* _____

Directions

Evaluate yourself using the scale in Table 5.4 by circling the number under the letter which most closely approximates your behavior for each of the seven statements. The key to each letter is as follows:

    A Very atypical of me
    B More-or-less atypical of me
    C Neither typical nor atypical of me
    D More-or-less typical of me
    E Very typical of me

Scoring Procedure

Add the numbers that you have circled for the seven statements to get a total score. Drop-out prone behavior is suggested by a score equal to or less than 24. If your score falls in this category, make a special effort to employ some of the motivational techniques presented in this chapter. Remember, each time you drop out before completing a task, the easier it gets to drop out of the next one.

*Adapted from R. K. Dishman and W. J. Ickes, in B. Falls, et al *Essentials of Fitness* (Philadelphia: Saunders College, 1980).

TABLE 5.4 Assessing Exercise Adherence

A	B	C	D	E	Adherence Issue
		Scale			
5	4	3	2	1	1. I get discouraged easily.
5	4	3	2	1	2. I don't work any harder than I have to.
1	2	3	4	5	3. I seldom if ever let myself down.
5	4	3	2	1	4. I'm just not the goal-setting type.
1	2	3	4	5	5. I'm good at keeping promises, especially the ones I make to myself.
5	4	3	2	1	6. I don't impose much structure on my activities.
1	2	3	4	5	7. I have a very hard-driving, aggressive personality.

POINTS TO PONDER

1. *Identify and discuss the various motivational strategies which may be employed to enhance starting and/or continuing in an exercise program.*
2. *Give some examples of specific and behavioral fitness objectives.*
3. *How would you respond to someone who says that they don't exercise because they don't have enough time?*

Chapter Highlights

The initiation of and compliance with an exercise regiment is dependent upon education and motivation. There must be sufficient motivation to sustain the program during the crucial first six months in order to attain long-term compliance. Both internal and external sources of reinforcement contribute to habitual physical exercise.

Human behavior is goal-directed but the goals that are selected must be realistic. Psychologists have determined that moderate levels of motivation are most effective in working toward and achieving our goals.

People exercise for reasons of health, social experiences, "the pursuit of vertigo," aesthetics, catharsis, and ascetic experiences. For exercise to be sustained, it must fulfill our needs but at the same time it must be fun. Exercise enhances body image and self-concept.

Motivational strategies include (1) defining and setting realistic goals, (2) exercising with a group, (3) obtaining the support of people who are important to you, (4) keeping a progress chart, (5) exercising to music, (6) setting a definite time and place for exercise, (7) exercising with a buddy, (8) associating with other exercisers, (9) dwelling on the positive, (10) not becoming obsessive about exercise, (11) there are no failures, and (12) selecting activities that you enjoy. Doing these things won't guarantee adherence but the application of these strategies will increase the probability of adhering to the program.

References

1. J. H. Wilmore, "Individual Exercise Prescription," *American Journal of Cardiology*, 33, (1974): 757.
2. R. K. Dishman, "Exercise Compliance: A New View for Public Health," *The Physician and Sportsmedicine*, 14, (1986): 127.
3. R. J. Sonstroem, "Psychological Models" in R. K. Dishman (ed.) *Exercise Adherence*, Champaign, Ill.: Human Kinetics Books, 1988.
4. M. L. Pollock, "Prescribing Exercise for Fitness and Adherence," in R. K. Dishman (ed.) *Exercise Adherence*, Champaign, Ill.: Human Kinetics Books, 1988.
5. J. M. Rippe (Moderator), "The Health Benefits of Exercise (Part 2 of 2)," *The Physician and Sportsmedicine*, 15, (1987): 120.
6. B. Ketchum, "Fit for the Fast Lane," *The Walking Magazine*, (March/April, 1989): 4.
7. Louis Harris and Associates, Inc. *The Prevention Index: A Report Card on National Health*, Emmaus, Pa.: Rodale Press, Inc., 1988.
8. "Report of the Secretary's Task Force on Black and Minority Health," U.S. Dept. of Health and Human Services, Publication No. 0–174–719: Government Printing Office, August 1985.
9. D. Giel, "Fitness and Exercise Issues for Black Americans," *The Physician and Sportsmedicine*, 16, (1988): 162.
10. T. Monahan, "Is Fitness Reaching Only the Wealthy?" *The Physician and Sportsmedicine*, 17, (1989): 200.
11. G. Sage, Motor Learning and Control: A Neuropsychological Approach, Dubuque, Iowa: Wm. C. Brown, 1984.
12. R. J. Shepard, "Motivation: The Key to Compliance," *The Physician and Sportsmedicine*, 13, (1987): 88.
13. B. A. Franklin, "Motivating and Educating Adults to Exercise," *Journal of Physical Education and Recreation*, 49, (1978): 6.
14. J. H. Buffington, "Getting Going," *Sky*, 112, (1985):
15. D. Greene and M. R. Lepper, "How to Turn Play into Work," *Psychology Today*, 8, (1974): 49.
16. F. Levine and G. Fasnacht, "Token Rewards may Lead to Token Learning," *American Psychologist*, 29, (1974): 816.
17. P. Klavora, "Customary Arousal for Peak Athletic Performance," in P. Klavora and J. V. Daniel (eds.) *Coach, Athlete and Sport Psychologist*, Champaign, Ill.: Human Kinetics Publishers, 1979.
18. G. S. Kenyon, "A conceptual Model for Characterizing Physical Activity," *Research Quarterly AAHPER*, 39, (1968): 566.
19. T. G. Harris and J. Kagan, "The Fitness Advantage," *American Health*, 4, (1985): 12.
20. National Center for Health Statistics, Vital and Health Statistics: Current Estimates from the National Health Interview Survey, United States 1985, Series 10, No. 160 DHHS Pub. No. (PHS) 86–1588, 1986.
21. W. P. Morgan and S. E. Goldston (eds.), *Exercise and Mental Health*, Washington, D.C.: Hemisphere Publishing, 1987.
22. C. H. Folkins and W. E. Sime, "Physical Fitness Training and Mental Health," *American Psychologist*, 36, (1981): 380.
23. K. E. Callen, "Mental and Emotional Aspects of Long-Distance Running," *Psychosomatics*, 24, (1983): 145.
24. T. Monahan, "Exercise and Depression: Swapping Sweat for Serenity?" *The Physician and Sportsmedicine*, 14, (1986): 192.
25. R. A. Hayes, "Relating Physical and Psychological Fitness: A Psychological Point of View," *Journal of Sports Medicine and Physical Fitness*, 18, (1978): 399.
26. G. R. Leonardson, "Relationships Between Self-Concept and Perceived Physical Fitness," *Perceptual and Motor Skills*, 44, (1977): 62.
27. G. R. Leonardson and R. M. Garguilo, "Self-Perception and Physical Fitness," *Perceptual and Motor Skills*, 46, (1978): 338.
28. S. Blair, "Values of Physical Activity as Expressed by Physical Education Majors," *The Physical Educator*, 41, (1984): 186.
29. T. R. Trimble and L. D. Hensley, "The General Instruction Program in Physical Education at Four-Year Colleges and Universities, 1982," *Journal of Physical Education, Recreation, and Dance*, 59, (1988): 28.
30. R. E. Koslow, "College Fitness Courses—What Determines Student Interest?" *Journal of Physical Education, Recreation, and Dance*, 59, (1988): 28.
31. B. A. Franklin, "Program Factors that Influence Exercise Adherence: Practical Adherence Skills for the Clinical Staff," in R. K. Dishman (ed.) *Exercise Adherence*, Champaign, Ill.: Human Kinetics Books, 1988.
32. L. M. Wankel, "Decision-Making and Social-Support Strategies for Increasing Exercise Involvement," *Journal of Cardiac Rehabilitation*, 4, (1984): 124.
33. D. N. Knapp, "Behavioral Management Techniques and Exercise Promotion," in R. K. Dishman (ed.) *Exercise and Adherence*, Champaign, Ill.: Human Kinetics Books, 1988.
34. G. Anderson et al., "Occurrence of Athletic Injuries in Voluntary Participants in a 1-Year Extensive Newspaper Exercise Campaign," *International Journal of Sports Medicine*, 7, (1986): 222.

35. F. J. Keefe and J. A. Blumenthal, "The Life Fitness Program: A Behavioral Approach to Making Exercise a Habit," *Journal of Behavioral Therapy and Experimental Psychiatry*, 11, (1980): 31.

36. M. L. Pollock et al., "Effects of Frequency and Duration of Training on Attrition and Incidence of Injury," *Medicine and Science in Sports*, 9, (1977): 31.

37. J. F. Massie and R. J. Shephard, "Physiological and Psychological Effects of Training—A Comparison of Individual and Gymnasium Programs, with a Characterization of Exercise Drop-Out," *Medicine and Science in Sports*, 3, (1971): 110.

38. G. M. Andrew et al., "Reasons for Dropout From Exercise Programs in Post Coronary Patients," *Medicine and Science in Sports and Exercise*, 13, (1981): 164.

39. D. Knapp et al., "Exercise Adherence Among Coronary Artery Bypass Surgery (CABS) Patients," *Medicine and Science in Sports and Exercise*, 15, (1983): 120.

40. A. C. King and L. W. Frederiksen, "Low–Cost Strategies for Increasing Exercise Behavior: Relapse Preparation Training and Social Support," *Behavior Modification*, 8, (1984): 3.

41. J. E. Martin et al., "Behavioral Control of Exercise in Sedentary Adults: Studies 1 Through 6," *Journal of Consulting and Clinical Psychology*, 52, (1984): 795.

42. R. O. Nelson et al., "Self-Reinforcement: Appealing Misnomer or Effective Mechanism?," *Behavior Research and Therapy*, 21, (1983): 557.

43. R. J. Trotter, "Maybe It's the Music," *Psychology Today*, 8, (1984): 19.

44. J. M. Rippe, "29 Tips for Staying With It," *Annual Edition—Health 89/90*, Guilford, Conn: The Dushkin Publishing Group, 1989.

45. G. McGlynn, *Dynamics of Fitness: A Practical Approach*, Dubuque, Iowa: William C. Brown, 1987.

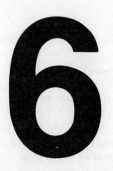

6

Developing the Cardiovascular Component:

Guidelines for Exercise

Chapter Outline

Mini Glossary

Active warm-up: dynamic movements for the purpose of readying the body for activity.

Adenosine Diphosphate (ADP): a complex, high-energy compound from which ATP is resynthesized.

Adenosine Triphosphate (ATP): a complex, high-energy compound stored in the cells from which the body derives its energy.

Aerobic: literally means "with oxygen."

Anaerobic: literally means "without oxygen."

Anaerobic Threshold: that point where exercise cannot be totally sustained by the aerobic processes. Anaerobic processes contribute to the production of ATP and lactic acid begins to accumulate in the blood.

Baroreceptors: sensory nerve endings which respond to stretching of the walls in which they are embedded.

Conduction: transference of heat from one object to another by means of physical contact.

Convection: transfer of heat from the body to a moving gas or liquid.

Creatine Phosphate (CP): a chemical that donates its phosphate to ADP for the resynthesis of ATP.

Cross-training: selection and participation in more than one physical activity on a consistent basis.

Dehydration: excessive loss of body fluids.

Dynamic stretching: stretches that involve bouncing and bobbing movements.

Electrolyte: any solution that conducts an electrical current through its ions.

Evaporation: the loss of heat by changing a liquid to a vapor.

Glycogen: the stored form of sugar.

Heat exhaustion: a condition characterized by a buildup of body heat. Symptoms include dizziness, fainting, rapid pulse, and cool skin.

Heat stroke: the most dangerous of the heat stress illnesses. Symptoms include a temperature of 106°F and above, absence of sweating, dry skin, and often delirium, convulsions, and loss of consciousness.

Hemoglobin: iron pigment of the red cells that combines with O_2.

Hyperthermia: overheating; abnormally high body temperature.

Hypothermia: abnormally low body temperature.

Lactic acid: a fatiguing metabolite resulting from the incomplete breakdown of sugar.

Passive warm-up: inactive means of preparing for physical activity; may include massage and dry and wet heat.

Proprioceptive Neuromuscular Facilitation (PNF): a group of stretching techniques involving the alternation of contraction and relaxation of various muscles.

Radiation: transfer of heat from the body to the atmosphere by electromagnetic waves.

Introduction

In this chapter, the definition and the differences between aerobic and anaerobic exercise will be presented. The production of energy in the form of ATP (adenosine triphosphate) generated by each of these metabolic pathways will be discussed in an elementary way.

Suggestions for exercise based upon guidelines developed by the American College of Sports Medicine as well as other sources in current literature will be presented. Exercises which currently meet the criteria for safety and effectiveness as well as those which are not recommended because they are potentially hazardous will be presented.

Environmental conditions have an impact on the exerciser. Guidelines are presented for exercising safely in hot and cold weather.

Retro walking and retro running are being used by some people as an adjunct to their stretching program. Information is presented on the efficiency of this technique along with a few tips on how to perform backward locomotion.

The effects of exercise on prepubescent children and pregnant women and their fetuses are also examined in this chapter.

Aerobic Versus Anaerobic Activities

The energy for muscular contraction comes from the foods that we eat, but our muscles cannot directly use carbohydrates, fats, and proteins for fuel. Protein liberates only a very small portion of its energy to generate human movement. Its primary function centers on building and repairing bodily tissues as well as synthesizing hormones and enzymes. No other food source can perform these functions. Protein becomes a substantial energy source only under conditions of starvation. Instead, carbohydrates and fats are metabolized enzymatically in a series of complex chemical stages to provide the fuel for movement. The chemical processes by which this is accomplished are very complex and beyond the scope and purpose of this text, but we will cover the anaerobic and aerobic operations associated with metabolic processes in order to emphasize the major differences between aerobic and anaerobic exercise.

Carbohydrates are broken down to water and carbon dioxide, which releases the energy needed to form **adenosine triphosphate (ATP).** The energy for muscular contraction occurs when ATP splits into **adenosine diphosphate (ADP)** and phosphate (P_1). A small quantity of ATP is stored in the muscles, along with **creatine phosphate (CP),** to provide an instant source of energy for muscular contraction. The splitting of CP to creatine and inorganic phosphate provides the energy to resynthesize ATP from ADP, thus restoring ATP levels in the muscles.

Fats are also oxidized to yield energy to form ATP. The type of fuel, carbohydrate or fat, used to manufacture ATP depends upon the intensity or the amount of effort required to perform an exercise or activity. Exercise and physical activity—indeed, all movement—may be categorized as being predominantly, if not exclusively, anaerobic or aerobic. **Anaerobic** literally means "without oxygen." Anaerobic activities, then, are high-intensity movements that can only be continued for a matter of seconds. Sprinting 100 yards, lifting a heavy weight, shot-putting, and running up two flights of stairs are some examples of anaerobic activities. The oxygen demand of these activities is higher than that which can be supplied by the body during their performance. As a result, these events rely on the short-term fuel supplies of ATP or CP stored in the muscles that can be mobilized rapidly in the absence of adequate oxygen. Sugar in the form of **glycogen** (the stored form of glucose) is broken down to pyruvic acid, which is temporarily shunted to **lactic acid** (a fatiguing metabolite that results from the incomplete breakdown of sugar) when oxygen cannot be supplied rapidly enough for processing by the muscle cells (see Figure 6.1). This process produces a very small quantity of ATP and a large quantity of lactic acid. The cells cannot tolerate high levels of lactic acid; therefore, performance must cease until it is removed. In the anaerobic cycle, one molecule of glucose yields only two molecules of ATP.

Fat is not utilized as a fuel source during high-intensity anaerobic activity because lactic acid blocks the action of epinephrine, a fat-mobilizing hormone produced by the adrenal glands. Epinephrine makes fat available from its storage depots for use as a fuel during low-intensity exercise where lactic acid production is inconsequential. Anaerobic activities are fueled entirely by carbohydrate metabolism. The limited production and storage capacity of ATP in this process dictates that high-intensity exercises can be sustained for only a matter of seconds.

Aerobic means "with oxygen." Aerobic activities depend on a continuous and sufficient supply of oxygen in order to burn fats and carbohydrates to support endurance or sustained activity. For exercise to be aerobic, the level of intensity is such that the oxygen needs of the activity can be adequately supplied by the body during the activity; in other words, the participant achieves a balance or "steady state" between oxygen supply and demand (see Figure 6.2).

Walking, jogging, biking, swimming, and aerobic dancing are some of the most popular forms of aerobic exercise. Carbohydrates and fat supply large quantities of ATP aerobically to fuel these activities. Walking, slow jogging, and prolonged exercises that are performed at less than 70 percent of one's oxygen utilization capacity rely primarily on fat for ATP production. Those activities that are sustained above 80 percent of one's capacity depend upon carbohydrates as the predominant source of ATP production.

When sufficient oxygen is available, carbohydrates are broken down to pyruvic acid which in turn is converted to carbon dioxide and water through a series of intermediate stages without the production of lactic acid. This process

---

FIGURE 6.1

Simplified Schematic of the Anaerobic Pathway
Without sufficient O_2 pyruvic acid is converted to lactic acid and ATP production stops. No O_2 is required for glycogen to break down to pyruvic acid.

Glycogen
↓
Glucose
↓
ATP
+

$$\frac{\text{Pyruvic acid} \rightarrow \text{Lactic acid}}{\text{Insufficient } O_2}$$

FIGURE 6.2

Oxygen Demand
This is a typical curve representing the achievement of a steady state between the O_2 demand of exercise and the exerciser's ability to meet it.

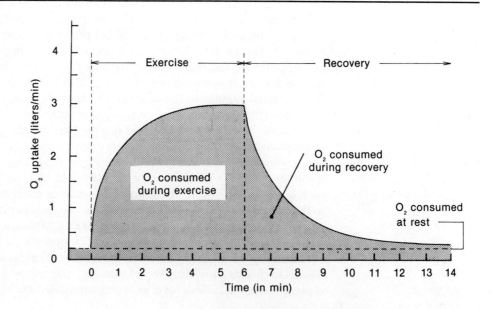

FIGURE 6.3

Simplified Schematic of the Aerobic Pathway
When sufficient O_2 is present, pyruvic acid is broken down to carbon dioxide and water and ATP is produced in large quantities. Once again, the breakdown of glycogen to pyruvic acid requires no O_2.

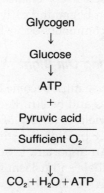

is accompanied by the systematic production of large quantities of ATP—19 times the amount produced anaerobically (see Figure 6.3). Fats make their contribution to ATP production by entering the cycle below the level of pyruvic acid.

In terms of ATP production, it is readily apparent why aerobic exercise can be prolonged and anaerobic activities cannot. Sharkey summarizes this way: "Aerobic pathways must be used if we are to delay fatigue. They are more efficient and the fuels are more abundant. As exercise intensifies from a walk to a jog we switch from fat as the predominate source of energy to a fat-carbohydrate (glycogen) mixture. Switch from a jog to a run, and glycogen becomes the main source of energy. Sprint and glycogen is the sole source of energy."[1]

Aerobic activities, which are dependent upon a constant supply of oxygen, stress the cardiovascular and respiratory systems. In this manner, they increase the aerobic capacity and produce the training effect that enables people to improve their performance in endurance-type activities while concomitantly attaining the health-related benefits covered in Chapters 4 and 5. On the other hand, anaerobic activities apply their stress for periods of time which are too short to enhance the aerobic system unless they are employed in circuit or interval training. These training systems will be discussed in Chapter 7.

Guidelines for Exercise

Many beginners approach the development of physical fitness with little knowledge and in a frenzied fervor. Guidance for the program emanates from their recollections of physical education classes or varsity athletics. Those experiences, regardless of their efficacy and/or lack of physiological soundness, become a frame of reference for the development of current programs. What has been forgotten is filled in through trial and error. Participants who begin in this manner may build on an unsound framework and/or fail to realize that they are no longer 17 years of age. The science and philosophy of physical fitness has changed in important ways since they were last involved.

This chapter will attempt to provide the type of information needed by beginners to intelligently assess their fitness needs and then develop a sound program to meet those needs. A sound program will avert many of the pitfalls that have beset and curtailed thousands of fitness programs. Start right and give

Choose what is best; habit will soon render it agreeable and easy.
Pythasoras

yourself every chance to succeed. Optimal benefits accrue by regular participation beginning early in life and continuing without the years of interruption that commonly occur between graduation from school and middle age.

Starting Out Right

Exercise must become habitual if it is to make an optimal contribution to physical fitness and health. Regular and consistent participation for three to six months will yield a variety of physiological and psychological benefits that may ultimately provide the stimulus for lifetime continuation.

An important lesson that prospective fitness devotees must learn is to contain their enthusiasm in the initial stages of the exercise program. Ten years of inactivity cannot be expunged with ten furious days of activity. Impatient beginners, overeager to attain fitness rapidly, tend to exercise beyond their capacity. Such efforts are predictably doomed to fail because the usual results are a profusion of aches, strains, pains, and no enjoyment of exercise. As exercise becomes a chore, enthusiasm subsides and the program, with all of its good intentions, will be discarded.

The Medical Exam

The American College of Sports Medicine (ACSM), in conjunction with the American Medical Association (AMA), has established guidelines for medical screening prior to starting an exercise program. These guidelines apply to three major categories of individuals who may be candidates for medical screening and testing: (1) apparently healthy individuals, (2) those at higher risk, and (3) individuals with a disease.[2] Individuals under the age of 45, who are apparently healthy, may begin exercising without an exercise stress test as long as they realize that they must start at a low level and progress slowly. Also, these individuals should be knowledgeable of and alert to the development of unusual signs or symptoms. Individuals who are older than 45, regardless of their exercise habits, should have a maximum exercise test. Individuals who are at higher risk—those having at least one major coronary risk factor and/or symptoms which suggest the possibility of cardiopulmonary or metabolic disease (diabetes, thyroid disorders, kidney and liver disease, etc.,) should have a maximum exercise test regardless of age prior to participation in vigorous activity. Persons of any age with known cardiovascular, pulmonary, or metabolic disease should have a maximal exercise test before they are cleared for exercise. This test is absolutely necessary to determine the individual's functional capacity and to establish a safe level of exercise. It is imperative that a physician be present for tests such as these.

Per-Olaf Astrand, a Swedish physician, is amused by our conservative approach to exercise. From his perspective, the medical exam should be used to determine whether we are healthy enough *not* to exercise; his point being that the unhealthy need exercise more than the healthy and that exercise is less of a risk than inactivity.

Aims and Objectives

Most people begin exercising because of dissatisfaction with their current status: their appearance, low fitness level, lost vigor, lost youth, compromised health, and so on. Regardless of the stimulus, beginners should attempt to articulate their reasons in one or two specific objectives. Defining objectives or what is hoped to be accomplished through exercise enables one to develop a realistic program to achieve the desired fitness goals.

Program objectives should be reflected by the manner in which the principles of intensity, frequency, duration, progression, overload, specificity, and type of exercise are manipulated by the participant. The degree to which each of these factors is emphasized or deemphasized is the key to accomplishing specific objectives. Exercises that are not targeted to program objectives will not produce desirable results. Knowing your objectives and goals is a very important first step if an appropriate exercise program is to be developed. Without objectives, the exercise program becomes a hit-and-miss proposition that might be analogous to sightseeing in Chicago with a map of Philadelphia. You may reach your destination, but the odds are against it. At the end of this chapter is an assessment instrument (The Physical Activity Questionnaire) which will help to clarify your present exercise status, your reasons for exercising, and your attitude regarding regular participation in exercise.

Warming Up for Exercise

Warming up, or getting the body ready for exercise, is one of the often slighted and sometimes neglected phases of a workout. The major reasons for engaging in a warm-up prior to exercise are to prevent injury and enhance performance. The efficacy of warm-ups for preventing injury and enhancing performance is theoretical and, as yet, unsubstantiated experimentally.[3] It is practically impossible to find people who are willing to put forth a maximum performance effort in the absence of warm-up because they feel intuitively that an injury will occur if muscles are stressed in this manner. Even if they agree to participate in such an experiment, they are not psychologically ready to produce a maximal effort.

Warm-up may be passive, active, or a combination of the two. **Passive activities** include massage, steam or sauna, hot towels, hot showers, and whirlpool baths. These might alleviate the stiffness and soreness that may carry over from the previous workout. A passive warm-up might be an adjunct to, but not a replacement for, an active warm-up prior to exercise. Passive warm-up may be counterproductive because it increases surface temperature by dilating the blood vessels in the skin. The result of this is the diversion of blood to the skin rather than to the muscles which will be involved in the activity.

An **active warm-up** usually includes a general and a specific component. The general component consists of stretching and large muscle activities designed to slowly raise the heart rate while increasing muscle temperature. Some typical activities appear in Figure 6.4 through 6.13.

The specific component of warming up involves participation in the activity to be performed or a related activity. For example, subsequent to the completion of the general phase of warm up, joggers might run in place or jog the first half mile of the workout at a leisurely pace slowly increasing to the desired speed. In this way, the body is allowed to selectively and gradually adapt to the specific stress to be imposed upon it. The concepts of general and specific warm up apply to most activities—swimming, biking, rope jumping, racquetball, tennis, and many others.

FIGURE 6.4

Groin Stretch
Lean forward from the hips until you feel a stretch in the groin area. Hold for 30 seconds and do one set.

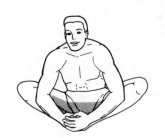
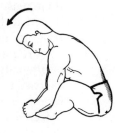

FIGURE 6.5

Trunk Rotation
Follow the number sequence to loosen the trunk and hamstrings.

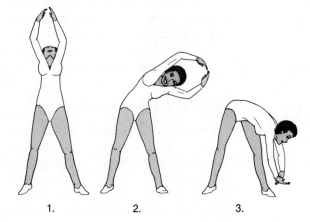

1. 2. 3.

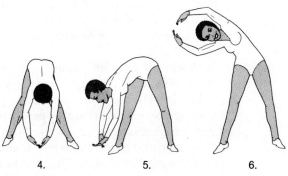

4. 5. 6.

FIGURE 6.6

Hamstring Stretch
Stand with your legs straight, clasp hands behind your back, and bend from the waist while raising your arms. This stretches the hamstrings. To intensify the stretch, rock back on your heels. Hold 15 to 30 seconds.

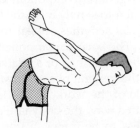

FIGURE 6.7

Quadriceps Stretch
Lean against a wall or other stable object and pull the heel close to the buttocks using the alternate arm. **Do not** overstretch the knee—it is not necessary to touch the heel to the buttocks. This stretches the quadriceps group. Alternate legs and hold each stretch for 15 to 30 seconds.

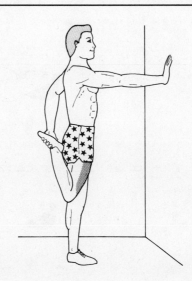

FIGURE 6.8

Calf and Achilles Stretch
Assume a stride position with the forward leg bent at the knee and the rear leg straight with the heel planted firmly on the floor. Lean forward until discomfort is felt in the calf and Achilles tendon.

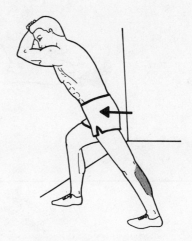

FIGURE 6.9

Low Back Stretch 1
Alternate pulling one leg and then the other to the chest. This stretches the low back. Place your hands under the knee.

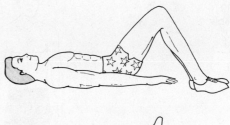

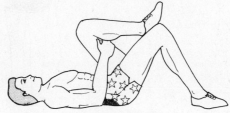

FIGURE 6.10

Low Back Stretch II
Pull both legs to the chest simultaneously. This stretches the low back. Place your hands under the knees.

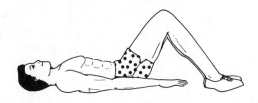

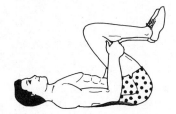

FIGURE 6.11

Curl-Up
Bring the heels close to the buttocks. With the arms crossed on the chest sit up until the shoulder blades clear the floor. Develops the abdominal muscles.

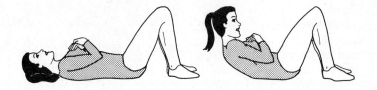

FIGURE 6.12

Jumping Jack
From the standing position, jump to a straddle position with the feet apart while throwing the arms overhead. Follow by jumping to an erect position with both feet together while returning the arms to the sides. Repeat 10 to 20 times.

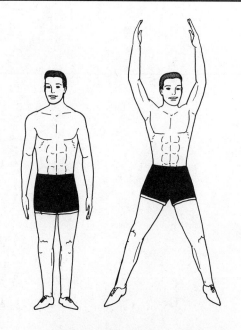

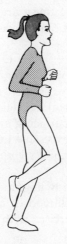

FIGURE 6.13

Jogging in Place
Jog slowly in place for 1
to 2 minutes.

Static stretching is the preferred method for enhancing and maintaining flexibility and suppleness. This involves slow stretching, holding terminal positions for 10 to 30 seconds, and then repeating the movement at least one more time. Muscles should be stretched slowly and progressively to the point of discomfort, not pain. This method does not stretch the tissues beyond their limits, is economical in terms of energy expenditure, helps prevent muscle soreness, alleviates soreness should it already exist, and does not require the assistance of a partner.

Static stretching should be preceded by large muscle activities such as rhythmic calisthenics, running in place and slow jogging. These activities raise muscle temperature and gently raise the heart rate toward that expected during the exercise session. An increase in muscle temperature facilitates muscular stretch, which results in an increase in flexibility in the long term and it theoretically reduces the likelihood of injury.

Dynamic stretching, consisting of bouncing movements, has been largely discarded because it stimulates specialized receptors located in the muscles that respond to fast bouncing movements. When these receptors are activated, the muscles being stretched are signaled to contract, resisting the stretch effect. The simultaneous action of stretching and contraction in the same muscles produces soreness and possible injury. These receptors are not stimulated to the same extent by slow, static stretching.

A third form of stretching, **proprioceptive neuromuscular facilitation (PNF)** has been slowly infiltrating the fitness movement as a technique for increasing flexibility. Physical therapists have been employing PNF stretching techniques for patients with neuromuscular disorders for many years. These are inappropriate for people who exercise on their own because the performance of these stretches requires a partner. It appears that PNF stretching techniques produce slightly better results immediately after their use when compared to other stretching methods but the long term results are probably no better than those that are attained with static stretching. As a result, we will recommend static stretching for practicality and effectiveness in enhancing flexibility.

There are many exercises that stretch the major muscle groups of the body. Some of these are inherently dangerous while others are dangerous because they are often performed incorrectly. Movements that are potentially hazardous involve:

1. overflexing a joint
2. excessively arching the back or neck
3. sudden twisting or flexing
4. bouncing and bobbing
5. excessive jumping or hopping
6. rapid swinging of the arms or legs

Poor body alignment during the performance of some exercises also increases the likelihood of injury. Table 6.1 presents some of the commonly used high risk exercises with safer alternatives for each.

Exercise Survival Guide

The following are some exercise tips to assist you in evaluating exercise programs, exercise leaders, and exercises.

1. If you opt for a supervised exercise program, check the credentials of the instructors who teach the classes. Ask if they have a college degree in fitness management or physical education. If not, are they certified by the American College of Sports Medicine (ACSM), as Health/Fitness Instructors or Aerobics Instructors? If no to both, have they had college courses in anatomy, physiology, exercise physiology, and kinesiology. Ask if they are certified in CPR (cardiopulmonary resuscitation). If the answer is no to all or most of the questions look for another program.
2. Check the facility and the surface on which you will exercise. Look for a suspended wooden floor as opposed to a carpet over a concrete floor.
3. Find out if exercise is monitored by target heart rate and perceived exertion. Do they periodically interrupt exercise to let you check your heart rate to determine if you are in the exercise target zone? Is the program primarily aerobic or is it predominantly muscular work?
4. Find out if the room is climate controlled.
5. Check to see if the equipment is maintained in good repair and that it is of the type that will enable you to achieve your exercise objectives.
6. Find out if and how you will be evaluated upon your entrance to the program and is exercise prescribed for you based upon this data.
7. Find out if individual attention is continuous or if it occurs only during the initial stages of the program.
8. Ask if your exercise program is updated as you become more physically fit.
9. Find out what their policy is on medical screening prior to entering the program and/or do they ask you to sign waiver forms.

After selecting the program you should

1. Control your movements while exercising. Avoid rapid, jerky movements because these can lead to injury.
2. As you move your limbs, keep the muscles slightly contracted as if you are pushing or pulling against resistance. This will keep you from flailing your limbs and help to control the movements.
3. Pay attention to your posture while exercising. Proper posture involves keeping your back straight with abdominal muscles contracted, buttocks tucked in, and knees slightly bent. This is important when jumping or reaching overhead.

TABLE 6.1   High Risk Flexibility Exercises: Dont's and Do's

Don't	Do

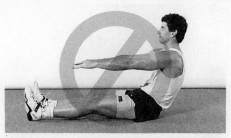

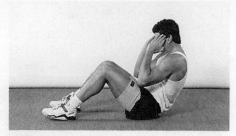

Straight-leg sit-up. Sit-ups done in this manner stress the low back by forcing it to arch. Muscles other than the abdominals do a significant amount of the work.

Bent-leg sit-ups. Keep your knees bent and your feet flat on the floor. Sit-up 30 to 45 degrees and keep your low back pressed to the floor.

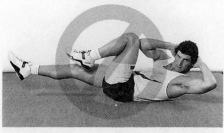

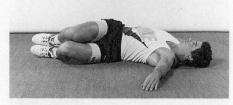

Alternating bent-leg sit-ups. Asymmetric pull on the pelvis occurs when you hold one leg straight out and touch the elbow opposite to the bent knee. This puts a strain on the low back.

Knee rolls. This exercise strengthens the oblique abdominal muscles more safely. Lie on your back with knees tightly tucked, arms out flat at shoulder level. Slowly roll to the right, hold for 2–3 seconds, return to the starting position and then roll to the left and hold. All movements are to be done slowly and under control.

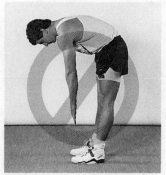

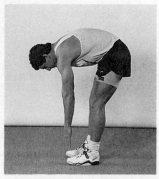

Toe-touches. Toe-touches with locked knees may overstress the back, hamstring muscles, and knees.

Bent-knee hang downs. Bend your knees slightly and slowly roll forward until stretch is felt in the hamstrings; hold for 10–15 seconds. Do not bounce or try to touch the floor.

Don't	Do

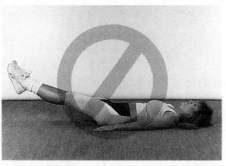

Double-leg lifts. This exercise forces the back to arch and increases the risk of injury.

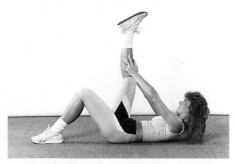

Raised-leg crunches. One leg is bent with the foot flat on the floor; the other leg is straight up. Raise your shoulders and upper back and reach toward the upraised ankle.

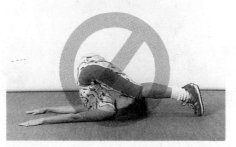

Yoga plow. Places considerable stress on the neck and its underlying structures. Any exercise that assumes this position is potentially hazardous.

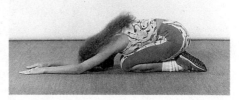

Fold-up stretch. Sit back on your heels, press your chest to the thighs, and reach forward with both hands. This is a safer way to stretch the upper and lower back.

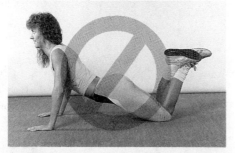

Arched-back push-ups. This incorrect method of doing push-ups will strain and possibly injure the low back.

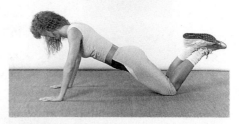

Straight-back push-ups. Hold your body in a straight line and slowly lower your chest to the floor by bending your arms and elbows. Provides greater workout for the arms, shoulders, and chest.

Don't	Do

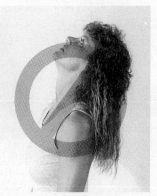

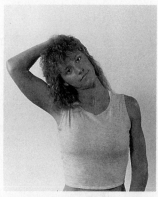

360° head rolls. Rolling the head in a full circle may injure the spinal disks in the neck.

Side neck stretches. Pull your head gently to one side, forward, to the other side, and back. You may also pull diagonally.

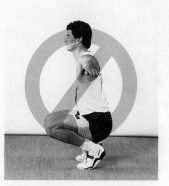

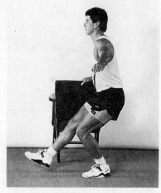

Full squats. Stretches ligaments in the knees and may result in injury.

Partial squats. Use the back of a chair or other object for balance and squat one-quarter on one leg while the other leg is extended forward.

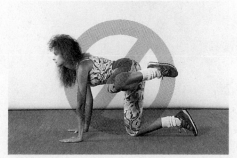

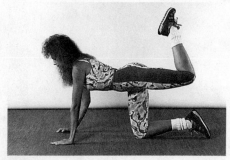

Donkey kicks. These force the back to arch and places the shoulders and neck in a contorted position.

Rear thigh lifts. Keep your back straight and slowly raise your leg straight up until the thigh is parallel to the torso.

Don't	Do

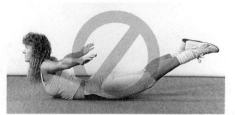

Swan stretch. Lifting your chest and legs simultaneously may put excessive stress on the low back.

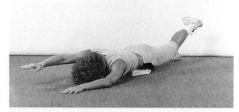

Prone arm/leg raise. Place one or two pillows under your stomach and raise the right arm and left leg 4 to 6 inches and hold for 5 seconds. Repeat with left arm and right leg.

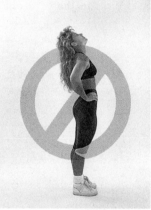

Trunk rolls. Puts pressure on the low back and sciatic nerve when knees are straight.

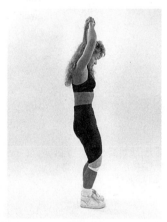

Bent knee trunk rolls. Bend your knees, pull in your stomach, and draw the pelvis forward. Slowly lean to the left, forward, and right.

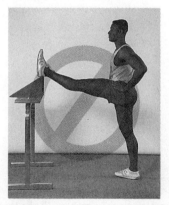

Hamstring stretch. When the foot is higher than the hips it excessively stretches the sciatic nerve, lower back, and muscles in the back of the leg.

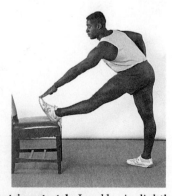

Hamstring stretch. Lead leg is slightly bent at the knee and the foot is well below the height of the hips. Bend forward slowly until stretch is felt in the hamstrings. Hold 15–20 seconds. Repeat with other leg.

Don't	Do

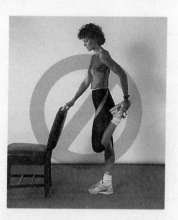

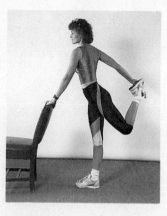

Quadriceps Stretch. If the ankle is pulled too hard there may be excessive pressure applied to the knee possibly resulting in ligament or muscle damage.

Opposite leg pull. Grasp one ankle with the opposite hand and attempt to straighten the leg.

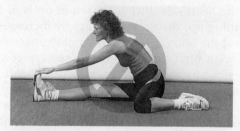

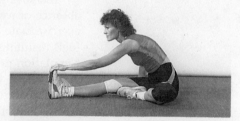

Hurdler's stretch. This position puts great stress on the hip, knee, and ankle.

Modified hurdler's stretch. Bend the right knee and place the right foot up against the left thigh. Lean forward until the stretch is felt in the left hamstring and hold for 15–20 seconds. Repeat with the other leg.

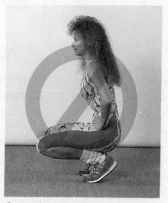

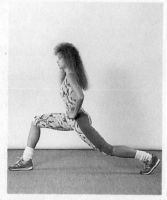

Deep knee bend. Places excessive pressure on the ligaments of the knee.

Single knee lunge. Place one leg in front and extend the other to the rear. Bend the lead leg 90° and hold for 5 seconds. Repeat with other leg.

Don't	Do

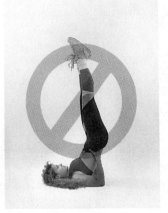

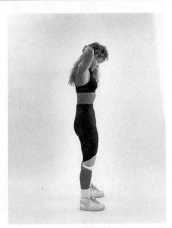

Shoulder stand. Excessive pressure on neck may cause injury to muscles or disks.

Neck stretch. Gently pull head forward and hold for 10 seconds.

Increasing the heart rate during the warm-up is of equal importance. In the absence of warming up, the heart rate rapidly increases from the resting to the exercise state and the body is forced to employ anaerobic processes to generate fuel, resulting in an undesirable and unnecessary accumulation of lactic acid. Circulation does not increase proportionately to heart rate, causing a brief interval when the heart is not fully supplied with oxygen. This delay can be hazardous for people whose circulation is compromised. Although the healthy, well-conditioned heart can usually endure such treatment, even a sound organ may be at risk. One study indicated that 44 healthy male subjects, ages 21 to 52, had normal electrocardiographic (EKG) responses to exercise which followed a warm-up consisting of two minutes of easy jogging.[4] But 70 percent of the group developed abnormal EKG responses to the same exercise when it was not preceded by a warm-up. You have probably warmed up sufficiently when you begin to sweat because this signifies that the core temperature is slightly elevated.

Intensity

Intensity refers to the degree of vigor associated with each bout of exercise. The American College of Sports Medicine recommends an exercise intensity level of 65 to 90 percent of the maximum heart rate.[2] This is roughly equivalent to 50 to 85 percent of aerobic capacity (the ability to take in, deliver, and extract oxygen for physical work). Cardiovascular endurance, functional capacity, and maximal oxygen consumption (max VO_2) are terms which have variously been used as a synonym for aerobic capacity.

Aerobic capacity is considered to be the best objective measure of endurance capacity and is defined as "the highest attainable oxygen consumption value in maximal or exhaustive exercise."[5] Since the training effect occurs at 50-85 percent of one's capacity, it follows that the intensity of exercise need not be maximum and rather nicely dispels the cherished myth that exercise must be painful to be beneficial. Exercising individuals who cannot talk without gasping for breath between each word are performing at a pace which is too vigorous for their fitness level. This is a good subjective check that lessens the probability of overexertion; however, it doesn't indicate whether the participant is exercising at the level needed to achieve optimal results. A more precise test utilizes the heart rate for calculating the upper and lower limits for exercise. It is fortunate that exercise programs can be gauged by using heart rate rather than aerobic capacity because the heart rate method is usually much easier for the average person to calculate and monitor. Maximal heart rate can be accurately determined by an exercise tolerance test to capacity on a treadmill, bicycle ergometer, and so on. Formulas based upon these tests have been developed to estimate maximal rate for the average person who does not have access to these sophisticated procedures. The formulas predict rather than assess maximal heart heart rate, so there is some measurement error associated with their use. The error factor must be considered when developing exercise programs.

The error of measurement for the assessment of maximal heart rate has been estimated to be a minimum of ten beats per minute. Based upon this estimate two-thirds of all people are within ten beats of their predicted maximal heart rate when using the formula, Maximum heart rate (Max HR) = 220 - age (see Figure 6.14).

The safety implications for developing exercise programs based on target heart rates are substantial. The upper limit serves as a barrier that need not be crossed by the person who exercises for health reasons. There are several methods for predicting maximal heart rate and exercise target heart rate. The following example is for a 20 year old:

$$
\begin{array}{rl}
220 & \text{(a constant)} \\
-\ 20 & \text{(subtract age)} \\
\hline
200 & \text{(predicted Max HR in beats per minute)}
\end{array}
$$

$$
\begin{array}{rl}
200 & \text{(predicted Max HR)} \\
\times\ .65 & \text{(65\% Max HR)} \\
\hline
130.00 & \text{(beats/min)}
\end{array}
$$

$$
\begin{array}{rl}
200 & \text{(predicted Max HR)} \\
\times\ .90 & \text{(90\% Max HR)} \\
\hline
180.00 &
\end{array}
$$

This method yields heart rates of 130 to 180 beats/min which form the lower and upper limits of exercise. It is desirable to select a ten-beat range within this continuum as the specific zone for exercise. A sedentary 20-year-old would select the lower end of the continuum (130–140) beats/min) as the target zone while a better conditioned individual of the same age would choose a ten-beat value closer to the upper end. The sedentary person would move the target zone in the direction of the upper portion of the continuum as fitness improves and his or her needs dictate.

A major advantage of this system of monitoring exercise is that the level of fitness can improve even though the participant may choose to remain in the same ten-beat range. As fitness improves, the heart rate for a given workload declines, so a lesser percentage of the aerobic capacity is required to do the same amount of work. For instance, jogging at a 10-minute-mile pace may elicit the target heart rate in the early days of the program when the individual is less fit. However, as fitness improves, the pace will need to be quickened to reach the target heart rate. Improvements will continue as the participant jogs faster and longer, all within the same target zone. Of course, remaining at the lower end of the continuum will limit the potential for improvement but the benefits that have been (and are being) attained may be compatible with the individuals objectives. Thus it may not be necessary to move the target zone upward. Maximal heart rate declines with age and with it the target zone for exercise (see Figure 6.15).

FIGURE 6.14

Possible Error Associated with Age-Related Prediction of Max HR

This figure indicates that 68% of the 20-year-olds will have a Max. HR between 190 and 210, 95% will be between 180 and 220, and the other 5% will be above and below these values.

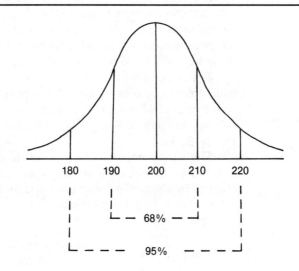

FIGURE 6.15

Maximal and Target Zone Heart Rates

This figure expresses average values by age for maximum attainable heart rate during an all-out effort. This value decreases approximately one beat/min/yr after age 20.

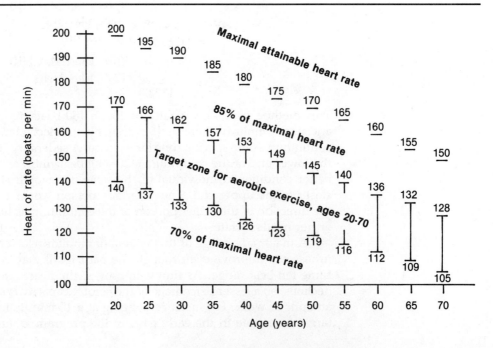

The Karvonen formula is also a popular and functional method for determining exercise heart rate (pulse rate). This method was developed by Karvonen in 1957 and validated by Davis in 1975.[6] The resting heart rate must be known in order to use this formula. Many factors (caffein, nicotine, environmental temperature, anxiety, eating a meal, etc) affect the resting heart rate therefore it is important to establish this parameter under standard conditions. The best time to determine the resting heart rate is in the sitting position after waking up in the morning.[7] You may need to empty your bladder first, then sit down and calm down for a few minutes prior to taking the pulse. Repeat this for four to five consecutive days and average the readings. This method should produce a good representation of the normal resting heart rate.

Now that the resting heart rate has been determined you may proceed to use the Karvonen formula to calculate the heart rate that should be maintained during exercise. The following example is for a 22-year-old whose resting heart rate is 72 beats/per min.

1. Calculate the max heart rate as before.

$$\begin{array}{r} 200 \\ \underline{-22} \quad \text{(age)} \\ 198 \quad \text{(predicted Max HR)} \end{array}$$

2. The Karvonen formula is

$$THR = (MHR - RHR) \times \text{Training Intensity (\%)} + RHR$$

where

    THR = Training heart rate
    MHR = Max heart rate
    RHR = Resting heart rate

therefore

$$\begin{aligned} THR &= (198\text{-}72) \times .70 + 72 \\ &= (126) \times .70 + 72 \\ &= (88.2) + 72 \\ THR &= 160 \end{aligned}$$

Table 6.2 presents guidelines which should help you select the proper training intensity to use in calculating the Karvonen formula based on your level of fitness.

Learning to take your pulse rate is a skill that you must develop in order to determine if the heart rate is within the prescribed zone. There are several sites

TABLE 6.2 Guidelines for Selecting Exercise Intensity Level

Fitness Level	Intensity Level (%)
Low	60
Fair	65
Average	70
Good	75
Excellent	80–90

in the body where the pulse can be felt. The two most practical sites are the radial pulse located in the wrist at the base of the thumb while the hand is held palm up and the carotid pulse that can be felt in the large arteries at either side of the neck (see Figure 6.16). Use the middle three fingers of the preferred hand to count the pulse. To locate the carotid pulse slide your fingers down from the angle of the jaw below the earlobe to your neck. Remember to start counting the pulse as soon as possible after exercise to get an accurate indication of the exercise heart rate because it declines rapidly when activity ceases. It takes some practice to quickly locate the pulse, begin the count, and count accurately.

The carotid pulse may not be the most appropriate site for estimating exercise heart rate because these arteries contain pressure-sensitive baroreceptors. Pressure applied to the carotid arteries stretches their walls stimulating the **baroreceptors** which in turn signal the brain to slow the heart rate. This will result in an inaccurate, underestimated exercise heart rate. In order to minimize or possibly circumvent this effect, the pressure applied to the carotid should not exceed that required to obtain the pulse rate.

To calculate exercise heart rate, the participant should periodically stop exercising, immediately count the pulse rate for ten seconds, and multiply this figure by six to obtain heart rate per minute. The first pulse beat which is felt after timing has begun should be counted as "zero."

A perceived exertion rating of 12 to 13 corresponds to approximately 60 percent of the heart rate range. A rating of 16 corresponds to approximately 90 percent of heart rate range.
ACSM

Monitoring exercise by heart rate is generally an effective method but it is not without flaws. First, stopping to take pulse rates becomes tedious and tends to interrupt the workout. Second, unless the maximum heart rate is assessed by an exercise tolerance test there is the possibility of substantial error. Third, it might encourage slavish dependence upon heart rate to the exclusion of perceived exertion or one's subjective impression regarding how difficult the workout feels. It is important that you tune into your body and that you learn to recognize and pay attention to the signals it gives. Some of the notable signals that form our perception of exertion during exercise include rate and depth of breathing, heart rate, body temperature, musculoskeletal stress and pain, and overall discomfort. Gunnar Borg has developed a rating scale that predicts actual exercise heart rate rather accurately.[8] See Figure 6.17.

You will note that the scale ranges from 6 to 20, with 6 being very, very light and 20 corresponding to very, very hard. When multiplied by a factor of 10, the numbers on the scale represent heart rates. A rating of 6 is translated

---

FIGURE 6.16

Common Sites for Taking Pulse Rate
Locating the pulse at the carotid artery (a) and at the wrist (b).

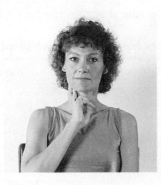
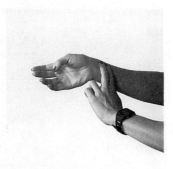

The Perceived Exertion Scale
This scale and the target heart rate during exercise are excellent ways to monitor physical activity.

6
7 Very, very light
8
9 Very light
10
11 Fairly light
12
13 Somewhat hard
14
15 Hard
16
17 Very hard
18
19 Very, very hard
20

as a heart rate of 60 and a rating of 20 is translated as a heart rate of 200. Published data indicate that the rating of perceived exertion not only correlates quite well with actual exertion as exhibited by exercise heart rate, but is oftentimes a better criterion measure since it considers more than just the exercise heart rate.[9] It encompasses sensory input from all of the systems associated with the generation of energy for movement. Perceived exertion is an excellent technique for monitoring exercise, particularly when maximal heart rate is estimated. If the heart rate maximum is overestimated, so too will the exercise target rate. Perceived exertion may be used to compensate for the error, thus averting overwork and its consequences. Also, we all experience days when exercise is more difficult. As Dishman stated, "there are days when the track just seems longer, and the hills are definitely steeper."[10] Much like a sputtering auto engine, our body is trying to tell us something. When we experience such feelings we should adjust the intensity downward and shorten the duration of the workout instead of pressing on as usual. Tomorrow will probably be a better day. The point is that we should not neglect what our body is attempting to communicate and we should capitalize upon this source of feedback to make adjustments when needed.

Frequency

The American College of Sports Medicine recommends that exercise be pursued three to five times per week.[2] A position paper produced by the ACSM regarding frequency of training stated, "the amount of improvement in $VO_{2\ max}$ tends to plateau when frequency of training is increased above three days per week. For the nonathlete, there is not enough information available at this time to speculate on the value of added improvement found in programs that are conducted more than five days per week."[11] However, evidence is available which indicates that susceptibility to injury increases as the frequency of exercise increases above five days per week.[12, 13]

The frequency of exercise should vary according to the objectives you are attempting to achieve. Those of you who are interested in weight loss and altering body composition would do well to exercise five or possibly six days per week, whereas three to four days would suffice for those who are lean and whose major concern is the development of more energy or endurance. The intensity and duration of exercise should have some bearing upon its frequency. Low-intensity exercise of moderate duration (20 to 40 minutes), such as walking, could be pursued every day without producing physiological or orthopedic problems, but high-intensity, longer-duration exercises such as jogging, biking, aerobic dancing, and the like need to be performed only three to five days per week. Days of rest are an important part of the training programs of people who exercise for health-related reasons—even world class competitive athletes need to take an occasional day off to recharge the physiological and psychological batteries. Rest days should be spaced rather than taken consecutively. However, the results of one study indicated that three consecutive days of exercise followed by four days of rest produced a training effect that was similar to a program featuring alternate days of work and rest.[14] A regimen such as this is not preferred because the cardiovascular benefits of exercise begin to regress 48 hours after the last bout. Two weeks of inactivity produce a significant reduction in exercise capacity and ten weeks to eight months without exercise will return the individual to pretraining levels.[11] Exercise should be performed at least every other day to maintain fitness. Also, data indicate that triglyceride levels in the blood are reduced for 48 to 72 hours subsequent to the last bout of aerobic exercise. Keeping this risk factor for heart disease continuously suppressed requires that the next exercise session occur prior to the elapse of that time. Periodic rest days also make sense in regard to lowering the likelihood of incurring an injury and combating the possibility of becoming "stale."

Recognizing the Signs of Overtraining

There is a fine line between the amount of exercise that produces maximum gains and the amount that results in the negative effects (staleness) associated with overtraining. Overtraining occurs when exercisers do too much too often. The signs of this phenomenon are

- a feeling of chronic fatigue and listlessness
- inability to make further fitness gains (or there may be a loss of fitness)
- a sudden loss of weight
- an increase of five beats or more in the resting pulse rate, taken in the morning prior to getting out of bed
- loss of enthusiasm for working out (the exerciser no longer looks forward to the workout).

Staleness may be both psychological (lack of variety in the program or boredom after years of training) and physiological. It is probably a combination of both, but the treatment is the same: either stop training for a few days to a few weeks (depends upon the severity of staleness) or cut back substantially. In either case, rebuild and regain fitness gradually. Prevention is the best treatment. Recognize the signs and adjust accordingly before staleness becomes a problem.

Duration

Duration and intensity are inversely related; the more intense the exercise, the shorter its duration and vice versa. Intensity is always an important consideration, but for people who exercise for health enhancement it is best to sacrifice some degree of intensity for duration. In essence, the total amount of work done as measured by calories expended appears to be the salient factor in achieving the health benefits of exercise. Three hundred calories per exercise session seems to be the lower limit for achieving these ends. In other words, decreasing the intensity to just above minimal threshold while increasing the duration will produce the same results as a higher intensity/shorter duration bout of exercise. The advantages of the former strategy are that exercise is performed comfortably and the probability of injury is diminished. For example, the caloric difference between jogging a mile in seven minutes versus a mile in nine minutes is insignificant; however, the slower pace is much more easily tolerated and produces similar cardiovascular training effects as the faster pace. For a 154 pound male, cycling at 9.4 miles per hour for 43 minutes, jogging at a nine-minute-mile pace for 32 minutes, swimming a slow crawl for 34 minutes and walking at a normal pace for 54 minutes all will use approximately 300 calories. For an estimate of the caloric cost of selected activities for your sex and weight, see Table 11.1.

The American College of Sports Medicine recommends that the length of each bout of exercise should be 15 to 60 minutes of continuous or noncontinuous aerobic activity.[2] Several epidemiological studies have shown that mileage run, or duration of activity, was the most significant cause of running injuries.[15,16,17]

Progression, Overload, and Specificity

When people attain a level of fitness which meets their needs and satisfies their objectives and further improvement is no longer desired, the program switches from the development of fitness to the maintenance of fitness. The principles of progression and overload are no longer needed at this point, but both are extremely important during the development or improvement phase of the program. Overload involves subjecting the various systems of the body to gradual and unaccustomed stresses. It is only through overload that the body adapts and improvements occur in strength, cardiovascular endurance and flexibility. Without overload, no adaptation or improvement occurs.

The principle of progression actually functions as the schedule for the application of overload. The key to overloading the body is to apply stress slowly and progressively but only when it is warranted and not before. Overloading too soon will probably culminate in injury to both body and ego. Be realistic—exercise is a lifetime endeavor; there's plenty of time for improvement. Slow down, enjoy it, and do not tear grimly and hastily through the exercise session. From a health standpoint, exercise is as important as anything you will do during the day, so give it the attention that any important and necessary activity deserves.

Weight training and jogging will be used to exemplify the principles of overload and progression. You should be able to generalize from these examples to the activity in which you participate. In weight training, overload consists of a combination of the amount of weight lifted (the resistance) and the number of times in which it is lifted (repetitions). A participant selects a weight that can be lifted a maximum of 10 times and remains with this weight until enough strength and endurance have been developed to lift it 15 times. At that point, the weight (resistance) is increased to reduce the number of repetitions back to ten. This process is repeated until the training objectives have been achieved.

In jogging, overload is applied by increasing the distance or decreasing the time required to cover the distance. Heart rate can be used to indicate the appropriate time to apply overload. A jogger aspires to cover a distance of five miles but is currently capable of jogging only two miles with a heart rate of 160 beats per minute. With training, the heart rate for covering that same two miles reduces to 150. At this point one-quarter to one-half mile is added to the distance. When the new distance is tolerated comfortably with a comparably low heart rate, more distance is added. The process is repeated until the goal is reached.

Three observations might be noted regarding the application of overload and progression:

1. patience is necessary
2. improvements occur in small imcrements but the greatest amounts occur during the first six to eight weeks of the exercise program[2]
3. overload should be applied only when certain criteria are met which indicate that the individual is ready to accept a newer challenge

There is ample evidence to support the contention that the body adapts according to the specific type of stress placed upon it. The muscles used in any given activity are the ones that adapt and they do so in the specific way in which they are used. Jogging does not prepare one for swimming and swimming does not prepare one for cycling. The legs are stressed in jogging in a manner indigenous to that activity. Those adaptations which occur from jogging provide very little carry-over to the leg kick for swimming.

Specificity of training was demonstrated in a study in which subjects pedaled a bicycle ergometer with only one leg.[18] Of course, the training effect occurred solely in the muscles of the exercised leg and the cardiovascular system responded with a lower heart rate when the trained leg was exercised. The heart rate did not respond in this manner when the untrained leg was exercised. The researcher hypothesized that exercise produced muscular changes in the trained leg that accounted for the lowered heart rate. In another study, two groups of subjects were tested maximally on a treadmill and then in the swimming pool.[19] One of the groups then received 12 weeks of swim training, while the other group was excluded from this activity. Both groups were retested at the end of the 12 weeks. The swim-trained group improved significantly in swimming capacity as indicated by the difference between their pretest and posttest scores and they were also significantly better than the nontrained group on the posttest. However, the swim-trained group did not improve on the treadmill test, indicating that specific adaptations were made to the training program. In yet another study, identical twin girls were subjected to a battery of maximal tests.[20] Both of the girls were outstanding swimmers but one of them had retired from competition three years prior to testing. The other twin continued training and competing. The retired twin remained physically active by participating in sports other than swimming. The swimming tests showed that the competitive swimmer achieved a much higher $VO_{2\ max}$ than her retired sister but treadmill values were identical for the two.

Specificity of training is also discernible at the biochemical and histochemical levels as the types of muscle fiber and their associated enzymes respond selectively to certain modes of training.[5] Slow-twitch muscle fibers and the enzymes involved in aerobic metabolism respond to endurance training, while fast-twitch muscle fibers and the enzymes involved in anaerobic metabolism are responsive to anaerobic training.

The application of specificity is extremely important for competitive athletes who are attempting to maximize the returns from their investment in training. Therefore, swimmers must train by swimming, distance runners must run, and cyclists must cycle in order to train the body in the specific manner in which it is to perform. This locks athletes into set training programs, but people who exercise for health reasons are not under such constraints. They can vary the activities in their program, averting the boredom and tedium of doing the same thing week after week.

Exercise heart rate is the key for the person who exercises for health. Any activity that elevates the heart rate sufficiently enough, often enough, and long enough will train the cardiovascular system. This allows participants the opportunity to inject elements of fun and diversity into the program. Cycling, jogging, swimming, racquetball, cross-country skiing, rope jumping, weight training, and so on, may be employed in the development of fitness and in any combination or order dictated by the participant. You may take into account weather conditions, availability of equipment and facilities, and what activity you feel like pursuing on any given day. You also might choose to combine two or more activities in the same exercise session.

Selecting and participating in more than one activity has come to be known as **cross-training.** It is possible that this form of training may reduce injuries but this has yet to be established. Even if it turns out that the injury rate does not decrease, cross-training injects some very important ingredients into the fitness program—fun, variety, and enjoyment.

Many people enjoy one activity more than others, while other people exclusively pursue one activity. Exercising for health does not preclude these approaches for those who desire it. More options are available to people who exercise for health purposes than for competitive athletes. The important point is to select an activity or activities that give both pleasure and the desired training effect.

Cooling Down from Exercise

Cooling down from exercise is as important as warming up. Just as the body was allowed to speed up gradually, it must also be allowed to slow down gradually. The body is not analogous to an auto engine that can be turned on and off with the twist of a key. Cool-down should last about 8 to 10 minutes. The first phase of cooling down should consist of walking or some other light activity to prevent blood from pooling in the active muscles. Five minutes of continuous light activity causes rhythmical muscle contractions that prevent the pooling of blood and helps to move blood back to the heart for redistribution to the vital organs. This boost to circulation after exercise is an essential component of the cool-down period. Inactivity during this time forces the heart to compensate for the reduced volume of blood returning to it by maintaining a high pumping rate. The exerciser runs the risk of dizziness, fainting, and perhaps more serious consequences associated with diminished blood flow. Light activity also speeds up the removal of **lactic acid** which has accumulated in the muscles.

**Deaths During
Cool Down**

A number of deaths during the cool down period after vigorous exercise have been documented. Many of these postexercise deaths have been attributed to hypokalemia (potassium depletion). People engaged in vigorous exercise lose potassium in both perspiration and urine. In one study, the lowest potassium levels recorded were at three minutes postexercise and this coincided with the time of death of several marathoners. Potassium depletion was implicated in the development of intractable rhythm disturbance. This strongly suggests that vigorous exercise should be accompanied by an increase in the consumption of potassium rich foods.

Bassler, T.J., "Deaths During the Cool Down Period," *American Medical Joggers Assoc. Newsletter*, March, 1984, p. 7.

The second phase of cool-down should focus upon the same stretching exercises that were used during the warm-up period. You will probably note that stretching is tolerated more comfortably after exercise due to the increase in muscle temperature. Stretching at this time helps prevent muscle soreness.

Backward locomotion is a new technique employed by some exercisers to supplement their stretching program. Backward walking (retro walking) and backward jogging (retro running) reduce the range of motion at the hip joint and increase it at the knee joint.[21] In backward locomotion, the maximum knee extension occurs late in the support phase (when each leg in turn supports most of the body weight). At this point there is substantial stretch of the hamstring muscle group (muscles located in the back of the thighs). The hamstrings tighten up when one walks, jogs, sits, and so on, therefore, it is important to engage in activities that keep them flexible.

Retro walking is currently being applied in the rehabilitation of hip and hamstring injuries, and in postsurgical knee therapy.[22] If you choose to experiment with retro walking or running, follow these guidelines.

1. Choose a flat smooth surface such as that found on running tracks or, if available, a treadmill.
2. Begin slowly in order to avert muscle soreness particularly of the calf muscle.
3. Walk or run backwards for brief periods—25 to 50 yards at a time and increase the distance slowly.
4. When looking over your shoulder, alternate sides to prevent cramping of the neck.
5. Retro activity should be a supplement to your usual stretching exercises.

POINTS TO PONDER

1. *Trace the production of ATP both anaerobically and aerobically. Which results in the development of the most ATP?*
2. *Discuss active versus passive warm-up, general versus specific warm-up, and the effectiveness of warm-up in enhancing performance and decreasing the incidence of injury.*
3. *What are some unsafe exercises and why are they unsafe?*
4. *Discuss the ACSM guidelines for frequency, duration, and intensity of exercise.*

5. *Compute a training heart rate for a 28-year-old man with a resting heart rate of 76 beats per minute by the Karvonen formula. Use 65 percent as the intensity level.*

Exercise During Pregnancy

Considerable controversy exists regarding the benefits and possible harmful effects of exercise to expectant mothers and their fetuses. Experts are lined-up on both sides of the issue because no difinitive study has occurred to provide substantive guidelines for maternal exercise during pregnancy. In lieu of such a study, the American College of Obstetricians and Gynecologists (ACOG) has developed guidelines for exercise during pregnancy. These are presented in Table 6.3. The ACOG guidelines have been criticized because they were written primarily by one physician, Raul Artal, based upon his research with little input from other experts. The major focus of criticism of the guidelines is that they are broad generalizations which are substantially without support from research. Mona Shangold, a physician who is director of the Sports Gynecology Center at Georgetown University is one of the major critics of the ACOG guidelines. Her concern centers upon the formulation of written guidelines which are not based upon research data.

The concerns for women who exercise during pregnancy are theoretical and include the following:

1. reduction of blood flow to the uterus
2. over heating of the fetus
3. reduction in maternal and fetal blood sugar levels
4. risk of musculoskeletal injury to the prospective mother.

Conversely, the advantages associated with maternal exercise include:

1. development and maintenance of physical fitness
2. avoidance of excess weight gain
3. reduction in the usual symptoms of pregnancy
4. less likelihood of complications during labor and delivery
5. faster recovery after giving birth[23]

While reduced blood flow to the uterus, elevated temperature during exercise, and lowered blood sugar levels in mother and fetus are genuine concerns, there are no hard data indicating that these have been harmful to the fetus or the mother. An additional source of concern is associated with pregnant women engaging in exercise while lying on their backs. The ACOG guidelines recommend that women refrain from this practice because the weight of the fetus in this position squeezes the aorta and causes a reduction in blood supply and therefore oxygen to the uterus. However, some gynecologists have noted that most pregnant women can tolerate lying on their backs unless they are at high risk for complications.

If all of this sounds confusing and contradictory, that's because it is. To this point, we have been examining the effects of aerobic exercise upon maternal and fetal well-being. Another issue involves the efficacy of weight training for

TABLE 6.3 American College of Obstetricians and Gynecologists Guidelines for Exercise During Pregnancy and Postpartum

Guidelines

1. Regular exercise (at least three times per week) is preferable to intermittent activity. Competitive activities should be discouraged.

2. Vigorous exercise should not be performed in hot, humid weather or during a period of febrile illness.

3. Ballistic movements (jerky, bouncy motions) should be avoided. Exercise should be done on a wooden floor or a tightly carpeted surface to reduce shock and provide a sure footing.

4. Deep flexion or extension of joints should be avoided because of connective tissue laxity. Activities that require jumping, jarring motions, or rapid changes in direction should be avoided because of joint instability.

5. Vigorous exercise should be preceded by a five-minute period of muscle warm-up. This can be accomplished by slow walking or stationary cycling with low resistance.

6. Vigorous exercise should be followed by a period of gradually declining activity that includes gentle stationary stretching. Because connective tissue laxity increases the risk of joint injury, stretches should not be taken to the point of maximum resistance.

7. Heart rate should be measured at times of peak activity. Target heart rates and limits established in consultation with the physician should not be exceeded.

8. Care should be taken to gradually rise from the floor to avoid orthostatic hypotension. Some form of activity involving the legs should be continued for a brief period.

9. Liquids should be taken liberally before and after exercise to prevent dehydration. If necessary, activity should be interrupted to replenish fluids.

10. Women who have led sedentary life-styles should begin with physical activity of very low intensity and advance activity levels very gradually.

11. Activity should be stopped and the physician consulted if any unusual symptoms appear.

Pregnancy only

1. Maternal heart rate should not exceed 140 beats min.$^{-1}$

2. Strenuous activities should not exceed 15 minutes in duration.

3. No exercise should be performed in the supine position after the fourth month of gestation is completed.

4. Exercises that employ the Valsalva maneuver should be avoided.

5. Calorie intake should be adequate to meet not only the extra energy needs of pregnancy, but also of the exercise performed.

6. Maternal core temperature should not exceed 38°C.

Reprinted with permission from the American College of Obstetricians and Gynecologists: Exercise During Pregnancy and the Postnatal Period (ACOG Home Exercise Programs) Washington, DC, ACOG, 1985 pregnant women. The same diversion of opinion exists.[24] Opponents state that the increased laxity (slackness) of ligaments and joints during pregnancy increases the probability of injury to these tissues. Weight training may be too stressful during this time particularly for those who have not participated in this activity prior to pregnancy. Proponents of weight training point out that it strengthens muscles, tendons, and ligaments thereby assisting pregnant women, to tolerate their altered center of gravity and increasing body weight more easily. Low-back pain is rampant during pregnancy. Strengthening the back muscles produces less discomfort.

The type of weight training suggested for pregnant women consists of lifting light to moderate weights three days per week. Weight machines and free weights are acceptable. Proponents also suggest that women who have never trained with weights may begin during pregnancy provided they receive instruction from someone who is qualified, for example, one who is a certified exercise specialist by the American College of Sports Medicine.[24]

Shangold has developed her own guidelines for exercise during pregnancy, some of which are at odds with the ACOG guidelines.[25] These include

1. Continue the same sport or activity at the same level of perceived exertion. Since exercise becomes more difficult as pregnancy progresses, the required level of perceived exertion will occur sooner at a lower level of intensity.
2. Body temperature should not exceed 101 degrees.
3. Maximal heart rate should be between, but not exceed 140 to 160 beats/min.
4. Total weight gain should be 20 to 30 pounds.
5. Adequate consumption of calories, vitamins, iron, and calcium is important.
6. Drink plenty of fluids.
7. Do not exercise at altitude or in high temperatures.
8. Consult a physician immediately if pain, bleeding, rupture of the membranes, or lack of fetal movement occur.

Two recent studies have shown that the physical fitness levels of pregnant women improved throughout their pregnancy.[26,27] In one study,[26] exercise for pregnant subjects was based upon the American College of Sports Medicine guidelines for exercise for healthy adults, that is, 3 to 5 times per week for 15 to 60 minutes at 65 to 90 percent of maximum heart rate. The exercising group participated in swimming, cycling, hiking, jogging, cross-country skiing, and aerobic dancing. A significant training effect occurred throughout the program. Additionally, there were no significant differences between the exercising and nonexercising groups in type of delivery, length of pregnancy, infant birth weight, and Apgar score. The Apgar score represents an evaluation of the physical status of a newborn infant by assigning numerical values (0–2) to each of five dimensions: heart rate, respiratory effort, muscle tone, response to stimulation, and skin color. The second study,[27] involved 845 pregnant subjects. The researchers concluded that exercise during pregnancy was beneficial rather than harmful. The women were divided into four groups based on the amount of exercise that they did during pregnancy. The groups were as follows: (1) a control group of

393 women who had few or no exercise sessions, (2) a low-exercise group of 82 women who participated in 11 to 20 exercise sessions, (3) a moderate-exercise group of 309 women who participated in 21 to 59 exercise sessions, and (4) a high-exercise group of 61 women who participated in 60 to 99 exercise sessions. Each session consisted of a 5-minute warm-up, 45 minutes of prescribed weight training, and a one to two mile ride on a stationary cycle. The groups were compared on length of hospitalization, incidence of cesarean section, and Apgar scores. The exercising groups, particularly the high-exercise group, fared much better than the controls on these parameters and they also experienced the greatest improvement in self-image, relief of tension, and reduction in the common discomforts of pregnancy such as low back pain.

This author suggests that exercise during pregnancy should be prescribed on an individual basis. Second, the benefits of sensible exercise, based upon individual needs are worth the effort. The evidence does not support the notion that exercise is harmful to the fetus and prospective mother. Third, for those who are ultra-conservative, walking is still an excellent choice for most women.

The Effects of Climate

Human beings are compelled to function in a variety of environmental conditions. People live and work in frigid, temperate, and tropical zones, at sea level and at high altitudes and have adapted and learned to tolerate extremes in temperature. In cold weather body temperature may be maintained by putting on more clothes or by increasing the body's production of heat through physical movement or shivering. In hot environments heat may be lost through sweating, increasing blood flow to the skin, and by wearing as little clothing as the law and culture will allow.

Humans are homeotherms (meaning "same heat") who are capable of maintaining the constant internal temperature necessary for the support of such life-sustaining processes as cellular metabolism, oxygen transport, muscular contraction, and so on. We exist within a relatively narrow band of internal temperature, ranging from 97 to 99 degrees, but our temperature (may and often) does rise to 104 degrees during exercise. Temperatures that rise above 106 degrees, if not rapidly reduced, often result in cellular deterioration, permanent brain damage, and death; while temperatures below 93 degrees slow metabolism to the extent that unconsciousness and cardiac arrhythmias (disturbances of normal heart rhythm that can be fatal) are likely.

Since many activities occur in the outdoors, participants are confronted with varying weather conditions. Their safety and comfort depend upon their knowledge of how the body reacts to vigorous exercise in different climate conditions.

Prepubescent children are more susceptible to heat stress than adults. Children who exercise continuously for 30 to 40 minutes become hyperthermic (overheated) much faster than adults exercising at the same rate in the same environmental conditions.[28,29] This is of interest because prepubescent children are participating in road races and triathlons where they are exposed to the possibility of **hyperthermia**. Children are at risk for a number of reasons. First, their sweat glands produce 40 percent as much sweat as adult sweat glands. The evaporation of sweat is the primary mechanizm for cooling the body during

Maximal aerobic power can be increased with training. However the degree of trainability in prepubescents seems somewhat lower than that of more mature age-groups.
Oded Bar-Or

exercise. The low sweat production of prepubescent children renders them more vulnerable to heat stress. Second, children absorb heat from the environment faster than adults through the mechanisms of convection, radiation, and conduction. Third, children produce more metabolic heat during exercise probably because their movements are not as refined or efficient as those of adults. Fourth, children acclimate more slowly than adults to hot weather.

Mechanisms of Heat Loss

Heat is generated in the body, at rest and during exercise, as a by-product of all of its biochemical reactions. Metabolism is the collective sum of these reactions. Exercise stimulates the metabolism and increases the amount of heat produced. Heat developed during exercise is positively related to its intensity and duration.

The efficiency of the body's machinery in the production of energy is considerably less than 100 percent; in fact, it varies from 10 to 30 percent depending upon the type of activity being performed. The majority of the energy produced to support physical activity is lost in the form of heat. This creates a substantial heat load in the body that must be dissipated for the safety of the participant. During exercise, the body's adaptive mechanisms, which are centered upon shunting blood to the skin, are mobilized for this purpose. The processes of heat removal involve conduction, radiation, convection, and the evaporation of sweat.

Conduction is the transfer of heat from the body to an object by means of physical contact between the two. Sitting in a chair or pressing one's back against a wall will transfer heat from the body to either object. Conduction contributes little to heat loss during most types of physical activity, but swimming is a notable exception.

Radiation involves the transference of heat from the body to the atmosphere by electromagnetic waves, providing the environmental temperature is below a skin temperature of 92 to 93 degrees. Heat travels on a temperature gradient from a warmer to a cooler object so the greater the difference between skin and environmental temperatures the greater the heat loss through radiation. Radiation occurs in the reverse direction when the environmental temperature is above skin temperature and the participant absorbs heat from the environment.

Convection involves the transference of heat from the body to a moving gas or liquid. Heat loss through convection occurs more rapidly and efficiently when the wind is blowing. Heat that is transmitted to the surrounding air is blown away, allowing for the additional transfer of heat to the newer surrounding air. Heat loss by convective processes occurs even more rapidly in the water.

Cooling results from the heat exchange that occurs when sweat evaporates—each liter of evaporated sweat removes 580 kcals of energy from your skin.
Bryant Stamford

The major means of ridding the body of the heat generated by exercise is through the evaporation of sweat. The loss of heat in **evaporation** occurs when the water in sweat is converted into gas. This mechanism is effective even in high temperatures provided the relative humidity is low. If both the temperature and humidity are high it is difficult to lose heat by any of these processes. Under these circumstances it is best to adjust the intensity and duration of exercise or to move the program indoors where the temperature and humidity can be controlled.

Exercise in Hot Weather

Hot, humid days present by far the greatest climatic challenge to the enthusiast who exercises outdoors. Humid air, which is very saturated with moisture, cannot absorb much more so sweat produced during exercise beads up and rolls off the body providing very little cooling effect. More blood than usual is diverted from the muscles to the skin in an effort to carry the heat accumulating in the deeper recesses of the body to its outer surface. The net result is that the exercising muscles are deprived of a full complement of blood and cannot work as long or as hard at a given task.

The high sweat rates which accompany vigorous exercise during hot and humid conditions promote the loss of a sizeable quantity of the body's fluid, some of which comes from the bloodstream. The blood becomes more viscous (sticky), lessening its ability to deliver oxygen to the active muscles. Fluid lost from the body is accompanied by the loss of the **electrolytes** sodium and potassium. If the participant continues to exercise strenuously, body temperature will rise and may exceed the capacity of the temperature regulating mechanisms to remove heat. **Heat exhaustion** or **heat stroke** occurs with the breakdown of the body's temperature regulating mechanisms. Both conditions require immediate first aid, but heat stroke is a medical emergency that poses an imminent threat to life. It is the most severe of the heat-induced illnesses. The symptoms include a high temperature (106° F or higher), generally the absence of sweating, and dry skin. Delirium, convulsions, and loss of consciousness often occur. The early warning signs include chills, nausea, headache, general weakness, and dry skin. The victim should be rushed to the nearest hospital immediately because death will probably occur without appropriate early treatment. Heat exhaustion, a serious condition but not an imminent threat to life, is characterized by dizziness, fainting, rapid pulse, and cool skin. The victim should be moved to a shady area or indoors, placed in a reclining position, and given cool fluids to drink.

Successful performance in a hot environment is dependent upon the temperature, humidity, air movement, the intensity and duration of exercise, the individual's level of fitness, previous exposure to heat (acclimatization) and whether the workout occurs in direct sunlight. Caution should be exercised when the temperature exceeds 83° F and the humidity rises above 60 percent. Sharkey has developed the following standards for work or exercise in hot weather:

1. Utilize discretion when the temperature is above 80° F
2. Avoid strenuous activity when the temperature is above 85° F
3. Cease physical activity when the temperature climbs above 88° F unless the individual is trained and heat-acclimated.[30]

Heat stress is precipitated by imprudent exercise in a hot and humid environment, but many incidents occur when the temperature is mild and the humidity is high. The latter weather conditions are deceptive and the possibility of the occurrence of heat illness at these times must be recognized. Heat illness may be prevented by adhering to a few simple guidelines. **Dehydration** (loss of water) can be avoided by liberally drinking water (or a beverge which is low in sugar and salt) 30 to 40 minutes prior to the workout, by drinking 8 ounces every 15 to 20 minutes during the workout, and by continuing to drink after the workout.

We do not voluntarily drink all that is needed to replace the fluid lost during exercise, so a good rule is to satisfy thirst and then drink some more. Research has shown that our thirst mechanism is not well attuned to our tissue needs and cannot be relied upon as a gauge for fluid replacement. The fluid we drink, preferably water, should be as cold as can be tolerated because it will absorb some of the body's heat as it is warmed to body temperature. There is no physiological data contradicting the use of cold water for the dual purposes of replacing fluid and lowering body temperature. A few people respond to cold water after exercise with nausea and headache. Should this occur it is advisable to drink slowly and/or drink tepid water.

Do not wear rubberized or plastic clothing while exercising because these garments promote sweating but retard its evaporation and seriously impede the cooling process. A supersaturated microenvironment is created between the skin and these garments which can lead very quickly to dehydration and heat illness.

Salt (sodium chloride) is lost in substantial quantities during the initial stages of the physical fitness program but as training continues, the body learns to conserve salt during exercise. This tends to increase its concentration in the body in relation to the fluid that remains while sweating is in progress. Taking salt during or after exercise is neither helpful nor desirable as it will interfere with the absorption of water from the gastrointestinal tract. The critical factor continues to be the replacement of water rather than salt.

The available evidence shows conclusively that Americans eat too much salt. It is used as an additive in most processed foods so a deliberate attempt to ingest more seems unnecessary. Salt tablets are unacceptable as a method of salt replacement for the following reasons: They are stomach irritants which may produce nausea and vomiting, they may perforate the stomach lining, they sometimes pass through the body undissolved, and they attract fluid to the gut from other tissues where it is needed and thereby enhance dehydration.

Potassium is also lost in sweat. Potassium and sodium are necessary for the contraction of muscles including the heart muscle. Studies have shown that exercise participants may become deficient in this electrolyte if they do not make an effort to eat potassium-rich foods daily. A severe deficiency can have serious consequences. Citrus juices, potatoes, dates, bananas, and nuts are excellent sources of potassium.

Modifications in the exercise program should be considered during hot weather. Participants should schedule their workout during the cooler times of the day. Shady locations where water may be obtained should be used. Clothing should be light, loose, and porous in order to facilitate the evaporation of sweat. It is wise to slow the pace and/or shorten the distance on particularly oppressive days. Be particularly alert for rapid weight loss because this may indicate an excessive loss of fluid. If you do not enjoy exercising in hot weather and cannot make the suggested schedule adjustments, try to move the program indoors into air conditioned comfort. The health benefits of exercise can be achieved there just as well. The important point is to continue to exercise to maintain what you have gained.

Exercise in Cold Weather

Problems related to exercise in cold weather include frostbite, **hypothermia** (abnormally low body temperature), and occasionally hyperthermia (abnormally high body temperature). The most frequently occurring cold-weather injury to young healthy adults is frostbite, which can lead to permanent circulatory damage and the possible loss of the frostbitten part caused by gangrene. This can be prevented by adequately protecting susceptible areas such as fingers, toes, nose, ears, and facial skin. Gloves, preferably mittens, should be worn to protect the hands and fingers. A stocking or toboggan type hat should be worn because it can be pulled down to protect the ears and to prevent significant heat loss through the bare head by radiation due to the poor vasoconstriction responses (clamping down of blood vessels) in the scalp. In very cold environments, participants may use surgical masks, ski masks, and scarves to keep facial skin warm and to moisten and warm inhaled air. All exposed flesh is vulnerable to frostbite when the temperature is very low and the windchill factor is high. (See Table 6.4.)

Hypothermia occurs when body heat is lost faster than it can be produced. Exposure to cold temperatures, pain, and wind chill combine with fatigue to rob the body of heat. The body reacts with vasoconstriction of peripheral blood vessels as it attempts to conserve heat for the vital internal organs. Shivering, an involuntary contraction of the muscles, increases body heat. The shivering muscles produce no work so most of the expended energy appears as heat.

TABLE 6.4 Wind Chill Index

Wind Speed in (MPH)	Actual Thermometer Reading (°F)											
	50	40	30	20	10	0	-10	-20	-30	-40	-50	-60
	Equivalent Temperature (F)											
Calm	50	40	30	20	10	0	-10	-20	-30	-40	-50	-60
5	48	37	27	16	6	-5	-15	-26	-36	-47	-57	-68
10	40	28	16	4	-9	-21	-33	-46	-58	-70	-83	-95
15	36	22	9	-5	-18	-36	-45	-58	-72	-85	-99	-112
20	32	18	4	-10	-25	-39	-53	-67	-82	-96	-110	-124
25	30	16	0	-15	-29	-44	-59	-74	-88	-104	-118	-133
30	28	13	-2	-18	-33	-48	-63	-79	-94	-109	-125	-140
35	27	11	-4	-20	-35	-49	-67	-82	-98	-113	-129	-145
40[1]	26	10	-6	-21	-37	-53	-69	-85	-100	-116	-132	-148

Little Danger (for properly clothed person)	**Increasing Danger—** Cover up fully (hands, ears, face, head, etc.)	**Great danger—** Exercise Indoors

[1]Wind speeds greater than 40 MPH have little additional effect.

Adapted from Sharkey, B.J. *Physiology of Fitness*, Champaign, Ill: Human Kinetics Publishers, 1979, p. 226.

Surprisingly, hyperthermia may occur when one exercises in cold weather. Such cases occur when too much clothing is worn. This problem can be avoided by wearing several layers of light clothing that will trap warm insulating air between the layers. Dressing in this manner allows the participant to peel off a layer or two as the metabolic heat produced by exercise increases. The amount and type of clothing worn should allow for the evaporation of sweat and help achieve a balance between the amount of heat produced and the amount of heat lost. Clothing that becomes saturated with sweat is rapidly cooled and can quickly chill a participant who is working or exercising in cold weather.

Very often people may experience a hacking cough for a minute or two following exercise in cold weather. This is a normal response and should not cause alarm. Very cold dry air cannot be fully moistened when it is inhaled rapidly and in large volumes during exercise, so the lining of the throat dries out. When exercise is discontinued, the respiratory rate slows and the volume of incoming air decreases, allowing the body to fully moisturize it. The lining is remoistened and coughing stops.

Some people develop chest pain while exercising in cold weather and fear that the blood vessels in the chest are being constricted or that the lungs are becoming frostbitten. But inhaled air is adequately warmed before it reaches the lungs. Data on armed forces personnel who were marched for several hours in subzero temperatures showed no ill effects to lung tissue. There is no evidence to support the notion that lung tissue is subject to frostbite in cold weather. Those who experience chest pain upon exertion in the cold should consult a physician to determine if an organic or physiological problem exists. If a medical problem is identified, the physician's recommendations regarding exercise should be followed. If a problem is not identified but chest pain in cold weather persists, the workout should be moved indoors. This simple act may be all that is necessary to continue the program during the winter months.

Exercise at Altitude

The major problem associated with the performance of physical activities at altitude is the reduced availability of oxygen at the cellular level. The percentage of oxygen at altitude is the same as it is at sea level (20.93%). The total pressure of atmospheric air reduces as altitude increases and so too, does the pressure of oxygen (commonly referred to as the partial pressure of oxygen). Atmospheric pressure at sea level is 760 mmHg and the partial pressure of oxygen is 159 mmHg (760 mmHg × .2093 = 159 mmHg). At 8200 feet of elevation the atmospheric pressure drops to 560 mmHg and the partial pressure of oxygen drops to 117 mmHg (560 mmHg × .2093 = 117 mmHg). Refer to Table 6.5 for the effect of altitude on the barometric pressure of the atmosphere and the corresponding partial pressure of oxygen.

Altitude produces physiological responses which reduce physical work capacity. For example, **hemoglobin** is 97 percent saturated with oxygen at sea level but this value drops to 92 percent at 8000 feet. This change is responsible for some of the decline in work capacity at altitude. The primary mechanism which seems to be responsible for the decline in performance relates to the decrease in the partial pressure of oxygen in arterial blood. At sea level, the arterial partial pressure of oxygen is 94 mmHg but this drops to 60 mmHg at 8000 feet. The partial pressure of oxygen in the tissues is approximately

TABLE 6.5 Barometric Pressure of the Atmosphere and Partial Pressure of Oxygen at Various Altitudes

Altitude		Atmospheric Pressure (mmHg)	Partial Pressure O_2 (mmHg)
Meters	*Feet*		
0	0	760	159
500	1,640	716	150
1,000	3,280	674	141
1,500	4,920	634	133
2,000	6,560	596	125
2,500	8,200	560	117
3,000	9,840	526	110
4,000	13,120	462	97
5,000	16,400	405	85
6,000	19,690	354	74
7,000	22,970	308	64
8,000	26,250	267	56
9,000	29,530	230	48
10,000	32,800	198	41
19,215	63,000	47	10

20 mmHg. The difference between the oxygen pressure in arterial blood and the oxygen pressure in the tissues is the pressure gradient. The pressure gradient produces the force which drives oxygen from the arteries to the tissues. The higher the gradient the more powerful the drive. At sea level, the pressure gradient is 74 mmHg (94 mmHg − 20 mmHg = 74 mmHg) but at 8000 feet the gradient drops to 40 mmHg (60 mmHg − 20 mmHg = 40 mmHg). This represents a 46 percent reduction in the driving force needed to deliver oxygen to the tissues resulting in a decrement in aerobic performance.

Acclimation to altitude begins within the first few days of exposure but it takes approximately three weeks to make a good adjustment[1] and full acclimation may take several months. The process of acclimation involves: (1) an increase in the number of red blood cells and an increase in hemoglobin which binds oxygen for transport in the circulatory system, (2) an increase in the number of capillaries in the lungs and skeletal muscles, and (3) increases in tissue myoglobin (the oxygen transporting protein of muscle). All of these changes enhance oxygen intake and carrying capacity so that the transport systems may facilitate the supply of oxygen to the muscles. While these adjustments ameliorate the effects of altitude, they never fully compensate for it. Endurance performance at altitude is never as good as that at sea level regardless of the degree of acclimation that has been attained. The adjustments to altitude reverse completely when one returns to sea level for a couple of weeks.

There are practical implications associated with the effects of altitude upon the human body. People with cardiovascular and/or respiratory disease who live at sea level need to understand the impact of altitude upon these conditions. People suffering from these conditions should seek medical advice prior to going to that mountain retreat, or on a skiing weekend. Even healthy young people

Prolonged exposure to extremely high altitudes (19,685 feet) leads to progressive deterioration that can eventually cause death unless the person is moved to a lower altitude.
George Brooks

need to reduce the intensity of exercise at altitude. Vacationers who go to the mountains must realize that they will be unable to perform as they did at sea level. Those whose cardiovascular and respiratory systems are compromised at sea level must be especially careful at altitude.

SELF-ASSESSMENT
The Physical Activity Questionnaire

Your answers to the following questions should help to: (1) quantify the amount of exercise that you are doing currently, (2) point out the types of exercise in which you are interested, (3) underline your reasons for participation, and (4) clarify your attitude regarding exercise.

1. Do you exercise regularly:
   a. 3 to 5 times per week? _____
   b. 30 minutes or more per session? _____
   c. at 65% of Max H.R. or greater? _____

2. Do you participate regularly in aerobic exercise (walking, jogging, cycling, swimming, and so on)? _____

3. Do you participate regularly in lifetime sports (racquetball, handball, tennis, badminton, and so on)? _____

4. Do you participate primarily in one activity or a combination of activities? _____

5. Do you participate regularly (at least 2 times per week) in resistance exercises (weight training, calisthenics, and so on)? _____

6. Do you compete in your event(s) or do you exercise for reasons other than competition? _____

7. Is competition, including competing with yourself, an important element of your exercise program? _____

8. Do you prefer to exercise with other people or by yourself? _____

9. Rank the following from the most important to the least important as a motive for you to exercise with 1 being the most important and 5 being the least important. If your most important reason is not listed below, add it to the bottom of the list and rank it 1.
   a. health _____
   b. physical appearance _____
   c. stress reduction _____
   d. fun and enjoyment _____
   e. competition _____
   f. other _____

10. Which of the following components is most important and which is least important as an outcome of your exercise program?
    a. muscular development _____
    b. cardiorespiratory endurance _____
    c. flexibility _____

11. Is becoming fit and maintaining physical fitness important to you? _____ If so, reflect on the reason.

12. Do you feel that one can achieve high-level wellness without being physically fit? _____ Think about why you feel the way you do.

POINTS TO PONDER

1. Why are prepubescent children at greater risk than adults when exercising in hot weather?
2. What are the potential harmful effects of exercise to pregnant women and their fetuses?
3. What are the benefits of exercise to pregnant women?
4. What are the mechanisms of heat loss? Define each of them.
5. What is the major mechanism through which we lose heat generated during exercise?
6. What is a heat stroke and what are its symptoms? How should it be treated?

7. *Should the fluid that exercisers drink during hot weather contain salt? Would you recommend salt tablets? Why or why not?*
8. *How should one dress for cold weather exercise?*
9. *Why does aerobic performance suffer at altitude?*
10. *What is the partial pressure of oxygen at a barometric pressure of 450 mmHg?*

Chapter Highlights

Carbohydrate and fat are the two major food sources which the body uses to manufacture ATP. Carbohydrate is the primary source of fuel when exercise is of high intensity; a mixture of carbohydrate and fat provide the energy in exercise of moderate intensity; and fat is the primary source of fuel during low intensity exercise.

The ACSM has established guidelines regarding medical clearance for exercise as well as guidelines for intensity, frequency, and duration of exercise. These include an intensity of 65 to 90 percent of the maximal heart rate, a frequency of 3 to 5 times per week, and a duration of 15 to 60 minutes. Each bout of exercise should be preceded by a warm up and followed by a cool down.

Two methods were presented for determining the training heart rate. These procedures, along with perceived exertion, may be utilized to monitor the intensity of exercise. Heart rates during exercise may be calculated by palpating the pulse at the wrist or neck. Care must be taken to locate the pulse rapidly and to count accurately. Caution must be used when palpating the pulse at the carotid arteries. Light finger pressure should be used at this site in order to inhibit the stimulation of the barareceptors.

Backward locomation is currently being employed by some exercisers to stretch-out the hamstrings after exercise. Retro movement has the support of some authorities who consider this technique to be a safe and effective procedure for stretching muscles and a effective treatment in the rehabilitation of some types of injuries.

The effects of exercise during pregnancy on maternal and fetal health were examined. The guidelines for maternal exercise written by the American College of Obstetricians and Gynecologists were presented. The major criticism of these guidelines is that they are broad generalizations which do not have adequate support form research.

Exercise performance is influenced by hot and cold weather. Heat presents the greater problem of the two and of the heat-related illnesses, heat stroke is a serious medical emergency. Frostbite is the most common injury associated with exercise in cold weather. Altitude presents some unique problems for exercisers all of which in some way center around the lowered partial pressure of oxygen. Acclimation to altitude improves aerobic performance.

References

1. B. J. Sharky, *Physiology of Fitness,* Champaign, IL: Human Kinetics Publishers, Inc., 1984.
2. American College of Sports Medicine, *Guidelines for Exercise Testing and Prescription,* Philadelphia: Lea and Febiger, 1986.
3. B. Stamford, "Warming Up" *The Physician and Sportsmedicine,* 15, (1987): 168.
4. R. J. Barnard et al., "Cardiovascular Responses to Sudden Strenuous Exercise—Heart Rate, Blood Pressure, and ECG," *Journal of Applied Physiology,* 34, (1973): 833.
5. J. H. Wilmore and D. L. Costill, *Training For Sport and Activity,* Dubuque, Iowa: Wm. C. Brown Publishers, 1988.
6. J. A. Davis et al. "A Comparison of Heart Rate Methods for Predicting Endurance Training Intensity," *Medicine in Science and Sports,* 7, (1975): 295.
7. M. L. Pollock et al. *Exercise In Health and Disease,* Philadelphia: W.B. Saunders, Co., 1984.
8. G. A. V. Borg, "Perceived Exertion: A Note on History and Methods," *Medicine and Science in Sports,* 5, (1973): 90.
9. W. P. Morgan and G. A. V. Borg, "Perception of Effort and the Prescription of Physical Activity," In *Mental Health and Emotional Aspects of Sport,* T. Craig (ed.), Chicago: American Medical Association, 1976.
10. H. B. Falls et al., *Essentials of Fitness,* Philadelphia: Saunders College, 1980.
11. "American College of Sports Medicine Position Statement on the Recommended Quantity and Quality of Exercise for Developing and Maintaining Fitness In Healthy Adults," *Medicine and Science in Sports,* 10, (1978): 3.
12. S. J. Jacobs and B. L. Bernson, "Injuries to Runners: A Study of Entrants to a 10,000 Meter Race," *American Journal of Sports Medicine,* 14, (1986): 151.
13. Y. Mutoh et al., "Aerobic Dance Injuries Among Instructors and Students," *The Physician and Sportsmedicine,* 16, (1988): 80.
14. R. J. Moffatt et al., "Placement of Tri-Weekly Training Sessions: Importance Regarding Enhancement of Aerobic Capacity," *Research Quarterly,* 48, (1977): 583.
15. J. P. Koplan et al., "An Epidemiological Study of the Benefits and Risks of Running," *Journal of the American Medical Association,* 248, (1982): 3118.
16. M. L. Pollock et al., "Effects of Frequency and Duration of Training and Attrition and Incidence of Injury," *Medicine and Science in Sports,* 9, (1977): 31.
17. S. N. Blair, "Risk Factors and Running Injuries," *Medicine and Science in Sports and Exercise,* 17, (1985): XII.
18. B. Saltin, "The Interplay Between Peripheral and Central Factors In the Adaptive Response to Exercise and Training," in *The Marathon* P. Milvy (ed.), N.Y.: New York Academy of Sciences, 1977.
19. J. R. Magalel et al., "Specificity of Swim-Training On Maximum Oxygen Uptake," *Journal of Applied Physiology,* 38, (1975): 151.
20. I. Homer and P. O. Astrand, "Swimming Training and Maximal Oxygen Uptake," *Journal of Applied Physiology,* 33, (1972): 510.
21. B. T. Bates and S. T. McCaw, "A Comparison Between Forward and Backward Walking," *Proceedings of the North American Congress On Biomechanics:* Human Locomotion IV, 2, (1986): 307.
22. C. Morton, "Running Backward May Help Athletes Move Forward," *The Physician and Sportsmedicine,* 14, (1986): 149.
23. M. M. Gauthier, "Guidelines for Exercise During Pregnancy: Too Little or Too Much?," *The Physician and Sportsmedicine,* 14, (1986): 162.
24. J. A. Work, "Is Weight Training Safe During Pregnancy?" *The Physician and Sportsmedicine,* 17, (1989): 256.
25. M. Shangold and G. Mirkin, *The Complete Sports Medicine Book for Women,* New York: Simon and Schuster, 1985.
26. P. J. Kulpa et al., "Aerobic Exercise in Pregnancy," *American Journal of Obstetrics and Gynecology,* 156, (1987): 1395.
27. D. C. Hall and D. A. Kaufmann, "Effects of Aerobic and Strength Conditioning on Pregnancy Outcomes," *American Journal of Obstetrics and Gynecology,* 157, (1987): 1199.
28. O. Bar-Or et al., "Voluntary Hypohydration in 10–12-Year-Old Boys," *Journal of Applied Physiology,* 48, (1980): 104.
29. O. Bar-Or, "Climate and the Exercising Child—A review," *International Journal of Sports Medicine,* 1, (1980): 53.

7

Developing the
Cardiorespiratory Component:
The Effects of Exercise

Chapter Outline

Mini Glossary

Aerobic capacity: the maximal ability to take in, deliver, and use oxygen; also referred to as cardiorespiratory endurance or Max VO_2.

Alveoli: tiny air sacs in the lungs that are richly perfused with blood. Gaseous exchange between the lungs and blood occurs at these sites.

Arterial-venous O_2 Difference (a-vO_2 diff): the difference between the oxygen (O_2) content of arterial and mixed venous blood.

Body composition: the amount of lean versus fat tissue in the body.

Cardiac output: the amount of blood pumped by the heart in one minute.

Coronary collateral circulation: the development of auxiliary blood vessels to enhance blood flow to cardiac muscle.

Double product or rate pressure product (RPP): heart rate multiplied by systolic blood pressure; it is an estimate of the oxygen required by the heart during aerobic exercise.

Metabolism: the sum of the chemical reactions and processes that supply the energy used by the body.

Mitochondria: organelles within the cells that utilize oxygen to produce the ATP needed by the muscles.

O_2 debt: the amount of oxygen needed in recovery from exercise, above that normally required during rest.

O_2 deficit: occurs at the beginning of exercise when the body does not supply all of the oxygen needed to support exercise.

Residual volume: The air remaining in the lungs following a maximal expiration.

Stroke volume: the amount of blood pumped by the heart with each beat.

Tidal volume: the amount of air inhaled and exhaled with each breath.

Ventilation: the amount of air inhaled and exhaled per minute.

Vital capacity: the amount of air that can be expired after a maximum inhalation.

Introduction

Exercise produces immediate but temporary physiological and metabolic changes. The acute effects of exercise are those that occur during and after every bout of exercise, regardless of whether or not the individual is trained. Physiology and metabolism return to normal when the bout of exercise is over.

When exercise becomes a habit and is pursued for months or years the physiological and metabolic changes that occur are longer lasting. These adaptations, which are the result of training, are the chronic effects of exercise.

Short-Term Effects of Aerobic Exercise

The short-term effects of exercise, also referred to as the acute adaptations, involve those physiological changes that occur during a single bout of exercise. It is important to recognize these adjustments and to understand that they are temporary.

Heart Rate

The heart's response to dynamic exercise is immediate. The rate of beating rises and continues to do so until a steady state has been achieved. Steady state occurs when the oxygen demand of the activity can be supplied by the body during the activity. If the exercise intensity is such that a steady state cannot be achieved, the heart rate (HR) will continue to increase until it reaches its maximum level. Elevating the heart rate represents the major vehicle for increasing blood flow, and therefore oxygen, to the muscles during moderate to intense exercise.

Stroke Volume

Stroke volume (SV) refers to the amount of blood that the heart can eject in one beat. The size of the stroke volume is dependent upon the amount of blood returning to the heart, the interior dimensions of the left ventricle, and the strength of ventricular contraction. Stroke volume rises linearly; that is, it is positively correlated with increases in workload up to 40 to 60 percent of capacity and then levels off.[1] From this point on, further increases in blood flow occur as the result of increases in heart rate.

The average male will have a stroke volume equal to 70 to 100 ml of blood, while well-endowed endurance athletes may reach values of 200 ml or more. The higher stroke volumes of trained people represent one of the major differences between them and the untrained and accounts for their ability to sustain endurance activities at a high level.

Cardiac Output

Cardiac output (Q) represents the amount of blood pumped by the heart in one minute. It is the product of heart rate and stroke volume ($Q = HR \times SV$). The cardiac output increases as the intensity of exercise increases. Initially, it increases because both heart rate and stroke volume increase. Stroke volume levels off when exercise reaches approximately 50 percent of capacity, therefore, further increases in cardiac output are a result of elevations in heart rate.

The average value for cardiac output at rest is approximately 4 to 6 liters of blood per minute with values reaching 20 to 25 liters during maximal exercise. Well-conditioned athletes can achieve as much as 40 liters during very high-intensity work.

Blood Flow

The body has the remarkable capacity to shunt blood to tissues that have the greatest need. For example, blood flow to the working muscles increases during physical activity. This is accomplished because blood flow to other tissues and organs such as the liver, kidneys and digestive system is reduced. In the competition for available blood, the muscles take precedence during physical activity. Blood flow to the digestive system is increased after a meal because this represents the greatest area of need. However, if physical activity occurs immediately after eating, blood will be shunted away from the digestive system to the muscles. Digestion will slow down or stop depending upon the severity of the exercise. This is one of the major reasons why a workout should not begin until at least one hour after a meal.

More blood than usual is shunted to the skin during hot weather to help cool the body. The skin competes with the exercising muscles for the available blood, which results in the muscles receiving slightly less than normal. Less blood means less oxygen and nutrients for exercise and the workout becomes more difficult. This is why exercise in hot weather should be less vigorous and last for a shorter period of time.

Blood Pressure

Systolic pressure, which is measured when the heart contracts and sends blood into the aorta, rises with exercise. It can increase from resting levels of 120 mm Hg to 200 mm Hg and beyond with very intense exercise. This is a normal response as long as the pressure does not get well above 200 mm Hg. The marked rise in systolic blood pressure is caused by the increase in cardiac output that is necessary to maintain blood flow to the heart and brain as well as supplying the needs of the working muscles and skin. The blood vessels in the working muscles dilate to accommodate more blood while the vessels in inactive tissues constrict. On the surface, this adjustment seems to indicate some reduction in blood pressure but the four- to five-fold increase in cardiac output overcomes the blood vessels' ability to distend and increases the systolic pressure.

The diastolic pressure during dynamic exercise changes very little (less than 10 mm Hg) or not at all. An increase of 15 mm Hg or more in the diastolic pressure indicates a greater likelihood of coronary artery disease.[2] However, static or isometric exercises, where forceful contractions are held in a fixed position for several seconds, increase diastolic as well as systolic pressures. The rise is caused by the increased resistance of statically contracting muscles.

Blood Volume

Fluid is removed from all areas of the body in order to produce the perspiration needed to cool the exerciser. Some of this fluid comes from the blood plasma, which reduces blood volume. The hematocrit, which is the volume percent of red blood cells, increases because of the reduction in blood volume. This increases the viscosity of the blood and inhibits the delivery of oxygen. The hematocrit returns to normal as fluids are consumed following the workout.

Respiratory Responses

The average person breathes 12 to 16 times per minute at rest and 40 to 50 times per minute during maximum exertion. **Ventilation (V),** the amount of air inhaled and exhaled per minute, is a product of the frequency of breathing (f) and the volume of air per breath or **tidal volume (TV).** At rest, the lungs typically ventilate 5 to 6 liters of air each minute. For example, 14 breaths per minute at 0.4 liter per breath results in a ventilatory rate of 5.6 liters of air per minute.

$$V = f \times TV$$
$$= 14 \times 0.4 \text{ liters}$$
$$= 5.6 \text{ liters}$$

Ventilation may escalate to 100 liters or more during maximal exertion. Large, well-conditioned athletes may move as much as 200 liters per minute.

The movement of large volumes of air from the lungs during exercise places a burden upon the respiratory muscles. The energy cost of breathing during rest represents 2 percent of the total oxygen consumed, but during vigorous exercise the cost may rise to 10 percent.[3]

Two respiratory phenomena, side-stitch and second wind, remain mysteries in terms of their etiology. A side-stitch is a pain in the side that may be severe enough to stop activity. Constant pressure applied with both hands at the site of the stitch may alleviate the pain and allow continued activity. Breathing deeply while extending the arms overhead may also provide some relief. Currently, there are two possible causes of side-stitch, spasm of the diaphragm caused by diminished blood flow, and trapped gas, decrease in blood flow, or a combination of both in the large intestine.

Second wind is an adaptation in which the perceived effort of exercise appears to become considerably lessened although there is no change in the intensity level. The mechanisms involved are not completely understood but when second wind is achieved, breathing becomes less labored and participants experience a sense of comfort and well-being. Wilmore states that "it is possibly a result of more efficient circulation to the active tissues or of a more efficient metabolic process."[1]

Metabolic Responses

Metabolism increases with the inception of exercise and continues to do so in direct proportion to increases in exercise intensity. **Metabolism,** the sum of the chemical reactions and processes that supply the energy used by the body, may be measured indirectly with appropriate equipment by the amount of oxygen consumed during exercise on a treadmill, bicycle ergometer, or other similar devices. When the intensity of exercise steadily increases the individual's ability to supply the oxygen needed to keep pace will eventually plateau. This plateau represents the upper limit of endurance and is referred to as maximal oxygen consumption (Max VO_2). Also known as **aerobic capacity** or circulorespiratory endurance, it defines a point where further increases in exercise intensity do not elicit further increases in oxygen consumption (see Figure 7.1).

FIGURE 7.1

Oxygen Uptake by Trained and Untrained People
This figure illustrates the difference in response to exercise between the trained and the untrained being exercised by a progressive treadmill protocol.

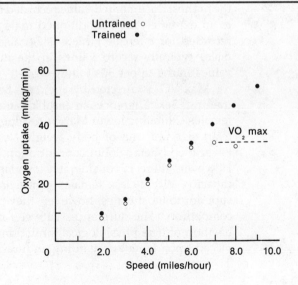

Max VO_2 represents the body's peak ability to assimilate, deliver and extract oxygen and it is considered to be the best indicator of physical fitness. It is a well-defined exercise endpoint that can be measured and reproduced accurately in the laboratory. These procedures are not generally available to the public, but fortunately field tests have been developed that correlate fairly well with the lab tests and may substitute for them. These will be discussed later in this chapter.

Max VO_2 is measured in liters of oxygen utilized per minute. This absolute value is influenced considerably by body size. Since oxygen is needed and used by all body tissues, larger people take in and use more oxygen both at rest and during exercise. Aerobic capacity, when expressed in liters of oxygen per minute, is not conducive to comparison as it will yield spurious results. To eliminate the influence of size, aerobic capacity must be considered in terms of oxygen utilization per unit of body mass. This is accomplished by converting liters of oxygen to milliliters and then dividing by body weight in kilograms. For example, a 220 pound subject uses 4.5 liters of O_2 per minute during maximum exertion, while a 143 pound subject's capacity is 3.5 liters of O_2 per minute. From these data it appears that the larger subject is more aerobically fit because of a greater capacity to use oxygen, but observe what occurs when these values are corrected for body size. Divide body weight in pounds by 2.205 to convert to kilograms:

Subject 1:

$$4.5 \ LO_2/min \ = \ 4500 \ mlO_2/min$$

$$4500 \ mlO_2/min \ \div \ 100 \ kg(220 \ lb.) \ = \ 45 \ mlO_2/kg. \cdot min$$

Subject 2:

$$3.5 \ LO_2/min \ = \ 3500 \ mlO_2/min$$

$$3500 \ mlO_2/min \ \div \ 65 \ kg(143 \ lb.) \ = \ 54 \ mlO_2/kg \cdot min$$

It's obvious from this example that the lighter subject can transport, extract, and use more oxygen per unit of body mass than the larger subject and is better equipped to perform endurance activities. Max VO_2 values expressed in ml $O_2/kg/min$ range from the mid-20s in sedentary older people to 94, which is the highest documented value recorded thus far. This enormous capacity belongs to an extremely well-conditioned male cross-country skiier. The highest value recorded for a female athlete is 74, also by a cross-country skiier. College-age males typically record values in the mid-40s, while college-age females have values in the upper 30s to low 40s.

Max VO_2 is affected by age, sex, body composition, heredity, and type of training. Sex differences in aerobic capacity become evident after puberty with females exhibiting lower Max VO_2 values. The difference is attributed to smaller heart size per unit of body weight, less oxygen-carrying capacity because of lower blood hemoglobin concentration, less muscle tissue, and more body fat. However, there is considerable overlap between the sexes regarding aerobic capacity. World-class females competing in endurance events are aerobically superior to most males, however, they have lower values than world class male competitors. The differences between males and females are probably a combination of true physiological limitations and cultural restraints that have been placed upon females regarding endurance training and competition. The influence of culture and biology on female performance will eventually become clearer as more females train and compete during the next decade.

Aerobic capacity increases with age to the late teens or early twenties and then begins to decline quite systematically by approximately 10 percent per decade for sedentary people and somewhat less for active people.[4] See Figure 7.2.

The decline in aerobic capacity with age may be partially attributable to the problems associated with the assessment of maximum performance in older people. Prudent exercise scientists who are reluctant to push elderly subjects to exhaustion as well as the fear of overexertion, lack of motivation, and muscular weakness experienced by many older people may operate together to cause underestimation of maximum capacity. Regardless of measurement problems, the decline in Max VO_2 seems to parallel the functional losses that occur as a result of the aging process. Maximum heart rate, cardiac output, and metabolism decrease during the adult years. **Body composition** changes as muscle tissue is lost, thus decreasing the body's energy-producing machinery. An increase in fat tissue is an impediment to physical performance. Ventilatory capacity decreases as the thoracic cage (chest) loses some of its elasticity caused by weakened intercostal muscles (muscles between the ribs), increased residual volume (air remaining in the lungs after expiration), and increased rigidity of lung structures. Many of these changes can be delayed or at least slowed down by a physically active lifestyle, as is exemplified by Figure 7.2. Active 60-year-olds exhibit Max VO_2 levels comparable to inactive 30-year-olds. The effects of training and heredity will be treated in greater detail later in this chapter.

When exercise begins, a short interval of time is needed for the body to adjust to the increased oxygen demand. This period, when the oxygen demand

---

FIGURE 7.2

Decline in Max VO₂ with Age
This figure illustrates the decline in Max VO₂ with age for active and inactive people.

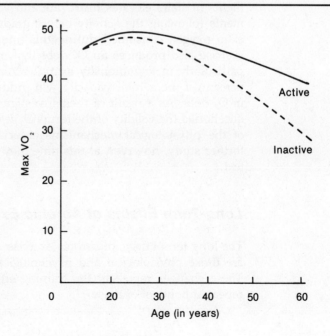

FIGURE 7.3

**O₂ Deficit and O₂ Debt
(Energy Debt)**

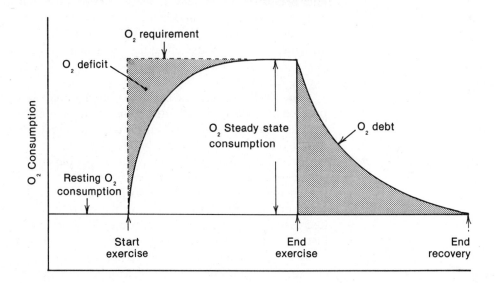

of exercise exceeds the body's transport capability, is referred to as the **O₂ deficit** (see Figure 7.3).

A second phenomenon, oxygen debt, occurs during both aerobic and anaerobic exercise (see Figure 7.3). **O₂ debt** refers to the amount of oxygen consumed during the exercise recovery period which is above that normally consumed while at rest. It is measured at the end of exercise and includes the O₂ deficit. During anaerobic exercise the body cannot supply all of the O₂ needed, resulting in a deficiency between supply and demand that must be repaid at the end of exercise. A ten-second sprint or a run up two or three flights of stairs elevates heart rate and ventilation. Both persist for a few moments following the activity before gradually returning to resting levels. The extra oxygen consumed during this interval represents the O₂ debt. Aerobic exercise also produces an O₂ debt that may be entirely due to the O₂ deficit, particularly in low-intensity exercise. Aerobic exercise that is in excess of 50 percent of the aerobic capacity will produce lactic acid and a further increase in O₂ debt. As a result of their investigations, Brooks and his associates have questioned the validity of the terms *O₂ deficit* and *O₂ debt* as well as the accuracy of the physiological mechanisms associated with each.[4] Both terms require further study, however, at this time they are adequate for the purposes of this text.

Long-Term Effects of Aerobic Exercise

The long-term effects of aerobic exercise, also referred to as *chronic adaptations*, are those physiological and psychological changes that result from training. These changes represent the training effect that is gradually developed after repeated bouts of exercise.

Heart Rate

A few months of participation in an exercise program will produce a decrease in the resting heart rate (RHR) by 10 to 25 beats per minute. This is accompanied by a decline in exercise heart rate for a given workload. For example, a bout of exercise that elicits a heart rate of 150 beats per minute prior to training may invoke a heart rate of 125 beats per minute after a few months of training. Five to six months of training will realistically lower the submaximum exercise heart rate by 20 to 40 beats per minute. Also, the exercise heart rate returns to resting level more rapidly as physical fitness improves.

The importance of lowered resting and exercise heart rates is that this allows more time for filling the ventricles with blood to be pumped to all of the body's tissues and more time for the delivery of oxygen and nutrients to the heart muscle. The delivery of these substances occurs during diastole (resting phase of the heart cycle) because relaxation of the heart muscle allows the coronary vessels to open up and receive the blood that it needs. Training substantially prolongs the heart's diastolic phase. The net result is that the heart operates more efficiently and with longer periods of rest.

Table 7.1 illustrates the differences between the trained and untrained heart. The efficiency of the trained heart at rest is readily apparent because it can pump the same amount of blood with fewer beats thereby reducing its energy requirements. During maximal exercise, even though the maximal heart rate is the same for the trained and untrained heart, the stroke volume is considerably higher for the former. The result is that more blood can be pumped per heart beat which increases the efficiency of the heart.

Stroke Volume

Stroke volume and heart rate are inversely related. The heart rate at rest and for a given workload is less because of the heart's enhanced ability to pump more blood per beat. This is accomplished because of more complete filling of the left ventricle combined with an increase in the contractile strength of its muscular walls resulting in a more forceful contraction and greater emptying of the blood in the chamber. This stronger, more efficient heart is capable of meeting circulatory challenges with less beats both at rest and during submaximum exercise.

TABLE 7.1 Comparison of Cardiac Efficiency—Trained versus Untrained

Efficiency Measurement	Rest		Maximal Exercise	
	Untrained	*Trained*	*Untrained*	*Trained*
Cardiac Output (ml)	5,200	5,200	22,000	34,000
Heart Rate (beats/minute)	74	52	200	200
Stroke Volume (ml)	70	100	110	170

Cardiac Output

Posttraining cardiac output is increased considerably during maximum exercise. However, there is little change during rest or submaximum work primarily because the trained individual is able to extract more oxygen from the blood. The oxygen concentration in arterial blood is essentially unchanged but the extraction rate (a-vO_2 difference) may be increased significantly. With training the **arterial-venous O_2 (a = vO_2) difference** is increased resulting in more oxygen being used as reflected by less oxygen in the venous blood.

Blood Flow

Although muscles receive almost 90 percent of the blood during vigorous exercise, they are not overperfused, since the increase in blood flow is proportional to the increase in oxygen utilization by the working muscles. Blood flow in a working muscle may increase eightfold; oxygen utilization rate may increase sixfold; and total oxygen uptake in the working muscle, thirtyfold.[5]

Training produces an increase in blood volume and a concomitant increase in the total number of red blood cells. However, the red blood cells do not increase proportionately to blood volume therefore, on a per-unit-of-blood basis, the red cells appear to have decreased in number. In fact many people who participate in vigorous physical activities may, on medical examination, appear to be anemic. They actually possess an above-normal total number of red blood cells but relative values per 100 ml of blood that are below normal. This adaptation to the stress of vigorous exercise is an important one because the lowered viscosity of the blood in the trained state facilitates the delivery of oxygen to working muscles.

Blood Pressure

The effect of exercise and training on blood pressure was discussed in Chapter 3. Training is a viable and effective adjunct in the control of blood pressure for many people. Particularly good are programs emphasizing jogging or walking/jogging combinations.

The oxygen demand of the heart during aerobic exercise may be estimated by multiplying the heart rate by the systolic blood pressure. This is referred to as the **rate pressure product (RPP)** or the **double product** and represents the volume of oxygen required by the heart muscle per minute. Training reduces the double product for a given amount of work. For example, an untrained individual may respond to a specific submaximal workload with a heart rate of 150 beats per minute and a systolic blood pressure of 160 mm Hg for a double product of 240 (150 × 160 = 24000). The last two zeros are dropped to produce a three digit, more manageable figure. After training, the same workload may provoke a heart rate of 130 beats per minute with a systolic blood pressure of 140 mm Hg for a double product of 182. This represents: (1) a reduced myocardial oxygen requirement for the same level of work, (2) an objective indication that aerobic conditioning has occurred, and (3) a response that implies the development of some degree of protection against ischemia.

Heart Volume

The heart responds to regular exercise in a similar manner as the other muscles of the body. It becomes stronger and oftentimes larger. The volume as well as the weight of the heart are increased with endurance training. The effects of bed rest and training upon heart volume have been determined. Prior to bed rest the mean heart volume of five young male subjects was 867 ml.[6] Twenty days of bed rest reduced the volume to 778 ml. Bed rest was followed by 50 days of training that increased the volume to 900 ml. Many other studies have confirmed the change in heart volume with aerobic training.

Aerobic exercise lowers the resting heart rate which allows more time for the ventricles to fill with blood. Since the ventricles are made of muscle, they respond to the extra blood by stretching. Stretching the muscle fibers in this manner produces a recoil effect resulting in a stronger contraction therefore, more blood is ejected per beat. The ventricles adapt to the stimulation by enlarging and growing stronger as training continues. The weight as well as the volume of the heart increases.

In the not-so-distant past, these exercise-induced changes in the heart were considered to be pathological. The term "athletes' heart" was assigned to describe the cardiac hypertrophy (heart enlargement) seen in many athletes and the connotation was that such a heart was harmful to health and longevity. Today, the medical community accepts these changes as normal responses to endurance training that have no long-term detrimental effects. In fact, it would be beneficial to maintain such a heart for as long as possible. Six months of inactivity following a training program will reduce heart weight and size to pretraining levels. The atrophy associated with inactivity is unavoidable.

Respiratory Responses

Some training-induced adaptations also occur in the respiratory system. The muscles that support breathing improve in both strength and endurance. This increases the amount of air that can be expired after a maximum inspiration **(vital capacity)** and decreases the amount of air remaining in the lungs **(residual volume).** Ventilation decreases slightly for a given workload and increases significantly during maximum exercise as a result of training. This indicates an improvement in the efficiency of the system. The depth of each breath (tidal volume) also increases during vigorous exercise.

Training increases blood flow in the lungs. In the sitting or standing position, many of the pulmonary capillaries in the upper regions of the lungs close down because gravity pulls blood down to the lower portions of the lungs. Exercise forces blood into the upper lobes and creates a greater surface area for the diffusion of oxygen from the **alveoli** (air sacs) to the pulmonary blood. Perfusion of the upper lobes of the lungs is improved with training.

Metabolic Responses

Training may improve aerobic capacity by 15 to 20 percent in a previously untrained healthy young adult. The improvement is caused by a combination of physiological adaptations resulting from several months of aerobic training.

First, the number and size of mitochondria increase. The **mitochondria** (often referred to as the cells' powerhouse) are organelles within the cells that utilize oxygen to produce the ATP needed by the muscles. Second, enzymes that are located within the mitochondria that accelerate the chemical reactions needed for the production of ATP are increased. These increases in the mitochondria and their enzymes produce greater amounts of energy and an improvement in physical fitness. Third, there is an increase in maximal cardiac output and local blood perfusion in the exercising muscles. Training increases the arterial-venous oxygen difference (a-vO_2 diff), which reflects the ability of the muscles to extract oxygen from the blood. At rest the oxygen content of arterial blood is approximately 20 ml per 100 ml of blood, while the oxygen content of venous blood is approximately 14 ml per 100 ml of blood. The O_2 difference between the two is 6 ml (20 mlO_2 − 14 mlO_2 = 6 mlO_2) representing the amount of oxygen that was extracted (the a-vO_2 diff) by the body at rest.

Exercise of increasing intensity results in a progressive widening of the difference as the body uses more of the delivered oxygen. The amount of O_2 in the venous blood decreases while the amount in arterial blood remains relatively unchanged. During strenuous exercise the oxygen content of venous blood approaches zero in the exercising muscles but it rarely drops below 2 ml when mixed venous blood is sampled in the right atrium of the heart. The reason for this phenomenon is that blood from the exercising muscles mixes with blood coming from inactive tissues as it returns to the heart. The a-vO_2 diff during maximum exercise, when measured in the right atrium, can achieve a value of 18 ml O_2 per 100 ml of blood. Training increases the a-vO_2 diff during maximum exercise but may not increase it at rest and during submaximum exercise (see Table 7.2).

Aerobic capacity is finite. Each of us is endowed with an aerobic potential limited by our heredity. A small percentage of people inherit the potential to achieve amazing feats of endurance as exemplified by performances in marathons, ultramarathons, Iron Man Triathalons, cross-country runs lasting weeks or months, and long-distance bike races. Most of us are in the average category for aerobic capacity but all of us can achieve our potential with endurance training.

Researchers are studying identical twins in order to determine the genetic component associated with aerobic capacity, adaptability to training, the composition of muscle tissue, and personality traits relating to competitiveness and leadership.[7] Identical or monozygotic twins (MZ) are genetically identical, therefore differences between them are considered to be environmentally induced. Fraternal or dizygotic twins (DZ) are genetically different, being no more similar than any other siblings. There is much anecdotal evidence regarding the simi-

TABLE 7.2   Comparison of A-VO_2 Difference—Rest versus Maximal Exercise

	Rest		Maximal Exercise
arterial blood	20 ml O_2/100 ml blood	arterial blood	20 ml O_2/100 ml blood
venous blood	− 14 ml O_2/100 ml blood	venous blood	− 2 ml O_2/100 ml blood
	6 ml O_2/100 ml blood		18 ml O_2/100 ml blood

Performances of identical twins: Skiers Phil and Steve Mahre took the gold and silver medals in the slalom in the 1984 Olympics; the DiDonato twins have set records in long distance swimming; the Soh twins finished 6 seconds apart in the 1983 Japan marathon; the Pountous twins have finished at least 6 triathlons side-by-side.
–Virginia Cowart

Twenty-two years of continuous data on one exercising population makes the Adult Fitness Study a treasure chest of information on the effects of exercise.
–Lan Barnes

larity of athletic performance for identical twins. There are many documented cases of identical twins who train, compete, and finish within an eyelash of each other in varying athletic events.

The influence of genetics in athletic performance was examined two decades ago.[8,9] The conclusion of the early studies was that genetics was responsible for approximately 80 percent of the factors associated with aerobic capacity. More recent studies have confirmed a significant genetic effect, however, not quite as strong as that suggested by the original studies.[10,11] Identical twins in these later studies were always more alike than other siblings when environmental influences were controlled. They were more alike as well in their adaptability to a physical training program.[12] The researchers concluded that maximal aerobic power and its trainability were significantly influenced by genetics. Muscle enzymes which increase with training reached similar levels in identical twins after four months of training.[10] An increase in muscle enzymes was considered to be the result of genetics. Other researchers noted that maximal muscle power was substantially influenced by genetics.[13] Still other researchers noted that identical twins were much more similar in slow-twitch muscle fiber composition.[14] The implication of the research, both early and late, shows that genetics exerts a significant role in the possession and development of many of the physiological factors associated with aerobic capacity.

Max VO_2 reaches a peak with six months to two years of endurance training. At this point aerobic capacity will level off and remain unchanged even if training is intensified. However, aerobic performance will improve with harder training. The following example which applies to both sexes illustrates this point. Let's assume that a female jogger has achieved her aerobic potential of 60 ml/kg/min with two years of hard training. At this point she is able to jog a five-mile course at a 42 ml/kg/min pace, or 70 percent of her aerobic capacity. After three more years of vigorous training (Max VO_2 still at 60 ml/kg/min) she is now able to sustain a 53 ml/kg/min pace, or 88 percent of her aerobic capacity. The extra three years of training has permitted her to use more oxygen, thereby sustaining a faster pace for the course without dipping materially into anaerobic fuels that produce lactic acid and oxygen debt. The point during exercise where blood lactate begins to increase is defined as the anaerobic threshold. Training moves the anaerobic threshold closer to the Max VO_2 and allows the participant to exercise at a higher percentage of capacity. Two people with the same Max VO_2 will perform differently if one has an anaerobic threshold substantially higher than the other.

Although aerobic capacity decreases with age, data from the only available longitudinal study (The Adult Fitness Study) indicates that it decreases more slowly than that determined by cross-sectional studies.[15] Fifteen men walked, jogged, swam, and cycled an average of 3.6 days per week for 20 years. They burned an average weekly total of 2104 calories in these activities. Their aerobic capacity declined only half as much as subjects in cross-sectional studies. Their resting heart rates and blood pressures were essentially unchanged, and their average body weight decreased by about eight pounds during the 20 years. This important longitudinal study has provided evidence to support what many exercisers and researchers intuitively knew. This study gave credence to physical training delaying the deterioration of aerobic capacity at least until age 65.

Deconditioning—Loss of Training Effect _____

Deconditioning takes place when training is discontinued or significantly reduced. Coyle investigated the physiological changes that accompany detraining as well as the approximate time-table of their occurrence.[16] The subjects in this study had been actively training for ten years. They abandoned training for 84 days in order for Coyle to observe and measure the changes that took place. He noted that the systems of the body reacted variably, that is, some showed the effects of detraining rapidly while others reacted more slowly. Stroke volume declined substantially in the first twelve days and, as expected, this event was accompanied by a significant reduction in aerobic capacity in the first three weeks. Aerobic capacity declined 16 percent by the 56th day of the deconditioning period. The oxidative enzyme level in the muscles dropped 40 percent at the end of eight weeks. However, the capillary density of the muscles declined by only 7 percent below the trained state by the end of the detraining period.

Coyle also examined the effects of detraining on submaximal responses to exercise in the same group of subjects.[17] Most of the negative effects associated with detraining occurred during the first eight weeks. A submaximal exercise test during the trained state was more easily tolerated than the same exercise test after eight weeks of detraining. By comparison, eight weeks of deconditioning resulted in: (1) an 18 percent increase in oxygen consumption, (2) a 17 percent increase in heart rate, (3) a 24 percent increase in ventilation, (4) a 34 percent increase in perceived exertion, (5) a greater reliance on carbohydrate for fuel, and (6) a large increase in the production of lactic acid for the same level of physical exertion. However, muscle capillary density and mitochondiral enzymes remained 50 percent higher than that of sedentary control subjects. These two factors tend to persist despite many weeks of inactivity. This is caused by years of vigorous training and partially explains why physical fitness is regained faster than it is initially attained.

Are American Children Fit? _____

Although many American youngsters are training for and participating in road races and triathalons of varying distances and some are involved in organized sports (many of which do not develop health-related fitness), the majority of American youth are not physically fit. The following, entitled "The Fitness of American Children," presents excerpts drawn from the medical and sports science literature.

The Fitness of American Children

1. **The American Academy of Family Physicians**
   On the whole, children (American) are not physically fit. All children in all grades should have access to daily physical education, and to structured physical activity in the schools.
2. **American Academy of Pediatrics**
   Children are not as fit today as they were 20 years ago. Financial strains and the back to basics trend in the schools, the lure of television, and the difficulty in motivating children to exercise for their health all work against the health-related fitness movement.

3. North American Society of Pediatric Exercise Medicine

Children in North America are less fit than children in other countries, and they are less fit than their counterparts of ten years ago. Schools in the United States are neglecting children's fitness by cutting physical education requirements.

4. The American College of Sports Medicine

Physical fitness programs should encourage children and youth to adopt appropriate lifelong exercise behavior. School physical education programs should emphasize the importance of lifelong exercise habits and encourage participation in community activities outside of school. The recreational aspects of exercise should be emphasized.

5. American Alliance for Health, Physical Education, Recreation and Dance

The United States is experiencing a youth fitness crisis. Lifetime health-related fitness should be encouraged.

6. American Academy of Physical Education

Given the prevalence of heart disease, obesity, and musculoskeletal problems in American society, national youth fitness tests should be based on health criteria.

7. President's Council on Physical Fitness and Sports

Although there has been no basic change in children's fitness over the last ten years, children are still not as fit as they could be.

> **Young children watch television an average of two hours a day on school days and 3.5 hours a day on weekends.**
> –Kathryn Raithel

POINTS TO PONDER

1. Define the acute and chronic effects of exercise.
2. What is the expected blood pressure response during a bout of exercise?
3. What are side-stitch and second wind?
4. What is Max VO_2 and how is it measured?
5. What is oxygen debt and oxygen deficit?
6. How does stroke volume react during exercise?
7. What is the double product; what does it measure; and how is it measured?
8. What is the $a\text{-}vO_2$ difference?
9. Describe the physiological changes that occur with deconditioning?
10. Comment on the physical fitness status of American children.

Unsubstantiated Effects of Aerobic Exercise

Coronary Collateral Circulation

Coronary collateral circulation refers to the development of tiny blood vessels in the heart muscle. This network of new vessels can supply those portions of the heart muscle whose normal complement of blood has to some extent been reduced. The development of coronary capillaries can enhance the delivery of oxygen because more blood is coursing through the myocardium and the capillaries are closer to the muscle fibers, thus facilitating the diffusion of oxygen to the muscle cells. Theoretically, these new vessels would protect against a heart attack and enhance survival and recovery should a heart attack occur.

Coronary collateral circulation has been extensively studied in animals. Rats, dogs, and pigs have been the most frequently used subjects in these studies. Of the animals studied, pigs have coronary circulation which is most similar to that of humans, but rats and dogs respond most readily to the development of coronary collaterals through experimental intervention.

Most of the studies with rats and dogs showed the development of collateral circulation with exercise when arteries were partially or totally occluded. Studies of animals with normal coronary circulation did not result in the development of coronary collaterals from exercise. Exercise may not produce the threshold of stimulation required to develop collaterals in the absence of disease. At the end of four weeks of training, researchers were unable to detect collaterals in healthy dogs.[18] However, when researchers artificially induced ischemia and repeated the measurements, they found a significant increase in blood flow to various portions of the heart muscle.

Coronary collateral circulation has been increased in animals through exercise and experimentally induced occlusion of one or more coronary vessels. Eckstein surgically narrowed the coronary vessels of about 100 dogs.[19] Only those dogs that developed changes in their electrocardiograms were selected for the study and these were separated into exercise and nonexercise groups. Measurements made at the end of eight weeks indicated that both groups developed collateral circulation but that it was developed to a greater degree in the exercised dogs. Other investigators exercised dogs at 50 percent of their capacity, however, they waited three months after occluding one coronary artery to begin the exercise program.[20] They found that collateral circulation improved twice as much in the exercised dogs compared to the sedentary control dogs. In another study, collateral blood flow increased by 75 percent at rest and 78 percent during exercise for dogs who were exercised after surgical constriction of one coronary blood vessel.[21] The fitness program consisted of 75 minutes of daily aerobic and anaerobic exercises. No significant changes occurred in the sedentary control dogs.

One of the better studies showed a 20 percent increase in the collateral blood flow of trained versus untrained pigs.[22] The trained pigs exercised for five months after surgical narrowing of one of the coronary arteries. The length of time of this study seemed more suitable for the development of collateral improvement.

Working with guinea pigs, Jokl was able to demonstrate an increase in capillary density as a result of treadmill running.[23] He examined the muscles of the calf, heart, and jaw and found an increase in capillary density in the calf (this muscle is used in running), and the heart (which pumped the blood needed during exercise) but no increase in the jaw muscle, which is not exercised by treadmill running.

Coronary collateral circulation or accessory vessels cannot develop suddenly following an acute occlusion but may be lifesaving if already developed.
–Lauralee Sherwood

Today, most researchers agree that the development of coronary collateral circulation is triggered by myocardial ischemia because of progressive atherosclerosis. Exercise simulates the ischemia of atherosclerosis but only on a temporary basis and only while exercise is in progress. Does this constitute enough of a stimulus for the development of collateral blood flow in humans? The answer at this time is that the direct evidence needed to support this notion is lacking. Kavanagh, reviewing the literature pertaining to this matter, has pointed out many of the problems associated with this research in humans.[24] The major drawbacks include the following: Flaws in experimental design include the use of small groups, and low-intensity, short-term exercise training programs, and the inadequacy of coronary artery angiography for measuring collateral growth.

Better assessment techniques and more sensitive instruments are needed before a definitive statement can be made regarding collateral circulation. While we wait for this to occur, the best advice would be to begin exercising now. Don't wait for proof positive because it may be a long time in coming. The implications of collateral circulation development for heart health are enormous. Even if future research unequivocally shows that collateral circulation does not occur in humans, the other benefits of physical activity are reason enough to establish the exercise habit.

Coronary Vessel Size

A number of studies have demonstrated that rats that are subjected to treadmill running or swim training develop coronary arteries with larger diameters than sedentary controls. This is particularly true of rats who are exposed to exercise early in life. One of these studies found an increase in vessel size for all exercising groups but a surprising finding was that rats who swam eight hours per week developed larger vessels than those who swam sixteen hours per week.[25] The possibility exists that there may be a threshold for exercise above which no further increases in coronary vessel size occur.

Pigs who ran on a treadmill for ten minutes a day at 10 miles per hour, five days per week, for 22 months did not increase the size of their coronary vessels. The duration of each bout of exercise (10 min) may not have been a sufficient stimulus for increasing coronary vessel size.

Endurance training seems to enlarge the diameter of the coronary blood vessels of animals. This phenomenon is much more difficult to study in humans, but the implications of this adaptation for heart attack prevention is significant. Probably the case most often discussed regarding coronary vessel size is that of Clarence DeMar. He was a distance runner virtually all of his adult life and competed in more than 1000 distance races in his career. He ran the Boston Marathon 34 times and won 7 of these. He died of cancer at the age of 70. An autopsy revealed that while his coronary arteries exhibited some atherosclerosis, their diameters were so large—two to three times normal size—that blood flow through them would not have been impeded for decades. Many have speculated that his enlarged arteries were caused by a lifetime of running, but there is no way to establish that fact. The reason for his large vessels could conceivably be that he was born with that endowment although there was nothing in his family history to account for such an unusual physical development. Hutchins and his coworkers found that there was a positive relationship between the weight of the heart and the diameters of the coronary vessels that service it.[26] That being the case, it may be more than a reasonable possibility that DeMar's large arteries were related to his larger, heavier heart (which was probably the product of a lifetime of exercise).

Cause-and-effect relationships between exercise and coronary vessel size remain elusive in humans. Extrapolating from animal studies to humans is risky, but the fact that this phenomenon has occurred in animals raises hope for the same response in human beings.

Exercise and Infection: Help or Hype?

People who have exercised for years claim that they have less viral infections and colds compared to their sedentary days. Although this response is prevalent among exercisers, research evidence remains equivocal on this point. That physically active people are less susceptible to these infections is probably true, however, is it because of the natural build-up of antibodies as we age or is it because of the effect of exercise in boosting the immune system?

Lymphocytes are the most important link in the relationship between exercise and immune function.
–Harvey Simon

Support for enhancement of the immune system through exercise comes from the increased production of lymphocytes, interleukin-1, and interferon which has been observed in some studies. The lymphocytes are the primary cells involved in the immune response. Most studies have shown an increase in the number of circulating lymphocytes with strenuous exercise but the effects may be short-lived.[27,28] Moderate exercise has increased circulating levels of interleukin-1.[29,30] Interleukin-1 stimulates the immune system by increasing the activity of both T- and B-lymphocytes. It also exerts a pyrogenic effect (produces a fever) which is part of the body's natural defense in combating infections.

Moderate exercise also stimulates the production of interferons.[31] Interferons are a group of naturally occurring proteins that have antiviral properties. The response of interferons to viral infections is initiated only a matter of hours after an infection develops. Exercise-induced increases in interferons last for approximately two hours. First the effectiveness of this transient response is debatable, and second the amount of interferons produced by exercise is less than that which naturally occurs to the virus alone.

Persistent, strenuous exercise, may have the opposite effect by reducing the activity of the immune system. High-intensity exercise performed frequently tends to increase the likelihood of respiratory infection by supressing some components of the immune system for up to two hours after exercise.[32]

Is exercise a help or hindrance with regard to infection? The research shows that exercise of moderate intensity may enhance the immune system and that exhaustive exercise might supress it. The suggestion for those who exercise for reasons other than competition is quite clear: Exercise moderately and frequently.

Activities for Improving Cardiorespiratory Endurance _____

Cardiorespiratory endurance may be developed through participation in rhythmic and continuous activities that elevate the heart rate to desired levels at least three times per week for at least 15 minutes at a time. Any activity meeting these criteria will suffice. Remember, fitness cannot be developed or maintained without effort and consistent participation, therefore, it is very important that you select activities that are enjoyable and satisfying.

Many activities, some better than others, have the potential for developing cardiorespiratory fitness. Many of these are more amenable to regulation in terms of exercise intensity and do not require an opponent nor a companion. The frequency and duration of these activities, as well as their intensity, are under your control. Some events that fall into this category include fast walking, jogging, biking, swimming, rope jumping, fitness trails, cross-country skiing and skating (ice and roller). Competition in these activities is not precluded, but their nature is such that they allow for individual participation and latitude in scheduling plus control of the criteria that must be met to develop and maintain cardiorespiratory endurance.

Many sports and games also have the capacity to develop and maintain cardiorespiratory endurance but some flexibility and control is lost. For example, the intensity of a game is dependent upon the skill level and motivation of the players as well as the degree to which the action is continuous. Court games such as squash, racquetball, handball, badminton, and tennis are noncontinuous-type activities. Optimal fitness benefits from these games are attained when two highly skilled players of equal ability oppose each other in singles competition.

Team sports such as basketball, ice and roller hockey, lacrosse, rugby, soccer, and water polo have the potential to develop aerobic capacity. The action in these sports is also intermittent but they pose the additional obstacle of rounding up more people to play as well as gaining access to an appropriate facility. It becomes more difficult to schedule these activities three or more days per week.

A more serious problem associated with court games and team sports is that they may be too strenuous for sedentary beginners. A sensible approach for those who want to maintain fitness through sports and games is to first develop a fitness base through those activities where the pace, frequency, and duration can be controlled.

Aerobic dancing is usually performed with a group under the leadership of an instructor and probably involves traveling to the site. These are not insurmountable but it may become inconvenient three times a week. Another problem centers upon the format of group participation. Since the entire group participates in unison, it is left to the individual to try to regulate the intensity; that is, to exercise harder or easier than the group in order to accommodate his or her exercise heart rate.

The comparative value of various physical activities will be discussed in greater detail in Chapter 12.

SELF-ASSESSMENT
Assessing Cardiorespiratory Fitness

Field Tests

The field tests for measuring aerobic capacity are performed outside of the laboratory setting. Using simple equipment these tests, which estimate Max VO_2, have been validated by comparing their results to those achieved through conventional laboratory techniques. Although not as accurate as laboratory methods, these tests offer a convenient and inexpensive way to estimate cardiorespiratory endurance.

The Rockport Fitness Walking Test

This field test was developed to evaluate aerobic capacity (Max VO_2) without expensive equipment or test technicians.[33] This walking test was validated by testing 343 men and women between the ages of 30 and 69 in the laboratory with a maximal exercise tolerance test. This was followed by two brisk one-mile walks on a measured track on separate days. The results of the walks and the exercise tolerance test were correlated to determine the degree of relationship between the two. There was a high-positive correlation which led the researchers to conclude that aerobic fitness could be predicted quite accurately with the one-mile walking test. They calculated that this test has an estimated error of less than 12 percent.

This walking test has several advantages over other field tests for determining aerobic capacity. These include the following: (1) it employs a natural form of locomotion (walking) with which we are all familiar, (2) it is a low-impact activity, (3) it is appropriate for all ages and both sexes, and (4) there is minimal risk associated with taking this test.

Since there is some risk associated with virtually all physical activity it is important to review the guidelines established by the American College of Sports Medicine in Chapter 6 regarding medical clearance for exercise. Do this prior to taking this test.

The Rockport Fitness Walking Test estimates aerobic capacity based upon the variables of age, sex, time needed to walk one mile, and the heart rate achieved at the end of the test. The directions for taking the test are as follows:

1. Heart rate is counted for 15 seconds and multiplied by four to get beats per minute.
2. The course should be flat and measured, preferably a 440 yard track.
3. Be sure to have a stop watch or a watch with a second hand.
4. Warm up for 5 to 10 minutes prior to taking the test. Warm up should include a ¼-mile walk followed by the stretching exercises in Chapter 6.
5. When you take the test, walk at a brisk even pace and cover the distance as rapidly as possible.

6. Take your pulse rate immediately after the test and enter it in the appropriate graph (based upon your age and sex) in Table 7.3.
7. Draw a vertical line through your time and a horizontal line through your heart rate. The point where the lines intersect will determine your fitness level. See Table 7.3.

Rockport provides a series of 20-week walking programs based on the results of the walking test. These are available for a nominal fee ($1.00 at this writing) by sending a request to Rockport Fitness Walking Test, 72 Howe St., Marlboro, Massachusetts 01752.

TABLE 7.3   Relative Fitness Level Charts

These charts are designed to tell you how fit you are compared to other individuals of your age and sex. For example, if your coordinates place you in the "above average" section of the chart, you're in better shape than the average person in your category.

The charts are based on weights of 170 lbs. for men and 125 lbs. for women. If you weigh substantially more, your relative cardiovascular fitness level will be slightly overestimated. If you weigh substantially less, your relative cardiovascular fitness level will be slightly underestimated.

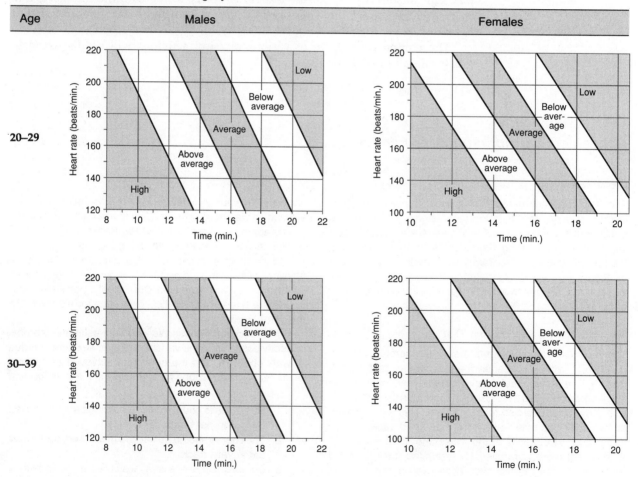

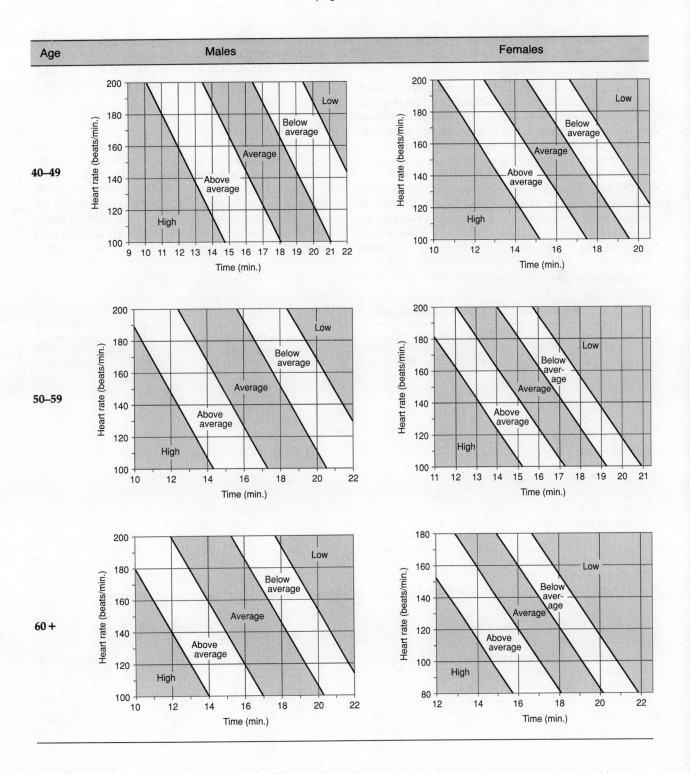

Running Tests

Running tests have become a very popular means for estimating cardiorespiratory endurance. A measured course, preferably a 440 yard track, and a stopwatch are required. Many people can be tested simultaneously. Running tests of sufficient length correlate quite well with treadmill values when subjects are allowed to practice running the course. Practice promotes familiarization with the test and provides an opportunity to develop the sense of pacing needed for optimum performance.

This writer recommends the Balke 1.5-mile run for adults and older teenagers. This is an adequate distance for the measurement of aerobic capacity. Children and young teenagers should be tested over a shorter distance such as a one mile or nine-minute run. The Balke Test covers a fixed distance making it easy to administer on a track because participants begin and end the test at the same place. The time taken to run or run/walk this test represents the score earned. Table 7.4 translates the time spent to cover the distance into estimated Max VO_2 in ml O_2/kg/min. Table 7.5 places the obtained Max VO_2 value into a fitness category.

Laboratory Tests

Laboratory procedures for testing aerobic capacity are quite sophisticated. The measurements are made under controlled conditions, are reproducible, and the data are comparable to those collected in any laboratory in the world. The tests and procedures employed in the laboratory are beyond the scope of this text. The two most common pieces of equipment for measuring Max VO_2 in the laboratory are the bicycle ergometer and the treadmill. A brief description follows.

TABLE 7.4   1½ Mile Run Test—Estimated VO₂ Max

Time in Minutes and Seconds	Estimated Max VO₂ (ml/kg/min)	Time in Minutes and Seconds	Estimated Max VO₂ (ml/kg/min)
7:30 or less	75	12:31–13:00	39
7:31– 8:00	72	13:01–13:30	37
8:01– 8:30	67	13:31–14:00	36
8:31– 9:00	62	14:01–14:30	34
9:01– 9:30	58	14:30–15:00	33
9:31–10:00	55	15:01–15:30	31
10:01–10:30	52	15:31–16:00	30
10:31–11:00	49	16:01–16:30	28
11:01–11:30	46	16:31–17:00	27
11:31–12:00	44	17:01–17:30	26
12:01–12:30	41	17:31–18:00	25

Adapted from K.H. Cooper, "A Means of Assessing Maximal Oxygen Intake," *Journal of The American Medical Association* 203 (1968): 201.

TABLE 7.5   1½ Mile Run Test—Estimated VO₂ Max Fitness Category

Age Group (yr) Males*	High		Good	Average	Fair	Poor	
10–19	Above	66	57–66	47–56	38–46	Below	38
20–29	''	62	53–62	43–52	33–42	''	33
30–39	''	58	49–58	39–48	30–38	''	30
40–49	''	54	45–54	36–44	26–35	''	26
50–59	''	50	42–50	34–41	24–33	''	24
60–69	''	46	39–46	31–38	22–30	''	22
70–79	''	42	36–42	28–35	20–27	''	20

*The average maximal O_2 uptake of females is 15 to 20 percent lower than that of males. To find the appropriate category for females, locate the score in the above table and shift one category to the left, e.g., the "Average" category for males is the "Good" category for females.

Adapted from J.H. Wilmore, *Training for Sport and Activity*, Boston: Allyn and Bacon, Inc., 1982.

Bicycle Ergometer

Bicycle ergometers are special types of stationary bikes in which a well-defined workload may be set to accurately measure work output. There are several advantages to using bicycle ergometers for measuring aerobic capacity. First, they are nonweight bearing activities that are appropriate for the overweight, the elderly, and those with lower body joint problems. Second, physiological measurements can be made during the test while the subject is pedalling. Third, they are portable and relatively inexpensive.

The major disadvantage is that most Americans are unaccustomed to bike riding leading to the development of local leg fatigue prior to cardiorespiratory fatigue. As a result, Max VO₂ is underestimated. Subjects must pedal at a prescribed rate in order to keep the workload constant for all subjects. Some subjects seem to lack the necessary rhythm to do this and other subjects lag behind the prescribed rate as they tire during the latter portion of the test.

Treadmill

Probably the most frequently used piece of equipment for measuring aerobic capacity in American physiology laboratories is the motor-driven treadmill. It accommodates walking, running, and walk/run tests. Belt speeds may reach 20 to 25 mph and the elevation of the bed may achieve a 40 percent slope. For Americans, the treadmill comes closer to eliciting a maximal aerobic response than any other piece of testing equipment. The selection of an appropriate treadmill test depends upon the purpose for testing and the population being tested.

POINTS TO PONDER

1. *What is coronary collateral circulation?*
2. *Does aerobic exercise develop coronary collaterals in humans?*
3. *Does exercise protect the individual against infection? Defend your answer.*
4. *Describe the Rockport Fitness Walking Test.*
5. *What is a bicycle ergometer and what problems does it present for Americans who are tested with this device?*
6. *Describe the Balke 1½-mile run test.*

Chapter Highlights

Physical activities may be categorized as aerobic or anaerobic. Aerobic activities require less than maximum effort and can be sustained in relative comfort for a period of time without causing significant increases in blood lactate and O₂ debt. On the other hand, anaerobic activities are high-intensity, short-duration exercises producing both lactic acid and O₂ debt. These activities do not train the cardiorespiratory systems unless they are performed in a circuit or in interval training.

A single bout of aerobic exercise produces some temporary changes in the body. These changes are referred to as the acute, or short-term, effects of exercise. The chronic, or long-term, effects of aerobic exercise are the result of training. These effects or adaptations persist if training is continued on a regular basis, but should the program be discontinued they are completely lost within six to eight months.

Genetics is a significant factor in the ability to perform endurance work. Studies with identical twins have confirmed the importance and influence of genetics in athletic performance.

The effects of deconditioning are discernible within the first few days after training has ceased. However, the systems of the body lose their level of condition at varying rates. Stroke volume is one of the first factors to be affected and muscle capillary density is one of the last. Most of the training effect is lost within the first eight weeks of inactivity.

Most medical and sport science organizations have stated that American children and youth are not as fit as they should be. Many cite cut-backs in physical education in the schools as the primary reason. Television is also cited as a major culprit.

Evidence exists to support the notion that both coronary collateral circulation and coronary vessel size increase in animals as a result of exercise, but this has yet to be established in humans. The best approach regarding exercise, given our current state of knowledge, is to establish the exercise habit while awaiting clinical proof because many other healthful changes, independent of collateral circulation and coronary vessel size, do occur.

Moderate exercise may help to ward off viral infections by boosting the immune system. Moderate exercise stimulates the production of the lymphocytes, interleukin-1, and the interferons. Exhaustive exercise, however, may suppress the immune system thereby lowering resistance to infection.

Cardiorespiratory endurance may be developed by participation in a variety of rhythmic and continuous activities. The pool of available activities presents enough diversification to appeal to almost everyone. Cardiorespiratory fitness may be assessed by field tests such as step tests and run/walk tests, and laboratory tests that employ bicycle ergometers and treadmills.

References

1. J. H. Wilmore and D. L. Costil, *Training for Sport and Activity*, Dubuque, Iowa: Wm. C. Brown Publishers, 1988.

2. D. Ships, "Exercise-Induced Increase in Diastolic Pressure: Indicator of Severe Coronary Artery Disease," *American Journal of Cardiology*, 43 (1979): 708.

3. P. O. Astrand and K. Rodahl, *Textbook of Work Physiology*, New York: McGraw-Hill Book Co., 1986.

4. G. A. Brooks and T. D. Fahey, *Exercise Physiology*, New York: John Wiley and Sons, 1984.

5. D. W. Eddington and V. R. Edgerton, *The Biology of Physical Activity*, Boston: Houghton Mifflin Co., 1976.

6. B. Saltin et al., "Response to Submaximal and Maximal Exercise After Bed Rest and Training," *Circulation*, 38, Supplement 7 (1968).

7. V. S. Cowart, "How Does Heredity Affect Athletic Performance?" *The Physician And Sportsmedicine*, 4 (1987): 134.

8. V. Klissouras, "Heritability of Adaptive Variation," *Journal of Applied Physiology*, 31 (1971): 338.

9. V. Klissouras et al., "Adaptation to Maximal Effort: Genetics of Age," *Journal of Applied Physiology*, 35 (1973): 288.

10. P. Hamel et al., "Heredity and Muscle Adaptation to Endurance Training," *Medicine and Science in Sports and Exercise*, 18 (1986): 690.

11. C. Bouchard et al., "Aerobic Performance in Brothers, Dizygotic and Monozygotic Twins," *Medicine and Science in Sports and Exercise*, 18 (1986): 639.

12. M. R. Boulay et al., "Sensitivity of Maximal Aerobic Power and Capacity to Anaerobic Training is Partly Genotype Dependent," in R. M. Malina and C. Bouchard (eds.), *Proceedings of the 1984 Olympic Scientific Congress, Vol. 4 Sport and Human Genetics*, Champaign, Ill.: Human Kinetics Publishers, Inc., 1986.

13. V. Klissouras and B. Jones, "Genetic Variation in The Force-Velocity Relation of Human Muscle," in R. M. Malina and C. Bouchard (eds.), *Proceedings of the 1984 Olympic Scientific Congress Vol. 4. Sport and Human Genetics*, Champaign, Ill.: Human Kinetics Publishers, Inc., 1986.

14. G. Lortie et al., "Muscle Fiber Type Composition and Enzyme Activities in Brothers and Monozygotic Twins," In R. M. Malina and C. Bouchard (eds.) *Proceedings of the 1984 Olympic Scientific Congress Vol. 4 Sport and Human Genetics*, Champaign, Ill.: Human Kinetics Publishers, Inc. 1986.

15. F. W. Kasch et al., "A Longitudinal Study of Cardiovascular Stability in Active Men Aged 45 to 65 Years," *The Physician and Sportsmedicine*, 16 (1988): 117.

16. E. F. Coyle et al., "Time Course of Loss of Adaptations After Stopping Prolonged Intense Endurance Training," *Journal of Applied Physiology*, 57 (1984): 1857.
17. E. F. Coyle et al., "Effects of Detraining on Responses to Submaximal Exercise," *Journal of Applied Physiology*, 59 (1985): 853.
18. D. R. Knight and H. L. Stone, "Alteration of Ischemic Cardiac Function in Normal Heart by Daily Exercise," *Journal of Applied Physiology*, 55 (1983): 52.
19. R. Eckstein, "Effect of Exercise and Coronary Artery Narrowing on Coronary Collateral Circulation," *Circulation Research*, 5 (1957): 230.
20. K. W. Scheel et al., "Effects of Exercise on the Coronary and Collateral Vasculature of Beagles With and Without Coronary Occlusion," *Circulation Research*, 48 (1981): 523.
21. M. V. Cohen et al., "Coronary Collateral Stimulation by Exercise In Dogs with Stenotic Coronary Arteries," *Journal of Applied Physiology*, 52 (1982): 664.
22. C. M. Cloor et al., "The Effects of Exercise on Collateral Development in Myocardial Ischemia in Pigs," *Journal of Applied Physiology*, 56 (1984): 656.
23. E. Jokl, *Heart and Sport*, Springfield, Ill.: Charles C. Thomas, 1964.
24. T. Kavanagh, "Does Exercise Improve Coronary Collateralization? A New Look at an Old Belief," *The Physician and Sportsmedicine*, 17 (1989): 96.
25. J. A. Stevenson et al., "Effect of Exercise on Coronary Tree Size in the Rat," *Circulation Research*, 15 (1964): 265.
26. G. M. Hutchins et al., "Correlation of Age and Heart Weight with Tortuosity and Caliber of Normal Coronary Arteries," *American Heart Journal*, 94 (1977): 196.
27. E. Soppi et al., "Effects of Strenuous Physical Stress on Circulating Lymphocyte Number and Function Before and After Training," *Journal of Clinical and Laboratory Immunology*, 8 (1982): 43.
28. L. S. Berk et al., "Lymphocyte Subset Changes During Acute Maximal Exercise," *Medicine and Science in Sports and Exercise*, 18 (1986): 706.
29. J. G. Cannon and M. J. Kluger, "Endogenous Pyrogen Activity in Human Plasma After Exercise," *Science*, 220 (1983): 617.
30. J. Cannon and C. Dinerello, "Interleukin-1 Activity in Human Plasma," *Federal Proceedings*, 43 (1984): 462.
31. A. Viti et al., "Effect of Exercise on Plasma Interferon Levels," *Journal of Applied Physiology*, 59 (1985): 426.
32. L. Sherwood, *Human Physiology*, St. Paul: West Publishing Co., 1989.
33. *Rockport Fitness Walking Test*, Marlboro, Mass: The Rockport Walking Institute. Pamphlet.

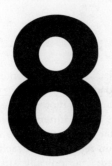

Developing the Muscular Component

Chapter Outline

Mini Glossary

Agonist muscle: the muscle that contracts to produce a specific movement; the prime mover.

Anabolic steroid: a drug with tissue-building or growth-stimulating properties.

Androgen: male sex hormone produced in the testes and to a limited extent, from the adrenal cortex.

Antagonist muscle: the muscle that stretches in response to the contraction of the agonist muscle.

Cardiac muscle: specialized muscle tissue found only in the heart.

Circuit training: a series of six to ten exercises performed in sequence and as rapidly as one's fitness level allows.

Concentric contraction: that phase of muscular contraction in which the muscle shortens.

Essentric contraction: that phase of a muscular contraction in which the muscle lengthens.

Fast-twitch muscle fiber: a type of muscle fiber which contracts rapidly but fatigues rapidly. Also referred to as "white" muscle fibers.

Hyperplasia: an increase in size caused by an increase in the number of cells.

Hypertrophy: an increase in size caused by an increase in the thickness of fibers.

Isokinetic contraction: a dynamic contraction in which the muscles generate force against a variable resistance that moves at a constant rate of speed.

Isometric contraction: a static contraction in which the muscles generate force against an immovable object with no observable shortening.

Isotonic contraction: a dynamic contraction in which the muscles generate force against a constant resistance; movement occurs as the muscles shorten and lengthen with each repetition.

Locomotor movement: movements that bring about a change in location and include walking, jogging, climbing, cycling, and swimming, to name but a few.

Lordosis: swayback; abnormal curvature of the low back.

Motor unit: a motor nerve and all of the muscle fibers that it innervates.

Muscular endurance: the ability of a muscle to sustain repeated contractions.

Overload: periodically stressing the body with greater loads than those that are usually experienced.

Periodization: a way to provide variety in training. The training period is divided into different cycles in which the volume is periodically reduced and the intensity is concomitantly increased.

Nonlocomotor movement: movements that take place around the axis of the body. The subject remains in one place creating dynamic movement by means of stretching, bending, stooping, pushing, pulling, and twisting, to name but a few.

Skeletal muscle: voluntary muscles whose attachments to the bones of the skeletal system provide the basis for human movement.

Slow-twitch muscle fiber: a type of muscle fiber that contracts slowly but is difficult to fatigue; referred to as "red" muscle fibers.

Smooth muscle: located in the blood vessels and digestive system; not under conscious or voluntary control.

Strength: the force exerted by a muscle or muscle group in a single maximal contraction.

Testosterone: a sex hormone appearing in much higher concentrations in males than females.

Valsalva maneuver: occurs when individuals lift heavy weights and hold their breath. The glottis closes and intrathoracic pressure increases, hindering the flow of blood to the heart.

Introduction

In keeping with the theme of this text—that physical fitness activities contribute positively to good health—strength training is presented as an adjunct to the aerobic program and not as a substitute for it. While strength training contributes to physical and mental health in the manner discussed in Chapter 3, its ability to affect health is not as profound or pervasive as that of aerobic activities. However, as an extension of the aerobic program, strength training uniquely promotes physical and mental health.

All human movement, locomotor and nonlocomotor, is dependent on appropriate muscular contractions and relaxations. **Locomotor movements** are those that bring about a change in location and include walking, jogging, climbing, cycling and swimming, to name but a few. **Nonlocomotor movements** are those that take place around the axis of the body. The subject remains in one place creating dynamic movement by means of stretching, bending, stooping, pushing, pulling and twisting, to name but a few. Movement may be categorized as fine or precision-oriented, such as typing or playing the piano; or gross (involving contractions of large muscles), such as punting a football or hitting a baseball. Movements may be job-related, recreational, rhythmical, athletic, or associated with daily living, but they all require the contraction and relaxation of appropriate muscles.

The muscular system consists of three types of muscle: smooth, cardiac, and skeletal. Smooth muscles, such as those which are located in the digestive system and blood vessels, are not under conscious control. These are involuntary muscles that are under autonomic neural control. Cardiac muscle, which appears in the heart only, is also under nonvoluntary control. Some practitioners of Yoga, the ancient philosophy of India that emphasizes mental attitude, diet, and posture, along with others who are trained in biofeedback, are able to influence their heart rate through meditation and will power, but by and large cardiac muscle responds to automatic control processes. The skeletal muscles, on the other hand, are voluntary muscles whose attachments to the bones of the skeletal system provide the basis for human movement. Their origins and insertions on the bones provide a lever system in which small contractions of the muscles produce large movements of the extremities.

The human body has over 600 muscles containing more than 6 billion microscopic muscle fibers. Each fiber is so strong that it can support more than 1000 times its own weight.
—C. Moore

Muscular Strength and Muscular Endurance

Muscular strength may be defined as the force exerted by a muscle or muscle group in a single maximum isotonic, isometric, or isokinetic contraction. Isometric strength is developed through muscular contractions against an immovable object (see Figure 8.1). The muscles contract statically for 6 to 10 seconds without shortening. Isometric strength is measured with dynamometers and cable tensiometers.

Isotonic muscular contractions consist of dynamic movement as a result of muscle shortening. Isotonic movements involve **concentric** and **eccentric muscular contractions**. The dumbbell curl in Figure 8.2 exemplifies both types of isotonic contractions. The concentric phase of this exercise occurs when the flexor muscles of the arm contract and lift the weight to the chest. The eccentric phase occurs as the weight is slowly lowered to the starting position against the force of gravity. Lowering the weight rapidly will limit the potential for strength development in the eccentric phase of exercise.

Most dynamic exercises consist of both types of contractions. **Strength** may be developed by either type of dynamic muscular contraction but little is known about the effects of exercise programs that feature eccentric movements exclusively. Systems of isotonic exercises (and most exercise equipment) involve both movements so for practical reasons these will not be treated separately.

FIGURE 8.1

Isometric Contraction
Force is exerted against
both sides of an
immovable door jam.

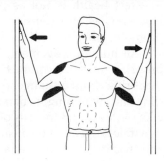

FIGURE 8.2

Isotonic Dumbbell Curl
Concentric phase—the
weight is lifted toward the
shoulder; eccentric
phase—the weight is
returned to the starting
position.

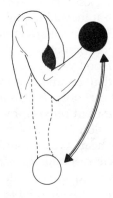

Isokinetic muscular contractions are dynamic movements requiring specialized equipment such as Cybex, Minigym, and so on, which adjusts the resistance so that it will be maximum throughout the full range of motion (see Figure 8.3). Regardless of the amount of force applied, these devices allow movement to occur at a constant rate of speed.

Muscles that are activated or in the process of contracting produce tension and may or may not react by changing their length. Contraction may produce a shortening of the muscle fibers (concentric movement) or a lengthening of the fibers (eccentric action) or no change in the length of the fibers (**isometric contraction**). Muscles that contract dynamically change their length because they are able to overcome a resistance. A muscle or group of muscles at a joint, that produce concentric movement, are the prime movers of the joint. For example, the prime mover in Figure 8.2 is the biceps muscle. Its contraction produces muscle shortening thereby moving the weight from thigh to shoulder. The prime mover is referred to as the **agonist**. In order for this movement to occur efficiently, the triceps muscle must relax and lengthen. In this exercise, the triceps is the **antagonist** of the biceps. The biceps and the triceps function synergistically so that as one muscle, the biceps, contracts and does the work, the other muscle the triceps relaxes and permits the work to occur. In Figure 8.3, the roles of these two muscles are reversed as the triceps becomes the prime mover or agonist and the biceps becomes the antagonist.

Muscular endurance is the ability of a muscle or muscle group to sustain repeated contractions (isotonic) or the ability to apply a constant force for a

FIGURE 8.3

Isokinetic Training and Testing Device

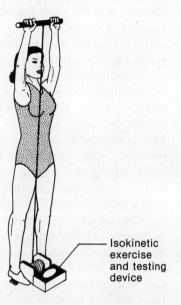

Isokinetic exercise and testing device

period of time (isometric). Muscular endurance is developed through exercise programs that emphasize many repetitions with relatively light weights. Muscular strength is highly correlated with "absolute" muscular endurance, which involves lifting a specified amount of weight a maximum number of times. This is dependent upon the maximum contractile force of the muscles involved. For example, two people of unequal strength attempt to lift 100 pounds as many times as possible. One is capable of a maximum lift of 200 pounds while the other can only lift 150 pounds. One hundred pounds represents one-half of the capacity of the first person but two-thirds of the capacity for the second person. Two-thirds of the weaker contestant's total strength must be used on every lift, while only one-half of the stronger contestant's total strength is used. Each lift is more difficult for the weaker person. A greater percentage of the weaker person's total number of motor units per lift must be used and will therefore fatigue more rapidly than the stronger contestant. (A **motor unit** is a nerve and all of the muscle fibers that it stimulates.) In order to increase absolute endurance, one must increase strength.

Muscular endurance can also be measured on a relative basis by testing people at a given percentage of their maximal strength for selected lifts. Returning to the two weightlifting contestants, if each were to be tested at 50 percent of their capacity, the stronger one would lift 100 pounds while the weaker one would lift 75 pounds. Under this protocol, it is conceivable that the weaker contestant could outperform the stronger one in muscular endurance.

The Muscular Component and the Wellness Connection

The relationship between strength training and wellness was discussed to some degree in Chapter 3. Progressive resistance exercises such as weight training with moderate loads produce several beneficial health effects. Hickson's study indicated that this type of program did not result in optimal strength development, but for participants whose major concern involves the health-related benefits of strength training, the gains will be sufficient.[1] His endurance-trained subjects may not have improved their strength to the same extent as the strength-trained group but they did improve.

Training with moderate weights increases muscle tissue while decreasing the amount of stored body fat. Several short-term studies have documented this occurrence. The largest increase in lean body mass was seven pounds and the largest decrease in the amount of fat in these studies was 9.4 percent.[2] This favorable change in body composition leads to an increase in the resting metabolic rate. Recall that this refers to the amount of energy used by the body during the resting state. The addition of muscle tissue increases the body's energy requirements because muscle uses more calories than fat tissue, both during rest and during physical activity. Since we spend more time resting than in activity, the increase in muscle tissue becomes an aid in the effort to control body weight. The change in body composition results in a restructuring of body contour as males and females acquire more muscle tissue, lose some fat, and develop more fit and trim silhouettes. This change in body composition occurs because muscle is denser than fat; one pound of muscle takes up less room in the body than one pound of fat. These changes in the body contribute to better mental health through the enhancement of a positive self-concept.

Fat Measures: A Pound of Lean— 18% Smaller

When you start to slide out of shape, you get to look really out of shape before your friends or your bathroom scales give you clear warning. That's because each pound of fat you put on bulges out 18% bigger than a pound of lean (1.1 liters compared with 0.9).

American Health, vol 1, no. IV, p. 17, Sept/Oct, 1982.

Appropriate resistance exercises develop the antigravity muscles of the abdomen and lower back, thereby decreasing the likelihood of back pain and injury. The development of these muscle groups provides the support needed by the spinal column to hold up the torso and to maintain good posture. Strengthening other antigravity muscles, (those of the hips, front and back of the thighs, and both calves) also helps maintain good posture. Proper posture reduces stress upon the spinal column and the low back. **Lordosis** (swayback) is an exaggerated curve of the lower back related to weak abdominals, poor posture, tight hamstrings, and excess weight—all of which lead to back pain and injury and all of which are beneficially affected by exercise.

Resistance training strengthens the ligaments, which attach one bone to another, and the tendons, which attach muscle to bone. Cartilage and connective tissue become thicker and stronger. The joints are better protected from injury and much more stable when their muscles and surrounding structures are well-developed and strong.

The poor physical condition of children participating in youth sports may be the leading cause of injury.
–The American Physical Therapy Association

Stiff Joints: Come Again to Cartilage

With a one-in-three chance of developing osteoarthritis by age 30, and a nine-in-ten chance by age 75, it's easy to assume that stiff, sore joints are an unavoidable part of aging. The cartilage slowly wears away—leaving bones to scrape against each other.

Not so, says Dr. John Bland, of the University of Vermont College of Medicine. Cartilage may be lost to injury, genetic defects and disease, but normally it's far too slippery to wear out. And so long as some healthy cartilage remains, exercise may bring it back.

A dozen years ago, researchers at the National Institutes of Health got rabbit cartilage to reproduce slowly in lab flasks. At first the cells wouldn't make collagen—the fibrous protein structure of ligaments, tendons and bones.

Proper amounts of vitamin C solved the collagin problem, and stirring things up speeded growth. Cartilage churned with a magnetic stir reproduced 20 to 50 times faster.

Next, Bland and fellow researchers at NIH turned to humans and found no gross difference in reproductive capability between the cartilage cells of children and those of elders (65–84). With proper nutrition and a little "stirring," Bland figured, old cartilage ought to rejuvenate.

Sure enough, in almost two dozen cases, Bland has shown that cartilage may grow again. In one case, after a year of aspirin, vitamins and exercise, a bedridden professor, 85, was able to walk again.

Surgery might have been faster, admits Bland, but "nothing beats your own joints." In any case, to keep moving late in life, keep on the move now.

By Barbara Kevles, "Come Again to Cartilage," *American Health: Fitness of Body and Mind,* July/August 1984, p. 25. Reprinted by permission of Barbara Kevles. Copyright 1984 by Barbara Kevles.

The bones, as living organs, also respond to resistance training in healthful ways according to the specific demands placed upon them. A study of 3000 adult laborers and sports participants showed that the characteristic shapes and structures of bones were significantly influenced by the stress placed upon them.[3] Changes in bone sizes and shapes were noted on shifts in occupation and sports participation. A classic example of the adaptation of bone to stress was reported by Ross.[4] A subject who had lost all but the little finger of his right hand showed remarkable hypertrophy of that digit. In the 32 years since the amputation, his little finger had grown in size to that of the middle finger of his left hand. This was measured and confirmed by x-ray examination of both hands. In another study, nationally ranked athletes were compared with nonathlete controls for bone mineral content.[5] The athletes had significantly more bone mineral content and they demonstrated bone hypertrophy consistent with the demands of their specific sport. The greatest amount of hypertrophy among the athletes was achieved by the weight lifters. The implications of studies such as these are that resistance as well as aerobic exercises strengthen and maintain the integrity of bony tissue.

Osteoporosis, a disease characterized by bone demineralization, may be prevented, delayed, or alleviated by long-term adherence to resistance exercises coupled with some form of aerobic training. "Regular exercise is essential. Bones that are not used are automatically thinned out by the remodeling process."[6]

Reporting on the effects of exercise for older people, the *Harvard Medical School Health Letter* indicated that, approached with caution, weight training can protect bone and soft tissue from injury.[7]

Weight Training for Children

Variety and innovation are important in training programs. Prepubescent children are immature psychologically and physiologically and need the elements of fun and play.
–L. Totten

What about the efficacy of resistance training for young children? Can they benefit from such training or are they exposing their immature musculoskeletal systems to possible harm? The American Academy of Pediatrics (AAP) developed a position paper on weight training and weight lifting for youngsters in 1983.[8] They essentially endorsed weight training for sports performance for adolescents but stated that pre-pubescent children would receive minimum benefits. This was based on the premise that circulating **androgens** in prepubescent children are not sufficiently high to stimulate muscle growth. A number of independent investigations since the publication of the AAP position have refuted the basic premise that strength cannot be attained by prepubescent youngsters with weight training.[9,10,11,12] These studies were well conceived; control groups were used used to account for the natural effects of growth; and weight training regimens which were similar in intensity, frequency, duration, and training techniques to those prescribed for adults were used. Each of these studies demonstrated significant strength gains for the exercised groups compared to nonexercising controls. These gains were even more remarkable considering the short length of training time in three of the four studies (5 to 9 weeks). These data, which are in conflict with the AAP position, prompted the National Strength and Conditioning Association (NSCA) to formulate a position endorsing weight training for prepubescent youngsters.[13] This group also addressed the need for precautions in developing and implementing weight training programs for this age group. Both organizations discourage weight lifting, (which is a sport in which contestants lift maximal weights) until the age of 16 or 17. At this time, the skeletal system is mature enough to withstand such loads. On the other hand, weight training is an activity in which light to moderate weights are used to exercise the major muscle groups of the body.

Nationwide samples of children typically show that they are poorly fit and particularly weak in upper body strength. This is often accompanied by excessive fat or poor body composition. Weight training programs guided by well-qualified instructors would help rectify this situation.[14]

Finally, weight training seems to increase the HDL fraction of cholesterol in the blood, as several well-conceived studies have indicated. Further investigation is needed in this regard but the initial data is promising. Twelve weeks of weight training produced some interesting changes in 34 healthy middle-aged males (average age 42).[15] They lost an average of 2.75 pounds of fat and gained an average of 4.88 pounds of lean tissue during the course of the study. Total cholesterol decreased, HDL-C increased, and LDL-C decreased. These changes are associated with a lower risk for coronary artery disease. Another short-term study with middle-aged male subjects produced similar results.[16] These subjects experienced significant increases in strength and lean body weight and a significant decrease in body fat. In addition, HDL-C increased "in a manner which would suggest a reduction in the risk for cardiovascular disease." Two studies in the Olympic Issue of the 1984 *Journal of the American Medical Association* have produced results which parallel these two studies regarding the health-related benefits of weight training. A-16 week program using sedentary men (average

age 33) and women (average age 27) yielded the following results: women demonstrated a 9.5 percent reduction in total cholesterol, a 17.9 percent decrease in LDL-C, a 14 percent reduction in the ratio of LDL-C to HDL-C, and a 28.3 percent reduction in triglycerides; and men demonstrated a 16.2 percent reduction in LDL-C, a 21.6 percent reduction in the ratio of total cholesterol to HDL-C, and a 28.9 percent reduction in the ratio of LDL-C to HDL-C.[17]

Eleven untrained, middle-aged (40–55), healthy males participated in 16 weeks of resistance training on Nautilus equipment and another 10 healthy same-aged males served as nonexercising controls.[18] At the end of the training period the exercising men improved significantly on the following: (1) LDL cholesterol decreased by 5 percent, (2) HDL cholesterol increased by 13 percent, (3) diastolic blood pressure decreased by 5 mm Hg, and (4) insulin response to glucose ingestion decreased. No comparable changes were observed in the nonexercising controls. The authors concluded that regular participation in resistance training can reduce the risk factors for cardiovascular disease regardless of whether there are accompanying changes in body weight and body composition.

Hurley and his associates investigated the effects of body building versus power lifting on selected blood lipids.[19] The subjects were young healthy males. The results indicated that the body builders, who are strength-trained athletes who typically employ moderate-resistance, high-repetition exercises with short rest intervals, had lipoprotein profiles that were characterized as protective against coronary artery disease. Their HDL-C values were high while their LDL-C values were low. On the other hand, the power lifters who used heavy resistance exercises with few repetitions and long rest periods between repetitions did not have favorable lipoprotein profiles. The type of strength training program appears to be an important variable regarding its potential for health enhancement. These studies support the notion that strength training programs featuring moderate resistance with high repetitions (10 to 12) produce desirable changes in body composition and lipoprotein-lipid levels in the blood. Animal and human studies have shown that the use of anabolic-androgenic steroids to increase muscle strength result in atherogenic lipoprotein profiles.[19,20,21] Steroid use has a particularly devastating effect on HDL cholesterol which reistance exercise is unable to overcome.

Several researchers have investigated the effect of weight training on resting blood pressure. One study found no change in blood pressure,[22] two studies found significant decreases in systolic pressure,[23,24] and another found a significant decrease in both systolic and diastolic pressures.[17] Weight training lowered resting blood pressure in the majority of the studies and did not negatively impact it in any of the studies.

From a health and aesthetic perspective it seems prudent to include resistance exercises in the fitness program because they increase strength, favorably change body composition, increase resting metabolism through the addition of muscle, contribute to the enhancement of self-concept, help prevent low back injury and joint injury, strengthen and thicken the bones (which may delay or prevent osteoporosis), they have the potential for favorably changing blood lipid and lipoprotein levels in ways consistent with lowering the risk for coronary artery disease, and they have produced beneficial changes in systolic and diastolic blood pressures.

Genetic and Gender Considerations _____

Several factors contribute to the differences in strength between males and females. Prior to puberty the differences between the sexes are small but they become substantially greater after puberty. The average male can generate 30 to 40 percent more force than the average female. The disparity is quite large when the sexes are compared for arm and upper body strength but much less when leg strength is compared. One factor responsible for the sex difference in strength is the male sex hormone **testosterone**. This substance stimulates the protein-synthesizing mechanisms and is responsible for the muscle **hypertrophy** seen in males. Females also produce testosterone but at a rate of one-tenth to one-twentieth of that of males, accounting for their lessened ability to gain substantial muscle size. Research has shown that females can make significant gains in strength without developing large muscles. The masculinizing effect of weight training is a myth that has persisted although there is much evidence to the contrary. It is a fact that women do develop muscle tissue with resistance exercises, but muscular development is limited by insufficient quantities of testosterone. Wilmore's study indicated quite nicely that college women could gain significant amounts of strength with ten weeks of weight training without significant increases in muscle size.[25] Male subjects in the same study improved significantly in both strength and muscle size. Cureton agrees that women's muscles don't grow as large as those of males but for a different reason.[26] He hypothesized that the, "absolute changes in muscle hypertrophy following weight training do tend to be larger in men than in women, probably because the initial size of the muscle fibers is larger and the number of fibers undergoing hypertrophy in some muscles is greater." He further indicated that women can and do get stronger and, on a percentage basis, they can achieve the same muscle hypertrophy as men without looking like men. Sex differences in muscle size are readily discernible by observing contestants in mixed pairs body building contests. Despite similar training philosophies and procedures, males develop extraordinary muscularity while females develop well-defined but significantly less muscularity. The differences between the sexes is considerable but when compared to the average woman, female body builders have more muscle tissue, much more muscle definition, and considerably less body fat.

Strength differences between the sexes essentially disappear when strength is measured by cross-sectional area of muscle tissue. Each sex is capable of generating a similar amount of force—3 to 4 kg/cm^2. Since the quality of muscle between males and females appears to be similar, the differences in strength seem to be due to the total muscle mass of males. Males may have as much as 50 percent more muscle tissue than females.

Hypertrophy of muscle fibers, total amount of muscle mass, and recruitment of motor units are associated with strength gains. Under ordinary circumstances, we are unable to mobilize all of the motor units in a given muscle. Training and emotionally charged situations increase our ability to recruit more motor units, thereby producing a more forceful muscular contraction.

Neural and cultural influences are also involved in the development of strength. According to Brooks, "old men and women of all ages seem to increase strength mainly by neural adaptation (with some hypertrophy), whereas young men rely more on increases in muscle size."[27] The evidence for the neural input to strength comes from cases of superhuman feats of strength that have been observed and documented from time to time. Workers trapped under heavy steel girders as a result of construction cave-ins or youngsters trapped beneath automobiles have provided some of the settings in which phenomenal feats of strength have occurred in both sexes. As a result of these extreme emotional conditions, rescuers have ignored body signals regarding their own safety and have been capable of expressions of strength which substantially exceed the ordinary. The victims of these unfortunate accidents are often spared by the heroic efforts of their rescuers. These efforts often result in muscle and skeletal damage because the average human is not trained or equipped to handle such heavy loads. People generally learn their strength limits through experience with heavy objects. But the urgency of rescue situations is characterized by a surge in the flow of adrenalin accompanied by suppression of the inhibitory neural impulses that formulate our safety system. A combination of both neural and chemical input produces superhuman strength for the brief interval needed for an extraordinary performance.

Neural factors are responsible for the rapid gains in strength achieved during the first two to six weeks of resistance training. These increases occur without muscle growth in fiber size or cross-sectional area and provide additional evidence supporting the neural influence associated with expressions of strength.[28,29] Some of the neural mechanisms include, (1) recruitment of motor units, (2) increased motor neuron excitability, (3) effective inhibition of antagonists, and (4) inhibition of neural protective mechanisms. The mechanisms designed to protect us from injury may be suppressed to some extent in highly emotionally-charged situations. Weight training is another vehicle through which the body is trained to inhibit the safety system. For example, untrained subjects were able to generate 17 percent more force in the muscles responsible for elbow flexion under hypnosis while trained subjects experienced no improvement.[30] The trained group was unable to improve because their weight training programs had already taught their bodies to repress the safety systems and hypnosis was unable to add to the effects achieved by training.

Sex role expectations and cultural dictates have discouraged women from participating in strength development programs. While the stereotypical image of the soft rounded female prevails, it has lost some if its appeal. Many of today's females, and indeed many female watchers, consider attractiveness to be synonomous with a firm, healthy-looking, fit body. It is indeed encouraging to find women, both young and old, in our Fitness Center who devote a portion of their fitness time to weight training because they have come to understand its contribution to physical appearance and health. Unfortunately, the myth that women will build masculine-type bulging muscles with resistance exercise persists in spite of evidence to the contrary. Proponents of this myth cite examples of female athletes who are muscularly well-developed as proof of the effect of training. In reality, these athletes are successful performers because they have the genetic endowment to capitalize upon training—they had a head start. All women—indeed, all people—respond to training but in differing degrees. Well-muscled female athletes might be producing above-average levels of testosterone which would account for their adaptation to training. Others might combine training with the ingestion of **anabolic steroids**. These are drugs that have similar muscle-building qualities as testosterone. The term "anabolic" implies that these substances promote the development of tissue, particularly muscle tissue. Because these drugs are considered to be harmful, the dosage that can be safely studied in laboratory experiments with humans is only a fraction of the dosage taken by competitive athletes. The laboratory experiments have not confirmed the alleged acceleration of muscle tissue growth with steroids, but many athletes attribute their muscle growth and strength increases directly to steroid use.

Steroids are a health hazard and illegal when used for the purposes of athletic enhancement. The medical risks associated with long-term usage include the possibility of contracting cancer, damage to the liver and kidneys, and sterility, to name a few. After studying the world-wide literature on this subject, the American College of Sports Medicine produced a position paper on the use and abuse of steroids.[31] The effect of steroid usage in men "often, but not always reduces the output of testosterone and gonadotropins and reduces spermatogenesis." The effects of steroids on females, particularly prepubertal adolescents or those who have not completed full growth, is especially hazardous. Steroid use disrupts the normal pattern of growth, promotes the development of acne, and produces such masculinizing effects as a deepening of the voice and growth of facial and body hair. These long-term risks far outweigh the short-term benefits that may be achieved. The purpose of this text is to present the necessity of exercise and physical fitness as an integral part of a wellness lifestyle. The use of steroids is to be deplored for competitors and noncompetitors alike because it is the antithesis of wellness.

In humans, it appears that the total number of muscle fibers and the fiber type is set genetically and that both are fully established at birth. Current research indicates that the number of muscle fibers probably cannot be increased nor can fiber type be changed. If this precept is accurate then the increases in muscle size resulting from training must be caused by hypertrophy of the existing fibers. However, a few studies have investigated the possibility that strength training might lead to an increase in the number of muscle fibers. Van Linge initiated this line of inquiry by transplanting a small rat muscle tendon into a position in the rat's body where it was obliged to exert unusual and unaccustomed amounts of force.[32] After several weeks of heavy work the muscle tendon was examined and found to be twice its original weight and three times its original strength. Unexpectedly, the heavy workload stimulated the development of new muscle fibers. Van Linge's study produced the first evidence of this phenomenon. More recent studies have indicated that heavy resistance training led to the formation of new muscle fibers in some animal species.[33] The existing muscle fibers split and each split fiber grew ultimately achieving the thickness of the parent fiber.[34]

One of the better studies from a research design perspective showed that heavy resistance training resulted in hyperplasia of muscle fibers in cats.[35] **Hyperplasia** is an increase in the number of muscle fibers in the affected muscle. This adaptation to strength training has not been verified in human subjects but it remains a possibility.

Muscle fiber type—red (**slow-twitch**) and white (**fast-twitch**)—seem to be unchangeable; that is, red fibers always remain red and white fibers remain white. There are marked differences between the fibers in terms of function. Red muscle fibers function aerobically, are richly supplied with blood, slow to fatigue, and relatively slow in contractile speed. White muscle fibers function anaerobically, are poorly supplied with blood, rapid to fatigue, and fast in contractile speed. White fibers are larger, contract with more force, and are well-equipped for short-duration, high-intensity work. On the other hand, red fibers, with their abundant blood supply, are well-adapted for endurance work. A motor nerve stimulates either all white or all red muscle fibers and when the impulse is delivered all fibers in the motor unit contract.

Muscle fibers do not cross over; that is, red fibers remain red and white fibers remain white regardless of the type of training to which they are exposed.[36] Heavy aerobic training will not cause the white fibers to become red but it will produce some degree of adaptation to aerobic work in these fibers. Conversely, weight training will produce adaptation of the red fibers without actual conversion from red to white. The ratio between red and white muscle fiber is set genetically and appears to be resistant to change. Changing one fiber type to another under natural conditions is probably impossible because the motor nerves which innervate the muscles determine muscle type. To produce a change in muscle fiber type would require a structural change in the motor nerve which supplies it with electrical impulses.

The ratio of red to white muscle fiber can be determined by examining muscle biopsies from selected sites. The world-class aerobic athletes (distance runners, cyclists, cross-country skiers, etc.) have predominantly red muscle fibers, while the world class power or anaerobic event athletes (shot-putters, hammer throwers, power and Olympic lifters) have a predominance of white muscle fibers. Knowing the ratio of fiber type could be important for these competitors but it is relatively unimportant when one exercises for health reasons. Health enthusiasts can participate in a variety of activities with some degree of success and satisfaction regardless of fiber type. When health is the objective, white-fiber people (a majority of fibers are white) can participate successfully in aerobic activities and, conversely, red-fiber people (a majority of fibers are red) can successfully participate in anaerobic activities. The connotation of success as it is used here refers to the amount of satisfaction and enjoyment derived by participants and does not refer to competitive success.

Training Considerations

Achieving optimum results safely with progressive resistance exercises requires some knowledge. You should know

1. how often to work out
2. the length of each workout
3. proper lifting and spotting techniques
4. the amount of weight with which to begin each lift
5. the number of times (repetitions) that the weight should be lifted
6. the number of times an exercise should be repeated (sets)
7. proper warm-up and cool-down procedures
8. the order of the exercises
9. the length of the rest periods between repetitions and sets.

The next step is to select the mode of training that best suits your needs. You may select from isometric, isotonic, or isokinetic training systems or combine two or more of these. The selection should be based upon your objectives, the availability of equipment and space, and the amount of time that you wish to invest.

Isometric Training

Isometric exercises train the muscular system by a series of static contractions, where no change in muscle length occurs. Force is applied against an unyielding object so that the affected muscles contract in a fixed position. An illustration of an isometric contraction appears in Figure 8.4. In this illustration, the top of the doorjam is the unyielding object. If this exercise is repeated regularly the affected muscles will gain in strength at the angle in which the joint is stressed. The development of strength through isometrics is joint angle specific, that is, maximal strength occurs at the angle of contraction.[37] There is a training carryover of approximately 20 degrees from that angle. Isometric contractions at four different angles throughout the range of motion of elbow flexion increases strength at each angle and significantly increases the dynamic power of the elbow flexors.[38] (See Figure 8.5.)

To optimize the results from isometric training, one should adhere to the following guidelines:

1. The total contraction time should be greater then 30 seconds. This can be accomplished by a few contractions of long duration or many contractions of short duration.[39]
2. Maximal contractions are superior to submaximal contractions.
3. Daily isometric training produces greater results.

FIGURE 8.4

Isometric Contraction

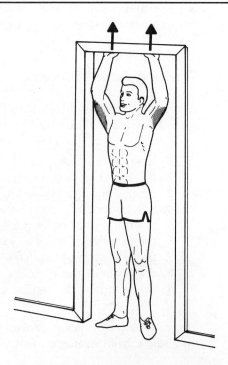

FIGURE 8.5

**Isometric Curl
Performed at Different
joint Angles**
Each dot represents a
joint angle where an
isometric contraction
should occur in order to
work the bicep muscle
through a full range of
motion.

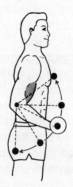

Isometrics may be performed quickly, with little or no equipment, and in very little space, but they tend to raise blood pressure by clamping down on the blood vessels. This increases the resistance to blood flow, forcing the heart to pump with greater force. These exercises are particularly unsuitable for older people, hypertensives, those with heart disease, atherosclerosis, or any form of compromised circulation. Since most Americans above age 35 have some degree of atherosclerosis, it would be wise to choose another means of developing the muscular system.

Improvement in strength is difficult to assess isometrically because the resistance does not change throughout the program. Knowledge of results remains a mystery unless you have access to equipment that records the amount of force exerted. Motivation is difficult to sustain in the absence of feedback.

The time savings associated with isometrics compared to other forms of resistance training diminishes when you attempt, and correctly so, to develop strength throughout the full range of movement for each exercise. This requires 5 to 10 sets of each exercise. The nature of isometric exercises is such that they stimulate the development of strength but they do not develop muscular endurance.

The disadvantages of isometrics tend to outweigh the advantages. There seem to be minimal health benefits associated with this type of exercise. However, this is the only type of exercise that may be performed to limit the muscular atrophy occurring when limbs are immobilized. The muscles of a leg placed in a cast because of a bone break may be exercised isometrically for the purpose of reducing atrophy with the approval of the physician.

Isotonic Training

Isotonic exercises feature dynamic muscle movement against a constant resistance. When executed correctly, the affected muscles shorten and move the resistance through a full range of motion around a joint. An isotonic muscular contraction is one in which the muscle exerts a constant force throughout the entire movement.[40] The term "isotonic" may soon be replaced by the term "dynamic constant external resistance" because lifting a specific weight through a range of motion is not truly isotonic.[41] The actual force exerted by the muscle is not constant. At some point in the movement the position of the joint will produce a mechanical advantage resulting in less force needed to overcome the resistance. For example, the two-arm biceps curl begins with a barbell held at arm's length resting on the thighs (Figure 8.6). The object is to lift the weight in a semicircular motion to the chest by contracting the biceps muscles. This constitutes the concentric phase of the two-arm curl. Slowly lowering the weight to the starting position represents the eccentric phase of the lift.

Both movements, concentric and eccentric, develop strength in the affected muscles. Researchers have investigated the effectiveness of each of the two movements in developing strength and found that neither was superior to the other.[42] Most dynamic exercises require both concentric and eccentric contractions and most training equipment incorporates both types of movement so participants receive the benefits of both. There is one negative feature associated with the eccentric phase of exercise: it appears to be responsible for the muscle soreness that occurs following a workout. Therefore, isotonic training sessions should be held every other day to allow for muscle recovery between sessions. Three to four workouts per week are sufficient for developing strength in the novice lifter. Frequency may be increased as one becomes trained and can tolerate the increased stresses.

Weight training is more effective for developing strength than calisthenics because the resistance can be adjusted as strength increases. Body weight is the resistance in calisthenic exercises. It can be increased by strapping on weight or by having a partner apply resistance and it can be reduced by modifying some of the exercises. These techniques tend to be too inconvenient for the average participant.

The starting weight in weight training is determined by trial and error. Find a weight which you can lift no more than 10 to 12 times (repetitions) and then perform three sets of each exercise. Add weight when you are able to execute 15 to 16 repetitions for three sets. At this point, add enough weight to bring you back to 10 repetitions and continue with that weight until you can perform 15 to 16 repetitions and repeat the cycle by adding weight once again. Each repetition should be executed slowly, rhythmically, and in strict form. You should not throw the weight during the concentric phase nor drop it rapidly during the eccentric phase. Move slowly enough (approximately 2 to 3 seconds for each phase) so as to maintain control of the weight and be sure to fully contract and extend the muscles during each repetition. Generally, the heaviest weight that can be lifted for 10 to 12 repetitions represents approximately 75

FIGURE 8.6

Isotonic Barbell Curl

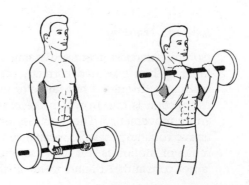

percent of one's maximum lift (1 Repetition Maximum-RM) and is a sufficient stimulus for developing muscles and improving strength. Bear in mind that the weight training program suggested here is a supplement to the aerobic program and it is not intended to produce a champion weight lifter or a Mr. or Miss Universe. It is intended to develop some strength and to increase muscle tissue. It should be explained that the optimum number of sets, repetitions, and amount of weight to be lifted are not fully known for meeting various objectives. The program suggested in this text is only one of many that has produced results.

For those who prefer to leave the health benefits to the aerobic portion of their training in order to concentrate on the strength development properties of weight training, the optimum routine is to lift heavy weights for four to six repetitions maximum, do more sets and take ample rest time (two to three minutes) between sets.[43] Since the optimum development of strength is not one of the major objectives of this book, interested students are directed to the following references:

T. L. De Lorme and A.L. Watkins, "Techniques of Progressive Resistance Exercise," *Archives of Physical Medicine* 29 (1978): 263.

W. L. Westcott, *Strength Fitness—Physiological Principles and Training Techniques*, Boston: Allyn and Bacon, Inc., 1983.

M.H. Stone and H. O'Bryant, *Weight Training: A Scientific Approach*, Minneapolis: Burgess Publishing Co., Inc., 1986.

Always warm-up prior to weight training or any other resistance exercises and cool-down after the workout. The warm-up should consist of stretching exercises and some activities that elevate the heart rate such as jogging in place, rope skipping, jumping jacks, and other calisthenic-type exercises. According to Westcott, programs that utilize sets of 10 to 12 repetitions do not require warm-up sets with lighter weights.[44] That is, it is not necessary to perform a set with a weight lighter than the weight that will ultimately be used for each exercise. He states that "under normal circumstances, a weightload that can be lifted ten times should not cause injury or require special preparation."

The cool-down procedure is important because what occurs during this time will affect recovery from the workout. Lactic acid produced during the workout seems to be most effectively removed from the muscles by 15 minutes of moderate aerobic activity. Rhythmic and continuous activities that stimulate circulation seem to accelerate the removal of lactic acid from the muscles. Quick removal allows the rebuilding process to occur and readies the individual for the next workout. The length of each workout will depend on program objectives, number of exercises, number of repetitions and sets performed, and the amount of rest taken between exercises. Beginners can benefit from one to two sets of each exercise.[45] The number of sets can increase to as many as five as fitness improves.

Rest periods less than one minute result in very high blood lactate levels and will impair one's ability to produce maximum force because the next exercise begins before recovery from the previous one is complete.[46]

There is some evidence indicating that large-muscle exercises should precede exercises affecting the smaller muscle groups. In that regard, bench presses, half-squats, and standing presses should precede dumbbell curls or lateral raises.[47] It may also be wise to alternate muscle groups with each exercise. The bench press should not directly follow the standing press because both exercises work the extensor muscles of the arms. You will be fresher if you separate these two exercises with one or two others for different muscle groups. Varying the training program may promote adherence and provide a measure of enjoyment. There are many ways of injecting variety but one of the latest of these techniques is "periodization." One of the basic concepts of **periodization** involves starting with high volumes of exercise at low intensity. The training period is divided into different cycles in which the volume is periodically reduced and the intensity is concomitantly increased. This system has been effective in developing strength. It may be accomplished by alternating light, moderate, and heavy workout days during the week. Another option is to perform light sets of 12 to 15 RM for two or three weeks; moderate sets of 8 to 10 RM for the next two or three weeks; and heavy sets of 3 to 5 RM for the last two or three weeks of the period.

Unlike isometrics, isotonic exercises develop strength throughout the full range of muscular movement. Progress is easily and objectively measured because a known quantity of weight is added as strength increases. Motivation is more easily maintained when results are readily available. One further advantage of isotonic training systems is that they are adaptable to free weights or exercise machines.

One of the disadvantages of isotonic exercise is that the maximum amount of weight that can be lifted is dependent upon the weakest point in the range of motion. This may be a limiting factor regarding optimum strength development throughout the range of muscle movement. A second disadvantage is that isotonic exercises produce muscle soreness because of their eccentric phase.

Isokinetic Training

Isokinetic training, which involves a unique system of dynamic exercises, was introduced in 1968 by James Perrine, a bioengineer who developed an exercise device that allowed for maximum resistance at a constant speed throughout the full range of movement. As a result, this revolutionary device theoretically improves upon traditional dynamic exercises where maximum resistance can only be experienced at the weakest point in the muscular contraction. Isokinetic devices accommodate to the applied force by adjusting the resistance to equal the force. The greater the application of force by the participant, the greater the resistance by the device. Highly motivated participants who apply maximum force throughout the full range of motion will be met with maximum resistance throughout. Isokinetic exercise's potential for strength development has generated much interest from athletes and the general public. Research in the next few years should determine the effectiveness of isokinetic training.

The early isokinetic devices could only load the muscles concentrically. The eccentric phase was passive or unloaded. This meant that strength was gained concentrically and there was no delayed muscle soreness. Today a new generation of isokinetic devices is capable of loading the muscle concentrically and eccentrically.

The major advantage of isokinetic training is that the resistance is maximum throughout the entire range of motion. Theoretically then, maximal strength may be obtained throughout the range of motion. The newer isokinetic devices allow one to select the speed of exercise movement. This has important implications for those who wish to develop strength for transfer to a specific sport or physical activity.

The disadvantage of isokinetic training is that it requires specialized equipment designed to produce isokinetic loading such as the Mini-Gym, or variable resistance equipment, such as Nautilus and Cam II. Some of this equipment is very expensive and is usually found only in health clubs, spas, and universities. However, there are some devices that cost no more than a good set of free weights.

In summary, all three exercise training systems—isometrics, isotonics and isokinetics—are effective in building and maintaining strength; however, static nature of isometric exercises limits their capacity to enhance muscular endurance. These three exercise systems are compared on ten factors in Table 8.1.

Circuit Training

Circuit training is a relatively new concept developed in England approximately 30 years ago. This versatile training method promotes the development of muscular strength and endurance as well as cardiorespiratory endurance. Training goals must be established in order to construct an appropriate circuit.

Typical circuits consist of a minimum of six to a maximum of twelve exercises. Each exercise represents a different station in the circuit. The object of this type of training is to complete each circuit rapidly. Each completion is followed by a short rest period of approximately two minutes. The entire workout includes three complete routes through the circuit.

Different components of fitness may be developed simultaneously with circuit training. The number of stations devoted to each component should be determined at the outset. The stations should be arranged so that the same muscle group is not exercised at two consecutive stations. When possible, exercises for each of the components of fitness should be alternated, that is, a cardiorespiratory exercise should not be followed by another cardiorespiratory exercise. For group participation, each station should be numbered and labeled with a concise set of instructions. A sample circuit combining the development

Eight to 12 weeks of circuit weight training increases VO₂ max 5 percent in men and 8 percent in women.
–L. R. Gettman

TABLE 8.1   Summary of Isometric, Isotonic, and Isokinetic Training Methods

Factors	Isometric	Isotonic	Isokinetic
1. Rate of strength gain	3[1]	2	1
2. Strength gain throughout the range of movement	3	2	1
3. Time per training session	1	3	2
4. Expense	1	2	2–3
5. Ease of performance	1	3	2
6. Ease of Progress Assessment	3	1	3
7. Probability of soreness	Little	Great	Little
8. Probability of musculoskeletal injury	Slight	Moderate	Slight
9. Cardiac Risk	Moderate	Slight	Some
10. Skill Improvement	None	Slight	Some

[1]A rating of 1 is superior; 2 is intermediate; 3 is inferior

Adapted from D. R. Lamb, *Physiology of Exercise*, New York: Macmillan Publishing Co., 1978.

of strength, muscular endurance, and cardiorespiratory endurance is presented in Table 8.2. The weights selected for each exercise should be heavy enough so that no more than 12 repetitions can be completed.

Table 8.2 illustrates the principles of circuit training. Improvement is reflected by the amount of time needed to complete each circuit or by the amount of work accomplished at each station or by both concurrently. Overload is initiated only when appropriate.

Circuit training has several advantages over conventional training systems. First, it is not boring because it incorporates a variety of activities. Second, different fitness components may be developed together. Third, circuits do not require large amounts of space nor are they confined to the indoors. Fourth, this system can accommodate groups of people since any station can be an entry point into the circuit. Fifth, the entire workout can be completed in less than 40 minutes.

Circuit training has few disadvantages for people whose major interest is the use of exercise for health enhancement. It may be employed as an adjunct to an aerobic program or it may be the primary vehicle for developing aerobic fitness. This is easily accomplished by loading the circuit with aerobic activities.

As with all forms of exercise, beginners should approach circuit training cautiously and slowly. It is best to utilize the circuit system after a degree of physical fitness has been developed through less demanding training systems. Enter circuit training with the following guidelines: (1) take at least one minute of rest between stations, (2) select weights which allow you to perform the suggested number of repetitions without straining, and (3) do the aerobic exercises slowly or reduce the suggested time for performing each. Training will result in progress and you will be able to reduce the rest period between stations to approximately 15 seconds, increase the weight and/or number of repetitions for each exercise, and increase the length and/or speed of the aerobic activities.

Overload, Progression, and Maintenance

Muscles grow in strength and size in response to the amount of overload placed upon them. **Overload** may be accomplished by increasing the resistance or by

TABLE 8.2 Circuit Training

Station	Exercise	Repetitions or Time
1	Bench press	12
2	Rope skipping	2 min
3	Two-arm curl	12
4	Half-squat	15
5	Stationary bike	2 min
6	Situps	20
7	Standing press	12
8	Running in place	2 min
9	Upright rowing	12
10	Toe raises	15

increasing the number of repetitions completed for each exercise. For strength development, maximum results are attained with few repetitions (4 to 6) and heavy weights. Muscular endurance occurs with 20 to 30 repetitions and light to moderate weights. Programs that attempt to develop both strength and endurance represent a compromise between the two, with resistance selected to elicit 10 to 12 repetitions per exercise. The resistance is increased when the number of repetitions increases to 15 to 16. This represents a safe and effective means of applying overload according to a set schedule of progression. This schedule may be continued until you reach a level of muscular strength and endurance that is satisfactory for your needs. At this point, a maintenance program should be initiated to preserve the gains that you have worked so hard to acquire. Two workouts per week are sufficient for maintenance.

Frequency, Intensity, Duration, and Rest

The optimum frequency of resistance training depends on the system selected. Isometric exercises may be practiced daily because muscle soreness does not occur, but because of motivational concerns and the need for muscles to recover, it would be best to take one or two days off each week. Isotonic training leads to considerable muscle soreness initially, so at least one day of rest is needed between workouts. Adequate rest is as important as consistent exercise because muscles need time to recuperate in order to meet the challenge of the next workout.

Muscle soreness which persists into the next scheduled workout reflects inadequate rest or an intensity of exercise which is greater than can be tolerated at this point in the training program. Isokinetic exercises which are eccentrically unloaded can be done every day, but the same motivational concerns would apply here as with any other daily activity—burn-out is a distinct possibility. If isokinetic exercises are loaded both ways then three to four sessions per week would suffice because muscle soreness would occur if the frequency were not reduced.

Exercise and Sore Muscles

Muscles may become sore during exercise (acute soreness) and/or one to two days later (delayed soreness). Acute soreness is probably the result of reduced blood flow to exercising muscles. When muscles contract vigorously—as in weight training—blood vessels constrict, inhibiting the delivery of oxygen and nutrients as well as the removal of waste products.

Delayed muscle soreness occurs 24 to 48 hours after a workout. There are several possible explanations for this phenomenon, but the most widely accepted of these is the tissue damage theory. Proponents of this theory state that exercise damages muscle fibers and connective tissue, which in turn respond by swelling and impinging upon nerves, resulting in soreness.

Lactic acid accumulation in the muscles was thought to be involved in delayed soreness, but this is unlikely because lactic acid is removed from muscles long before soreness occurs. Secondly, activities which produce lactic acid do not necessarily result in muscle soreness, while other activities produce no lactic acid but considerable muscle soreness.

Delayed muscle soreness occurs to untrained beginners, but it also occurs to trained participants who overload excessively or who change from one activity to another. It can be prevented or minimized by exercising within your capacity and by overloading in small increments. People trained in one activity should approach new activities cautiously because their previous training may not carry over to the new activity.

The antidote to delayed muscle soreness involves stretching exercises, light workouts, or complete rest. The best treatment is prevention.

Optimal gains in strength occur with high intensity training. This translates to near-maximum resistance for all exercises regardless of the training system. The duration of the workout will depend upon the program objectives, the number of exercises, and the training system. A well-conceived isometric or isokinetic program might take 30 to 45 minutes compared to an hour for isotonic programs. If maximal strength development is the goal, the workout may take two hours or longer.

Safety Tips

The risk of injury is increased when people progress from sedentary habits to vigorous physical activity. Karpovich studied the rate of injury associated with weight training and found it to be one of the safest forms of physical activity.[47] This study was completed more than 30 years ago but a European study in 1970 reaffirmed these results. Familiarization and practice of simple safety procedures will sharply minimize the incidence of injury.

The following suggestions will help to decrease the risk associated with resistance training:

1. Warm up prior to working out. The warm-up should include stretching and exercises of moderate intensity that cause sweating and an increase in muscle temperature (see Figures 8.7 through 8.20). The evidence regarding the effectiveness of warming up for improved performance and injury prevention is inconclusive, but it should also be emphasized that the evidence against it is not compelling.
2. Learn correct lifting techniques.
   a. Keep the weight close to your body during the lift.
   b. Lift all weights resting on the floor with your legs rather than with the lower back. This is accomplished by placing your feet close to the bar, bending your knees and lowering your hips into a half-squat position. Keep your back straight and your head up. This technique applies to lifting a barbell, a child, a piece of furniture, or any other object.
   c. Do not hold your breath during the lift. Breath holding can be dangerous, particularly if you are having difficulty pressing a weight overhead. If the breath is held during this time the chest compresses and the glottis (an opening between the vocal cords) closes, resulting in greatly elevated pressure within the chest cavity. The blood vessels returning blood to the heart may be shut down as the pressure in the chest exceeds that in the veins. This produces a sudden drop in blood pressure and a back-up in the flow of blood attempting to reach the heart. Dizziness, which may be followed by fainting, will occur unless you exhale. When exhaling, a surge of blood rushes into the

heart and blood pressure increases to well above normal values. These circumstances, collectively known as the **Valsalva** phenomenon, may be tolerated by young people with healthy circulatory systems, but it is an unwise and potentially dangerous practice. This is particularly hazardous for older people and people who have undetected weaknesses in the heart and circulatory system.

   d. Avoid excessive backward lean (hyperextension of the low back) when pressing a weight overhead.

3. Make sure that the collars securing the metal plates to dumbbells and barbells are tightly bound to the bar and that pins are fully inserted if you use weight machines.

4. Use rubber-soled shoes for secure footing.

5. Gloves are effective in protecting against blister and callouses and decrease the likelihood of slippage due to perspiration. Chalk dust can be used if you do not wish to wear gloves.

6. Work out with a partner for safety and mutual motivation. Partners are especially handy as spotters for such lifts as bench presses and half-squats.

FIGURE 8.7

Neck and Upper Back Stretch
Slowly pull your head forward until you feel a stretch in the back of the neck and hold for 5 to 10 seconds. Do 2 to 3 sets.

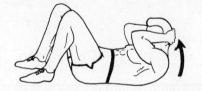

FIGURE 8.8

Elongated Stretch
Stretch by reaching in both directions. Extend your fingers and toes and hold for 5 to 10 seconds. Do 2 to 3 sets.

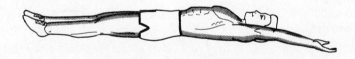

FIGURE 8.9

Low Back Stretch
Pull both legs to your chest and curl your head up to your knees. Hold 15 to 30 seconds and do one set.

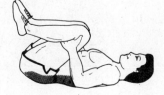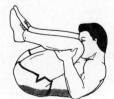

FIGURE 8.10

Calf and Hamstring Stretch
Straighten the extended leg and reach forward and pull back on your toes to increase the stretch on the calf muscle. Hold for 15 to 30 seconds and reverse legs. Do one set.

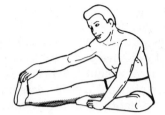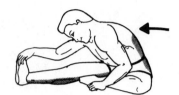

FIGURE 8.11

Triceps and Shoulder Stretch
Gently and slowly pull the elbow behind the head. Hold for 15 to 30 seconds and reverse arms. Do one set.

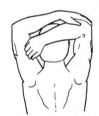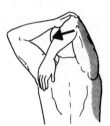

FIGURE 8.12

Arm, Shoulder and Chest Stretch
Interlace your fingers, straighten and lift the arms to produce a stretch in the arms, shoulders, and chest. Hold 15 to 30 seconds. Do one set.

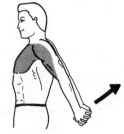

FIGURE 8.13

Groin Stretch
Lean forward from the hips until you feel a stretch in the groin area. Hold for 30 seconds and do one set.

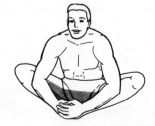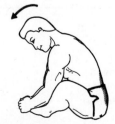

FIGURE 8.14

Calf Stretch
Keep the heel of the back foot on the floor and point this foot straight at the wall. Do one set of 15 to 30 seconds for each leg.

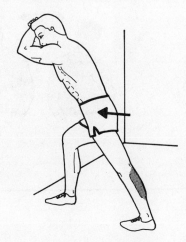

FIGURE 8.15

Achilles Tendon Stretch
Bend the knee of the extended leg in order to stretch the Achilles Tendon. Hold 15 to 30 seconds and repeat with the other leg.

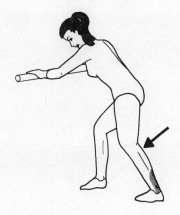

FIGURE 8.16

Side Stretch
Keep your hips facing front and bend to the left. Hold for 5 to 10 seconds and repeat on the right side. Do 3 repetitions on each side.

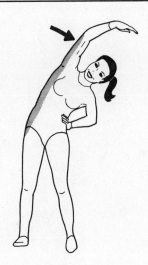

FIGURE 8.17

Neck Stretch
Bend your neck alternately to the left, right, front, and back. Hold each position for 5 seconds and do 2 repetitions. Do not rotate your neck—each movement should be distinct.

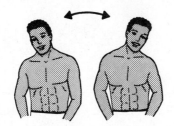
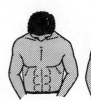
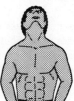

FIGURE 8.18

Jog in Place
Jog slowly in place for 30 to 60 seconds. Lift your knees as shown.

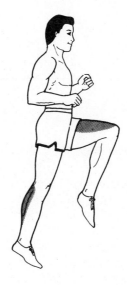

FIGURE 8.19

Rope Jumping
Jump slowly for 60 seconds. Keep your elbows close to your sides, turn the rope with small circular motions of your hands and wrists and jump high enough to clear the rope.

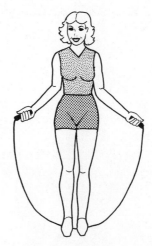

FIGURE 8.20

Quadriceps Stretch
Pull your right foot up to
the buttocks and bend
forward from the waist.
Hold 15 to 30 seconds
and repeat with the other
leg.

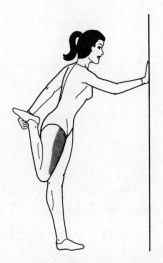

Exercises for Developing Strength and Endurance

Programs for developing muscular strength and endurance for health purposes differ significantly from those utilized by athletes preparing for competition. Athletes attempt to develop strength and endurance in a manner specific to the sport in which they participate. They train their muscles to apply force in a manner similar to the demands of their sport. These programs are highly structured and leave little room for variety and fun. Those who engage in resistance exercises for the health benefits have a wide variety of exercises and several systems from which to choose. Isotonic and/or isokinetic exercises using free weights and/or weight machines are recommended. The major muscle groups of the body should be exercised in each session. Figures 8.21 and 8.22 show some of the major muscles of the body.

Selected exercises for the major muscle groups are presented in Figures 8.23–8.32, illustrated with both free weights and machine weights. The muscles that are developed by each exercise are highlighted in the free weight figures through the use of shading. Refer to Figures 8.21 and 8.22 for the name and location of the muscles which are affected by each exercise. These exercises comprise a good basic program for developing strength and endurance. Three sets can be completed in 30 to 45 minutes and would be an excellent supplement to your aerobic program. Either the free weight or machine weight method will develop the muscular system, and both have advantages and disadvantages.

FIGURE 8.21

Selected Muscles of the Body—Front View (Shaded areas indicate bone).

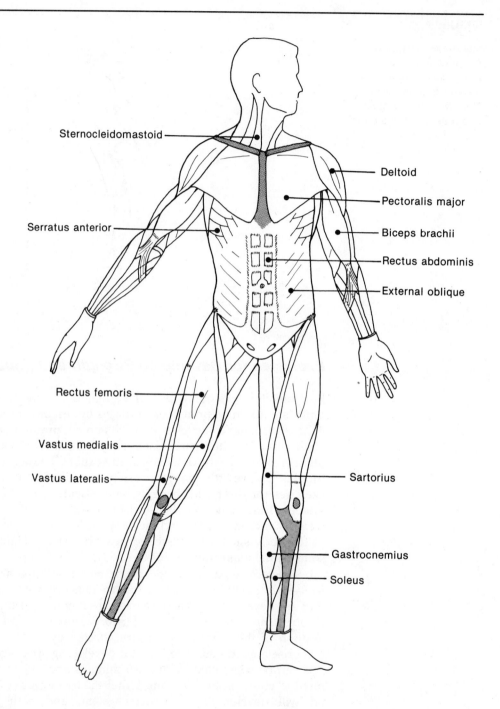

Sternocleidomastoid

Deltoid

Pectoralis major

Serratus anterior

Biceps brachii

Rectus abdominis

External oblique

Rectus femoris

Vastus medialis

Vastus lateralis

Sartorius

Gastrocnemius

Soleus

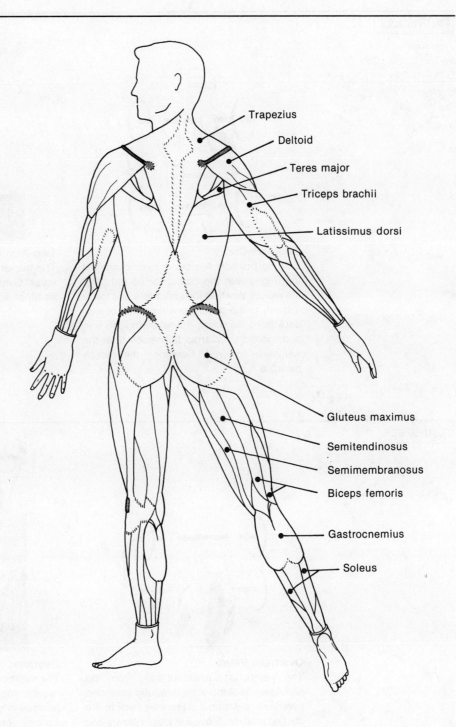

FIGURE 8.22

Selected Muscles of the Body—Back View (Shaded areas indicate bone).

Trapezius

Deltoid

Teres major

Triceps brachii

Latissimus dorsi

Gluteus maximus

Semitendinosus

Semimembranosus

Biceps femoris

Gastrocnemius

Soleus

FIGURE 8.23

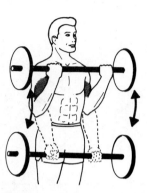

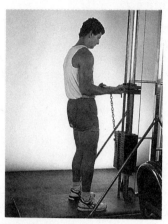

Two-Arm Curl

Starting position: the bar is resting against the thighs with the palms facing out. Curl the weight slowly to the shoulders and lower it slowly to the starting position. Do not lean back from the waist, do not swing the bar, and extend your arms fully each time the weight is lowered. Develops the biceps muscles.

Two-Arm Curl

The two-arm curl is performed on the Universal Gym by following the same directions as those for the free weights.

FIGURE 8.24

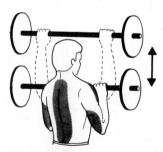

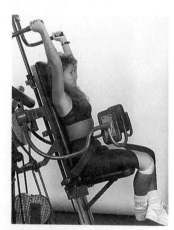

Overhead Press

The weight is pushed upward from the shoulders until the arms are fully extended overhead and then it is lowered back to the starting position. Move the weight slowly and rhythmically. Avoid excessive backward lean and do not jerk the weight by bending and extending the knees. Develops the triceps, deltoids, and trapezius.

Overhead Press

The overhead press on Nautilus equipment is performed in the seated position. Strap yourself in and adjust the height of the seat so that you can complete a full range of motion.

FIGURE 8.25

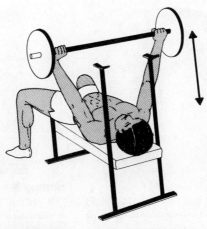

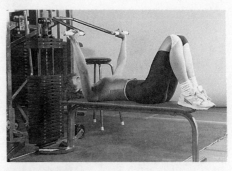

Bench Press

Lie on your back on an exercise bench and keep your feet flat on the floor for balance. Start with the weight on your chest, slowly push it to arm's length, and slowly lower it to the starting position. If you use free weights, it is best to have a spotter who can assist in returning the weight to the stand at the completion of the exercise. Develops the pectoralis majors, deltoids and triceps.

Bench Press

This exercise is performed on the Universal Gym by following the same directions as those for the free weights. One word of caution: if you have low back problems, or if your tendency is to arch your back in the lifting phase on either free weights or Universal, it would be advisable to bend your knees and place your feet on the bench.

FIGURE 8.26

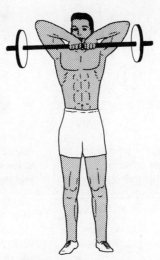

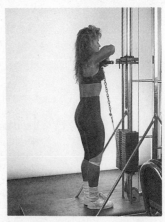

Two-Arm High Pulls

Starting position: the bar is held against the thighs, arms extended, palms facing inward, hands close together. Slowly pull the weight to the chin ending with elbows high and slowly lower to the starting position. Develops the trapezius, deltoids and biceps.

Two-Arm High Pulls

High pulls on the Universal follow the same directions as free weights.

FIGURE 8.27

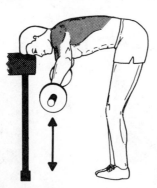

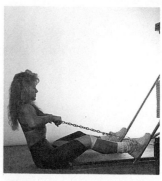

Bent-Over Rowing
Bend from the waist and rest your forehead on a table. This position minimizes the likelihood of back injury. Start with the weight held at arms length, bend your knees slightly and slowly pull the weight to your chest and lower to the starting position. Develops the latissimus dorsi, deltoids, and biceps.

Sitting Row
Sit on the floor, legs extended, facing the Universal and pull the bar back to your chest. Do not lean back as you pull.

FIGURE 8.28

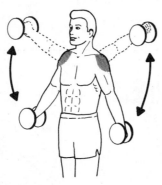

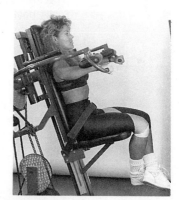

Lateral Raises
Start with the weights held at your sides, lift them laterally with straight arms to shoulder height, and lower them to the starting position. Both movements should be executed slowly. Develops the deltoids and triceps.

Lateral Raises
Adjust the seat so that you can raise your elbows to shoulder height or slightly higher, and then return to the starting position.

FIGURE 8.29

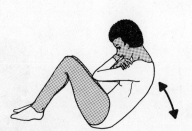

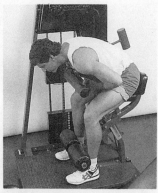

Bent Leg Sit-Ups

Lie on the floor with your knees bent as shown. Fold your arms across your chest and sit up until your elbows touch your thighs and return to the starting position. Develops the abdominals.

Abdominal Crunches

Sit in an upright position, place your chest against the padded bar, lean as far forward as you can, and then slowly return to the starting position.

FIGURE 8.30

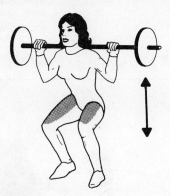

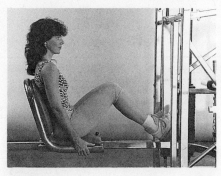

Half-Squat

Start in the standing position with the weight held across your shoulders behind the neck. Keeping your back straight and your head up, slowly bend your knees until you reach a half-squat position and then return to the starting position. Do not allow your hips to get lower than your knees. Develops the quadriceps.

Leg Press

Adjust the seat so that your knees are bent at approximately 90° when your feet are placed on the pedals. Slowly extend your legs fully, and return to the starting position.

FIGURE 8.31

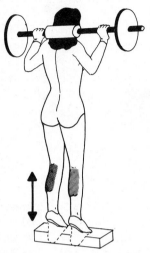

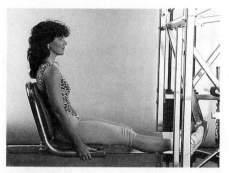

Heel Raises
With the weight across your shoulders, slowly raise and lower your heels. Develops the gastrocnemius.

Calf Press
Follow the same direction as for the Universal leg press, except that you should place the balls of your feet on the pedals, keeping the heels off the pedals. Extend your legs fully, press forward with your toes, and release. Repetitions are performed while the legs are fully extended.

FIGURE 8.32

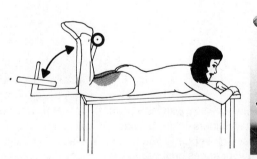

Hamstring Curl
Start with your leg extended then slowly bend your knee until your lower leg forms a 90° angle with your thigh and return to the starting position. Develops the hamstring group.

Assessing Muscular Strength and Endurance _____

Muscular strength is measured by the amount of force a given muscle or muscle group is capable of exerting in a single maximum contraction. A number of tests measuring the strength of different muscle groups must be administered if one wishes to estimate total body strength. Several tests are needed because strength is not a general component. If it were, total strength could be accurately predicted by measuring any muscle group, but in reality the strength of different muscle groups is often disproportionately unequal. This may be the result of body build, the physical demands of a person's occupation, or it might be due to fitness training that concentrates on particular body parts.

A good battery of strength tests should measure the strength of the arms, shoulders, back, abdomen, and legs. These measurements may be made isometrically, isotonically, or isokinetically. But a word of warning: measuring the strength of novices is potentially hazardous because they are not physically prepared to exert maximum force. The measurement of back strength is particularly perilous because of the body positions that must be assumed during these measurements. To help insure safety, strength measurement should not occur until participants have been actively involved in resistance training for several months. For those who are interested in the health-related benefits of resistance training, the measurement of strength is unnecessary. Those who train isotonically and isokinetically will see the improvement that occurs with time and effort. To them, the measurement of strength should be viewed as an unnecessary hazard.

Muscular endurance involves repeated contractions or positions held for a certain length of time. It is a function of how long or how many times a muscle can contract. Once again, several tests must be administered to determine the endurance of various muscle groups.

Isometric Assessment

The measurement of isometric strength requires devices that assess the tension exerted by different muscle groups in static positions. Back and leg dynamometers (Figures 8.33 and 8.34) measure leg and back strength. Cable tensiometers (Figure 8.35), used in conjunction with a specially constructed table, may be used to measure many muscle groups.

Figures 8.36 through 8.38 illustrate the measurements of the arm flexors, quadriceps, and hamstrings at specified angles using the cable tensiometer. The validity of these measurements is dependent upon the subject's ability to produce maximum exertions. All tests of strength, regardless of the method employed, should isolate the muscle or muscle group being tested. Precautions must be taken to minimize the possible assistance that might come from other muscle groups because this would overestimate the strength of the test group.

Isometric muscular endurance may be evaluated with the same devices by measuring the amount of time that a contraction can be maintained at a specific percentage of maximum strength.

FIGURE 8.33

Measurement of Back Strength with A Dynamometer

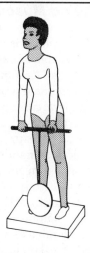

FIGURE 8.34

Measurement of Leg Strength with A Dynamometer

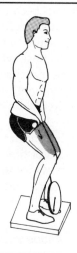

FIGURE 8.35

Cable Tensiometer

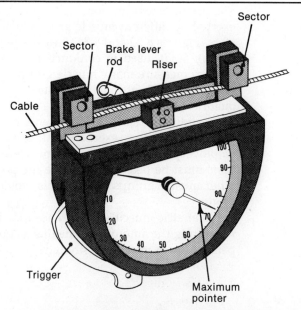

FIGURE 8.36

**Measurement of
Hamstring Strength with
Cable Tensiometer**

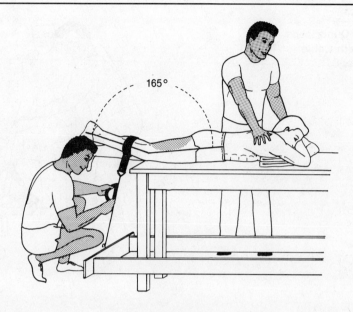

FIGURE 8.37

**Measuring Biceps
Strength with Cable
Tensiometer**

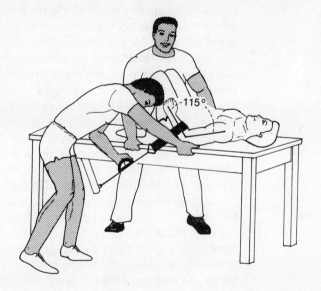

Isotonic Assessment

Isotonic or dynamic strength may be assessed by measuring the maximum amount of weight (1-RM) that can be lifted by different muscle groups. These measurements may be made with free weights or weight machines. Figure 8.23 illustrates the biceps curl, which is a measurement of arm flexor strength; Figure 8.25 illustrates the bench press, which measures the strength of the pectorals, deltoids, and extensors of the arms; Figure 8.24 illustrates the standing press which measures the strength of the extensors of the arms, deltoids, and trapezius; Figure 8.30 illustrates the half-squat, which measures the strength of the quad-

FIGURE 8.38

Measuring Quadriceps Strength with Cable Tensiometer

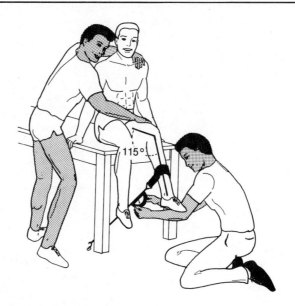

riceps and hip flexors; and Figure 8.32 illustrates the hamstring curl, which measures the strength of the hamstrings. The measurement of low back strength is not included for reasons alluded to earlier in this chapter.

If you are interested in assessing your strength in these categories, and comparing your performance to the values obtained from other college age students, see the Self-Assessment section in this chapter. A word of caution: Do not attempt to lift maximum amounts of weight until you have been in training for at least two months. It is not necessary to test yourself to achieve the health benefits of strength training.

The muscular endurance of these muscle groups is measured with the same exercises. The number of repetitions that can be performed at a selected percentage of 1-RM (70 percent is used in many cases) will provide this measurement.

Muscular endurance may also be measured with a variety of calisthenics. For males, the number of pull-ups (Figure 8.39), push-ups (Figure 8.40), parallel bar dips (Figure 8.41), and bent-leg situps in 60 seconds (Figure 8.42) are commonly used to measure muscular endurance. For females, muscular endurance is usually measured by the number of modified push-ups (Figure 8.43), bent-leg situps that can be done in 60 seconds (Figure 8.42) and the amount of time that the flexed-arm hang can be held (Figure 8.44).

Interested individuals can consult the Self-Assessment section in this chapter for selected muscle endurance tests of a practical nature along with standards of performance for comparison.

Isokinetic Assessment

Isokinetic strength is assessed with accommodating resistance devices equipped with indicators that measure the amount of force being generated (Figure 8.3).

Because of the nature of these devices (they allow the contraction to be completed at any percent of maximum) several trials must be allowed to ensure that a maximum voluntary contraction has been attained. Once this has been achieved, then muscular endurance can be measured by the number of repetitions performed at a specified percentage of maximum strength (70 percent of 1-RM is a common standard).

FIGURE 8.39

Chin-Ups
Measures Endurance of the Arm Flexors (primarily the biceps).

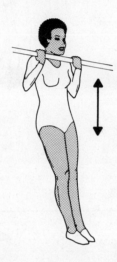

FIGURE 8.40

Push-Ups for Males.
Measures Endurance of the Arm Extensors (primarily the triceps).

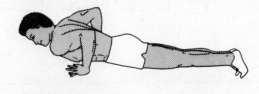

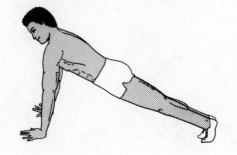

FIGURE 8.41

Parallel Bar Dips
An Alternative Way to
Measure Endurance of the
Arm Extensors.

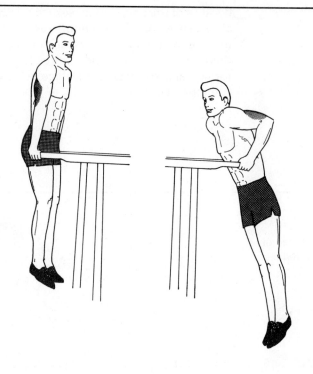

FIGURE 8.42

**Measurement of
Abdominal Endurance**

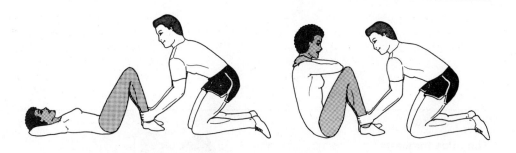

FIGURE 8.43

**Measuring Endurance of
the Arm Extensors**
This is one of the modified
versions of the push-up
which is commonly used
for female subjects.

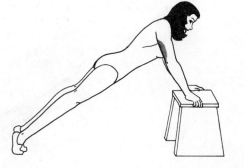
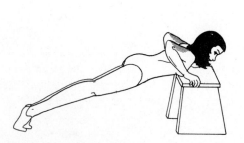

FIGURE 8.44

Flexed-Arm Hang
Measures Endurance of
the Arm Flexors. This is a
modified version of the
chin-up and is commonly
used for female subjects.

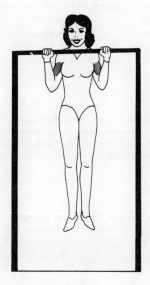

SELF-ASSESSMENT
Strength and Endurance Tests

Muscular Strength

Gauging relative muscular strength is not merely measuring the ability to manipulate a weight. A heavier individual may lift more weight than a lighter individual, but it may be proportionately less than the lighter person lifted relative to his or her body weight. To be more specific, a 150-pound subject bench presses 200 pounds, while a 250-pound subject bench presses 275 pounds. Who is stronger pound for pound? The answer is figured by dividing the body weight into the weight lifted. The calculations are:

For 150 lb subject:

$$\frac{200}{150} = 1.33$$

For 250 lb subject:

$$\frac{275}{250} = 1.10$$

You can see that the lighter subject can exert more strength per unit of body weight than the larger subject.

To determine your own strength-per-pound of body weight, test yourself in a one-trial maximum effort on the biceps curl, standing press, bench press, half-squat, and hamstring curl (Figures 8.23-8.25, 8.30, and 8.32), and calculate the ratio by using the pounds lifted ÷ body weight equation. To assess yourself in terms of averages, consult Tables 8.3 and 8.4 which present strength-to-body-weight standards for men and women.

Note: Do not attempt to lift maximum amounts of weight until you have been in training for at least two months. It is not necessary to test yourself to achieve the health benefits of strength training.

Muscular Endurance

This assessment will analyze muscular endurance of the arm flexors (chin-ups for men—Figure 8.39; flexed-arm hang for women—Figure 8.44) and the abdominals (bent-knee sit-ups—Figure 8.42). Gauge your abdominal endurance by the number of repetitions in 60 seconds. Arm flexor endurance should be measured by repetitions for men, and hang time for women.

Table 8.5 presents standards for these muscle endurance categories. Compare your results to the norms in this table to assess your muscular endurance status.

TABLE 8.3   Strength to Body Weight Ratio for Men

Biceps Curl	Standing Press	Bench Press	Half Squat	Hamstring Curl	Strength Category
.65 and above	1.0 and above	1.30 and above	1.85 and above	.65 and above	Excellent
.55–.64	.90–.99	1.15–1.29	1.65–1.84	.55–.64	Good
.45–.54	.75–.89	1.0–1.14	1.30–1.64	.45–.54	Average
.35–.44	.60–.74	.85–.99	1.0–1.29	.35–.44	Fair
.34 and below	.59 and below	.84 and below	Less than 1.0	.34 and below	Poor

Values adapted from B. L. Johnson and J. K. Nelson, *Practical Measurement for Evaluation in Physical Education*, Burgess Publishing, 1986 and W. W. K. Hoeger, *Lifetime Physical Fitness and Wellness*, Englewood, Colorado: Morton Publishing Co., 1989.

TABLE 8.4   Strength to Body Weight Ratio for Women

Biceps Curl	Standing Press	Bench Press	Half Squat	Hamstring Curl	Strength Category
.45 and above	.50 and above	.85 and above	1.45 and above	.55 and above	Excellent
.38–.44	.42–.49	.70–.84	1.30–1.44	.50–.54	Good
.32–.37	.32–.41	.60–.69	1.0–1.29	.40–.49	Average
.25–.31	.25–.31	.50–.59	.80–.99	.30–.39	Fair
.24 and below	.24 and below	.49 and below	.79 and below	.29 and below	Poor

Values adapted from B. L. Johnson and J. K. Nelson, *Practical Measurement for Evaluation in Physical Education*, Burgess Publishing, 1986 and W. W. K. Hoeger, *Lifetime Physical Fitness and Wellness*, Englewood, Colorado: Morton Publishing Co., 1989.

TABLE 8.5   Muscle Endurance Standards for Men and Women

Men			Women		
Bent Knee Sit-Ups (60 sec)	*Chin-Ups*	*Endurance Classification*	*Bent Knee Sit-Ups (60 sec)*	*Flexed-Arm Hang (sec)*	*Endurance Classification*
60 or more	20 or more	Excellent	52 or more	30 or more	Excellent
52–59	15–19	Good	44–51	24–29	Good
40–51	10–14	Average	35–43	15–23	Average
35–39	6–9	Fair	30–34	9–14	Fair
34 or less	5 or less	Poor	29 or less	8 or less	Poor

Values adapted from R. R. Pate, *Norms for College Students: Health Related Physical Fitness Test* (AAHPERD, 1985) and B. L. Johnson and J. K. Nelson, *Practical Measurement for Evaluation in Physical Education* (Burgess Publishing, 1989).

POINTS TO PONDER

1. Define isometric, isokinetic, and isotonic contraction.
2. Which of these is not dynamic and why?

3. *What are concentric and eccentric contractions? Which of the two is involved in delayed muscle soreness?*
4. *Discuss fully the relationship between resistance training and health.*
5. *What is responsible for the difference in strength and muscle size between males and females.*
6. *Respond to this statement: Several years of heavy resistance exercise will convert slow-twitch muscle fibers to fast-twitch muscle fibers.*
7. *Weight training for prepubescent children is ineffective for the development of strength. Do you agree or disagree and why?*
8. *Define hypertrophy, hyperplasia, and atrophy.*
9. *What seems to be most responsible for the delayed muscle soreness which accompanies resistance exercise?*
10. *What are the agonist and antagonist muscles for the push-ups?*

Chapter Highlights

Muscular strength is the ability to exert maximum force in a single contraction, while muscular endurance is the ability to sustain repeated contraction or to apply force for a period of time. Strength may be developed with isometric, isotonic, and isokinetic exercises. Isometric exercises do not seem to build muscular endurance; isotonic and isokinetic exercises do increase muscular endurance.

Isotonic and isokinetic exercises are excellent complementary programs to aerobic training. The disadvantages of isometric exercises tend to outweigh their advantages and their potential for health enhancement seems very limited. Several of the health benefits associated with dynamic programs are new and currently under investigation. They have great potential for strength development and future research will determine the validity of isokinetic training principles and procedures.

Circuit training is also relatively new. It seems to be an appropriate supplement to a good aerobic program. Depending upon the selection of exercises and resistances, circuit training may be used to develop muscular strength, muscular endurance, cardiorespiratory endurance, and flexibility.

Regardless of the training system, the principles of overload and progression must be applied in an appropriate manner and at the proper time. The number of workouts per week, the number of repetitions and sets, the length of each workout, and the amount of rest between workouts will depend upon the type of resistance training and the program objectives. Participants should be safety-conscious and follow generally accepted procedures for conducting a workout.

References

1. R. C. Hickson, "Interference of Strength Development By Simultaneously Training for Strength and Endurance," *European Journal of Applied Physiology,* 45 (1980): 255.
2. S. J. Fleck and W. J. Kraemer, "Resistance Training: Physiological Responses And Adaptations (Part 3 of 4)," *The Physician and Sportsmedicine,* 16 (1988): 63.
3. M. Prives, "Influences of Labor and Sport Upon Skeleton Structure in Man," *Anatomical Record* 136 (1960): 261.
4. J. A. Ross, "Hypertrophy of the Little Finger," *British Medical Journal,* 2 (1950): 987.
5. B. Nilsson and N. Westline, "Bone Density in Athletes," *Clinical Orthopedics,* 77 (1971): 179.
6. "Osteoporosis—A Silent Epidemic," *The Harvard Medical School Health Letter,* no. 2, (November, 1981): 4.

7. "Aging and Exercise," *The Harvard Medical School Health Letter*, no. 5 (April, 1983): 4.

8. American Academy of Pediatrics, "Weight Training and Weight Lifting: Information for the Pediatrician," *The Physician and Sportsmedicine*, 11 (1983): 157.

9. R. D. Pfeiffer and R. Francis, "Effects of Strength Training on Muscle Development in Prepubescent Males," *The Physician and Sportsmedicine*, 14 (1986): 134.

10. C. B. Rians et al., "Strength Training in Prepubescent Males: Is it Safe?" Paper presented at the annual meeting, American Orthopedic Society for Sports Medicine, Nashville, Tenn, 1985.

11. L. Sewall and L. J. Micheli, "Strength Training for Children," *Journal of Pediatric Orthopedics*, 6 (1986): 143.

12. A. Weltman et al., "The Effects of Hydraulic Resistance Strength Training in Prepubertal Males," *Medicine and Science in Sports and Exercise*, 18 (1986): 629.

13. National Strength and Conditioning Association, "Position Paper on Prepubescent Strength Training," *NSCA Journal*, 7 (1986): 27.

14. J. Siegel, "Fitness in Prepubescent Children: Implications for Exercise Training," *NSCA Journal*, 10 (1988): 43.

15. C. C. Johnson, "Diet and Exercise in Middle-Aged Men," *Journal of the American Dietetic Association*, 81 (1982): 695.

16. M. H. Stone and H. O'Bryant, *Weight Training: A Scientific Approach*, Minneapolis: Burgess Publishing Co., Inc., 1986.

17. L. Goldberg et al., "Changes in Lipid and Lipoprotein Levels After Weight Training," *Journal of the American Medical Association*, 252 (1984): 504.

18. B. F. Hurley et al., "Resistive Training Can Reduce Coronary Risk Factors Without Altering VO_2 Max or Percent Body Fat," *Medicine and Science in Exercise and Sports*, 20 (1988): 150.

19. B. F. Hurley et al., "High Density Lipoprotein Cholesterol in Body-builders Vs. Power Lifters, Negative Effects of Androgen Use," *Journal of the American Medical Association*, 4 (1984): 507.

20. E. M. Leeds et al., "Effects of Exercise and Anabolic Steroids on Total and Lipoprotein Cholesterol Concentrations in Male and Female Rats," *Medicine and Science in Sports and Exercise*, 18 (1986): 663.

21. H. M. Taggert et al., "Reduction in High Density Lipoproteins by Anabolic Steroid (Stanolozol) Therapy for Post Menopausal Osteoporosis," *Metabolism*, 31 (1982): 1147.

22. T. E. Allen et al., "Hemodynamic Consequences of Circuit Weight Training," *Research quarterly AAHPER*, 47 (1976): 299.

23. M. H. Stone et al., "Cardiovascular Responses to Short-Term Olympic Style Weight Training in Young Men," *Canadian Journal of Applied Sport Science*, 8 (1983): 134.

24. T. D. Fahey et al., "Body Composition and VO_2 Max of Exceptional Weight Trained Athletes," *Journal of Applied Physiology*, 39 (1975): 559.

25. J. H. Wilmore, "Alterations in Strength, Body Composition, and Anthropometric Measurements Consequent to a 10-Week Weight Training Program," *Medicine and Science in Sports and Exercise*, 6 (1974): 33.

26. K. J. Cureton et al., "Muscle Hypertrophy in Men and Women," *Medicine and Science in Sports and Exercise*, 20 (1988): 338.

27. G. A. Brooks and T. D. Fahey, *Exercise Physiology*, New York: John Wiley and Sons, 1984.

28. T. Moritani and H. A. de Vries, "Neural Factors Vs. Hypertrophy in the Time Course of Muscle Strength Gain," *American Journal of Physical Medicine*, 58 (1979): 115.

29. D. L. Costill et al., "Adaptations in Skeletal Muscle Following Strength Training," *Journal of Applied Physiology*, 46 (1979): 96.

30. M. Ikai and A. H. Steinhaus, "Some Factors Modifying the Expression of Human Strength," *Journal of Applied Physiology*, 16 (1961): 157.

31. American College of Sports Medicine, "Position Statement on the Use and Abuse of Anabolic-Androgenic Steroids in Sports," in R. H. Strauss (ed), *Sports Medicine*, Philadelphia: W. B. Saunders Co., 1984.

32. B. Van Linge, "The Response of Muscle to Strenuous Exercise," *Journal of Bone and Joint Surgery*, 44 (1962): 711.

33. A. Salleo et al., "New Muscle Fiber Production During Compensatory Hypertrophy," *Medicine and Science in Sports and Exercise*, 12 (1980): 268.

34. W. J. Gonyea, "Role of Exercise in Inducing Increases in Skeletal Muscle Fiber Number," *Journal of Applied Physiology*, 48 (1980): 421.

35. W. J. Gonyea et al., "Exercise Induced Increases in Muscle Fiber Number," *European Journal of Applied Physiology*, 55 (1986): 137.

36. J. H. Wilmore and D. L. Costill, *Training for Sport and Activity*, Dubuque, Iowa: Wm. C. Brown Publishers, 1988.

37. J. J. Knapik et al., "Angular Specificity and Test Mode Specificity of Isometric and Isokinetic Strength Training," *Journal of Orthopedic Sports Physical Therapy*, 5 (1983): 58.

38. J. Kanehisa and M. Miyashita, "Effect of Isometric and Isokinetic Muscle Training on Static Strength and Dynamic Power," *European Journal of Applied Physiology*, 50 (1983): 365.

39. M. J. N. McDonagh and C. T. M. Davies, "Adaptive Responses of Mammalian Skeletal Muscle to Exercise with High Loads," *European Journal of Applied Physiology*, 52 (1984): 139.

40. W. J. Kraemer et al., "A Review: Factors in Exercise Prescription of Resistance Training," *NSCA Journal*, 10 (1988): 36.

41. H. G. Knuttgen and W. J. Kraemer, "Terminology and Measurement in Exercise Performance," *Journal of Applied Sport Science Research*, 1 (1987): 1.

42. S. J. Fleck and R. C. Schutt, "Types of Strength Training," *Clinics in Sports Medicine*, 4 (1985): 159.

43. S. J. Fleck and W. J. Kraemer, *Designing Resistance Training Programs*, Champaign, Ill: Human Kinetics Publishers, 1987.

44. W. L. Westcott, *Strength Fitness—Physiological Principles and Training Techniques*, Boston: Allyn and Bacon, Inc., 1983.

45. W. J. Kraemer and S. J. Fleck, "Resistance Training: Exercise Prescription (Part 4 of 4)," *The Physician and Sportsmedicine*, 16 (1988): 69.

46. W. J. Kraemer et al., "Physiologic Responses to Heavy-Resistance Exercise With Very Short Rest Periods," *International Journal of Sports Medicine*, 8 (1987): 247.

47. P. V. Karpovich, "Incidence of Injuries in Weight Lifting," *Journal of Physical Education* 48 (March/April, 1951): 71.

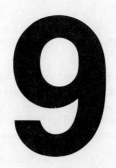

9

~~~ECG waveform~~~

Developing the
Flexibility Component

Mini Glossary

Dynamic Stretching: Also known as ballistic stretching, it employs bouncing and bobbing to stretch muscles.

Flexibility: The range of motion about a joint or series of joints.

Flexometer: An instrument for measuring static flexibility.

Goniometer: A protractor-like device used to measure static flexibility.

Static Stretching: Stretching that employs slow movements and positions that are held for 15 to 30 seconds.

Stretch Reflex: The myotatic reflex that responds to stretching of the muscle tissues.

Introduction

Flexibility is defined as "the range of possible movement in a joint (as in the hip joint) or series of joints (as when the spinal column is involved)."[1] Flexibility is not a general component; that is, the flexibility of one joint cannot be predicted accurately from a measurement made at another joint. This implies that the capacity for movement may differ from joint to joint. Flexibility, then, is specific to each individual joint.

Motion is limited at a given joint by its bony structure, accompanying muscle size, and soft connective tissues—the tendons, ligaments and joint capsules.[2] Additionally, the skin may be involved to some degree in the resistance to movement. The skeletal structure of joints constitutes one of the unalterable limitations to movement. It is not amenable to change. Therefore, improvement in flexibility is accomplished by increasing the elastic properties of the soft tissues—the muscles and their facial sheaths, tendons, ligaments, and connective tissue.

Flexibility and Wellness

Flexibility is recognized as one of the important health-related components of physical fitness. Its major contribution to health is related to the prevention of low back pain and injury. A healthy low back is dependent upon abdominal strength, good posture, and flexibility of the hamstrings and back extensors.[3] Flexibility wanes with age and inactivity. Active individuals tend to be more flexible than sedentary individuals.[4] Although range of motion diminishes with passing years, there appears to be no evidence that the biological processes associated with aging are responsible.[5] Inactivity, rather than aging, seems to be implicated in the loss of flexibility because muscles and other soft tissues lose their elasticity when they are not used. For example, a sedentary life characterized by sitting maintains the hamstrings in a shortened position which will lead to a loss in their range of motion and increases susceptibility to low back injury.

There is a theory that developing strength in the antagonistic muscles of the tight muscle or muscle group has the potential for increasing flexibility.[6] If the hamstrings are tight, their antagonists, the quadriceps muscles, are strengthened to provide for greater range of motion. Research evidence in support of this approach to the enhancement of flexibility is lacking at this time, however, greater elasticity is one of the properties of stronger muscles.

Flexibility appears to reach a peak in most of the joints at 24 years of age for males[7] and 25 to 29 years of age for females.[8] The range of motion for most movements begins to decline in the mid-twenties for males and about 30 years of age for females. As range of movement declines, so too does the quality of life. The ability to perform essential movements such as walking, bending, stooping, climbing stairs, as well as occupational and recreational movements, declines markedly with a decrease in physical activity and the absence of a planned program designed to increase and/or maintain flexibility.

Females of all ages were more flexible than males, but males outperformed females on strength tests.
–The Canadian Fitness Study

Developing the Flexibility Component

Flexibility may be improved through exercises that promote the elasticity of the soft tissues of the joints. Chapman showed that 20 young men (ages 15 to 19) and 20 older men (ages 63 to 88) responded similarly to an exercise program designed to enhance finger-joint flexibility.[9] The older subjects exhibited greater joint stiffness at the inception of the program but the amount of their improvement equaled that of the younger subjects. Munns evaluated the impact of a 12-week exercise-dance program on the flexibility of 40 adults aged 65 to 88.[10] Half of this group participated in the activity program (the experimental group), while the other half acted as nonparticipating controls. Munns measured the range of motion of six joints with a flexometer before and after exposure to the treatments. She found that the experimental group improved their range of motion significantly at all six sites while the controls lost some degree of their range of motion at every site. Lesser completed a similar study using 30 experimental and 30 control subjects ages 61 to 89.[11] The experimental group exercised two days per week for 30 minutes per session for 10 weeks. The experimental group improved significantly in 8 of the 12 measured sites despite the low frequency of exercise and the nonspecific nature of the program. The research data regarding the effectiveness of physical activity in improving and maintaining flexibility is limited. Some of the researchers did not employ a control group, while others did not develop exercise programs targeted specifically to improve flexibility in the joints that were measured. The studies presented here controlled all or most of the major limitations.

Prevention of back disorders should be the goal of all exercisers. Flexibility and muscle strengthening must be integral parts of the training program.
–Carl L. Stanitshi, M.D.

Static versus Dynamic Stretching

In the past, dynamic or ballistic stretching was used as a "loosening" procedure prior to physical activity. But today, dynamic stretching is recognized as being counterproductive and may actually be harmful. **Dynamic stretching** employs bouncing and bobbing movements. This technique is illustrated when individuals try to touch their toes by bending from the waist with a series of bobbing movements, each of which takes the finger tips closer to the toes. Most people have stretched in this manner and some continue to do so. It is counterproductive because dynamic movements stimulate the stretch reflex (the myotatic reflex originating in the muscle spindle), which responds by sending signals for the muscle to contract rather than stretch. Each bob or bounce stimulates the stretch reflex, which, in turn, signals the muscle to contract with a force which is proportional to the force generated by bobbing and bouncing.[12] If you have dozed off while sitting upright in a chair, you have experienced the results of the stretch reflex doing its work. Your head drops forward as you nod off causing the neck muscles to stretch rapidly and dynamically. This sudden and unexpected stretch stimulates the **stretch reflex** which signals the central nervous system to order those muscles to contract thereby snapping the head back to the upright position. Soreness may occur because the muscle is forced to pull against itself. Each bounce ends suddenly and forcefully, thereby applying substantial stress to muscle tissue. This technique may lead to injury because it is possible to exceed the elastic limits of the muscles. Such an occurrence is even more likely if cold muscles are stretched in this manner.

Toe-touching is used here for illustrative purposes only, to show the differences between dynamic and **static stretching,** because most people are familiar with this exercise. Toe-touching with straight legs is not recommended because it may lead to an injury of the low back and/or knees.

When a muscle is stretched, the muscle spindles (part of the stretch reflex) are also stretched, sending a volley of sensory impulses to the spinal cord that inform the central nervous system that the muscle is being stretched. Impulses return to the muscle from the spinal cord, which causes it to contract reflexively, thus resisting the stretch.
–William E. Prentise.

The Right Way to Warm Up

It is a crisp winter day, and before you begin your morning jog you lean against your favorite tree to begin your stretching. This is the way you always start off, and you're confident it's the right way. Well, you're wrong. Athletes and doctors are now convinced that stretching cold muscles, especially on a cold day, can lead to injuries. According to Dr. Fred Allman, Jr., past president of the American College of Sports Medicine, "You don't get as much benefit from stretching a cold muscle, and you might hurt it." And Daphne Barnes, head athletic trainer at Yale University says, "The thing about stretching is just to relax, and if you're really chilled while you're trying to relax you defeat the whole purpose of stretching."

The best way to prepare for jogging, bicycling, squash, or any other exercise is to warm up the muscles gently, and after that do your stretches. Dr. Allman recommends "a very mild form of exercise, something that will slowly cause the body to warm up—walking at a rapid pace, jogging at a slow pace, running in place, or utilizing a stationary bicycle. You can do this for 5 or 6 minutes, and after you begin to perspire, or after your heart rate is slightly increased and you're beginning to feel the warmth a little bit, then you should do your stretching exercises."

There are sound physiological reasons for getting yourself warmed up for stretching. A warm-up period increases the flow of blood, raises the temperature of the muscles and tendons and increases their flexibility, and releases synovial fluid, the body's natural lubricant for the joints. The heart also needs some time to get ready for stretching. Vigorous stretching without a gradual warm-up leads to temporary abnormalities in blood flow and blood pressure that can be dangerous, especially for middle-aged exercisers.

Wearing heavy sweat clothes does not help you warm up. Dress for the weather— if it's cold, wear warm sweats; if it's hot, wear shorts. Keeping a warm-up suit on while exercising on a hot day simply defeats the body's cooling mechanisms and does no good.

Not only should you warm up before stretching, but you should also perhaps discard some of the stretches you have been doing. The old keep-your-knees-stiff-and-touch-your-toes stretch is definitely out. It overextends the knees and back. And deep knee bends can damage ligaments and cartilage. Any kind of bouncing on cold muscles and joints to get them loose is very bad, since bouncing actually tightens cold muscles.

There are many beneficial stretching movements that athletes have adopted from ballet and yoga. These "static stretches" gradually loosen the muscles without straining them. In the static touch-your-toes, for example, you lock your knees and bend as low as you can until you feel your hamstring and back muscles start to stretch—and you hold that position for 10 to 15 seconds without fighting the muscles. When you stand up, bend your knees to ease the load on the back. Repeat this several times until you can reach the floor without strain. After 5 minutes of careful stretching, you're truly ready for a healthy workout.

"The Right Way to Warm Up," *University of California, Berkeley Wellness Letter*, p. 2, Feb., 1985. Reprinted permission of University of California, Berkeley Wellness Letter, P.O. Box 10922, Des Moines, IA 50340. Copyright © Health Letter Associates, 1985.

Stretching statically is the preferred method. **Static stretching** features slow movements leading to the desired position, which is then held for 15 to 30 seconds. The final position should produce a feeling of discomfort but not pain. When the position of mild discomfort is reached, it is held for 15 to 30 seconds and then slowly released. This technique does not stimulate the stretch reflex allowing the muscles to stretch essentially free of opposition. Each exercise may be repeated several times. Compared to dynamic stretching, static stretching is less likely to cause injuries, produces no muscle soreness (and is, in fact, advocated as an antidote to soreness), and consumes less energy. One must perform stretching exercises on a regular basis to receive optimal benefits.

The stretching component of the physical fitness program may be incorporated as a segment of the warm-up and cool-down phases of aerobic exercise. For the stretching exercises to be most effective, they should follow exercises in the warm-up phase that stimulate circulation and heat up the muscles. Stretching during cool-down should follow a few minutes of walking. Flexibility exercises performed at this time afford the best opportunity to stretch those muscles which have been contracting vigorously during the workout. Stretching after the workout is very important because it helps prevent the muscle shortening that is associated with loss of flexibility and it prevents or decreases muscle soreness.

Exercises to Enhance Flexibility

The exercises presented in this section are a sample of the many exercises that have been devised to enhance flexibility. Choose at least one exercise from each of the areas, and remember the following rules.

1. Warm up for a few minutes prior to stretching.
2. Stretch to the point of discomfort, not pain.
3. Hold each stretch for 15 to 30 seconds.
4. Move slowly from one position to the next.
5. You may perform each stretch more than once.
6. Stretching exercises may be performed daily.

See Figures 9.1 through 9.24 for samples of stretching exercises for the major joints and soft tissues of the body and select one exercise from each group.

FIGURE 9.1

Stretching the Neck
Rotate your head downward and to the extreme left. Hold this position for 5 seconds and then rotate your head upward and to the extreme right. Hold for 5 seconds and then look downward. Hold for 5 seconds and rotate your head upward and to the extreme left and hold for 5 seconds. Repeat the sequence in reverse order.

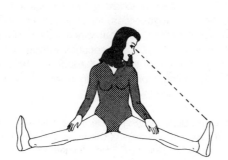
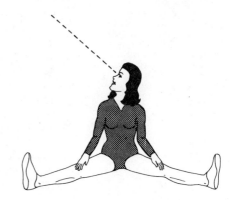

FIGURE 9.2

Stretching the Neck
Gently pull your head forward until a stretch is felt in the back of the neck and hold for 15 to 30 seconds.

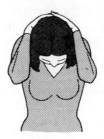

FIGURE 9.3

Stretching the Neck
Bend your neck from side to side and then from front to back. Do not roll your head in a circle.

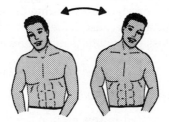
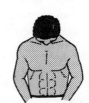
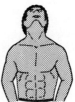

FIGURE 9.4

Stretching the Shoulders and Arms
With the left elbow up and the right elbow down, try to clasp your hands behind your back. If you cannot clasp then reach as far as possible and hold for 15 seconds and then reverse arms.

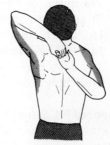

FIGURE 9.5

Stretching the Shoulders and Arms
Gently pull your right arm behind your head and hold for 15 seconds. Then pull the left arm in the same manner.

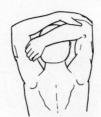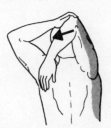

FIGURE 9.6

Stretching the Shoulders and Arms
Stretch your arms forward to full extension with both palms on the floor and press down with your chest. Hold 15 to 30 seconds.

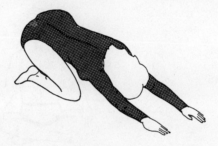

FIGURE 9.7

Stretching the Shoulders and Arms
Place your hands on opposite sides of a doorjam and lean forward and straighten your arms. Hold 15 to 30 seconds.

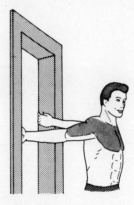

FIGURE 9.8

Stretching the Upper Back
Sit in a chair with feet separated greater than shoulder width. Place your arms to the inside of the thighs and bring your chest down toward the floor. At the same time, attempt to reach back as far as you can with your arms.

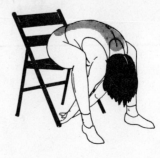

FIGURE 9.9

Stretching the Upper Back
Interlace your fingers behind your head and gently pull forward until you feel a comfortable stretch. Hold 15 to 30 seconds.

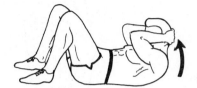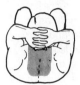

FIGURE 9.10

Stretching the Lower Back
Cross your legs and lean forward extending your arms to the front. Hold 15 to 30 seconds.

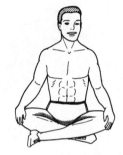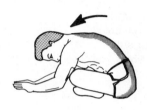

FIGURE 9.11

Stretching the Lower Back
Pull your left knee to your chest while simultaneously raising your head. Hold 15 to 30 seconds and repeat with the other leg.

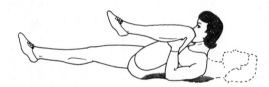

FIGURE 9.12

Stretching the Lower Back
Pull both knees to the chest while simultaneously raising your head. Hold 15 to 30 seconds.

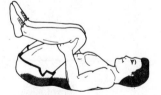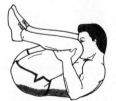

FIGURE 9.13

Stretching the Chest
Clasp your hands behind your back, straighten your arms, and lift them in the direction of the arrow.

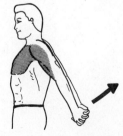

FIGURE 9.14

Stretching the Chest
Stretch your arms forward to full extension with both palms on the floor and press down with your chest. Hold 15 to 30 seconds.

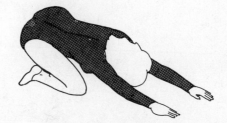

FIGURE 9.15

Stretching the Groin
Place the soles of your feet together and lean forward. Hold for 30 seconds. A variation of this exercise is to push down gently on both knees until a stretch is felt and hold 15 to 30 seconds.

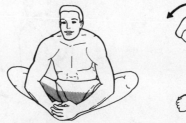
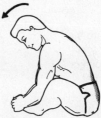

FIGURE 9.16

Stretching the Groin
Keep your legs straight, rest your heels against a wall, and slowly let your feet slide downward so that your legs spread apart. Stop when you feel a good stretch and hold for 15 to 30 seconds.

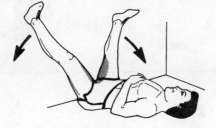
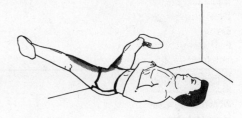

FIGURE 9.17

Stretching the Quadriceps
Bend your right leg and pull that foot upward toward the buttocks until a stretch is felt in the front of the thigh. Hold for 15 to 30 seconds and repeat with the other leg.

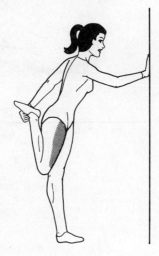

FIGURE 9.18

Stretching the Quadriceps

Assume the above position and lower your hips to create a stretch in the front of the thigh and hold 15 to 30 seconds. Repeat with the other leg.

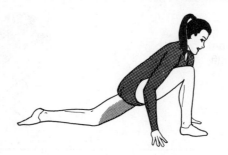

FIGURE 9.19

Stretching the Quadriceps

Extend your left leg to the rear and place your foot on a chair or other object at a comfortable height. Press downward until a stretch is felt. Hold 15 to 30 seconds and repeat with the other leg.

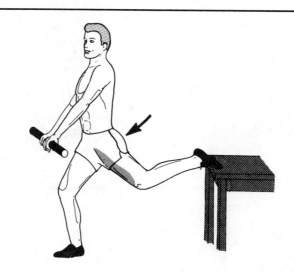

FIGURE 9.20

Stretching the Hamstrings

Extend one leg and place the sole of the other foot against the thigh of the extended leg. Lean forward and pull the toes back to exert a stretch in the calf and hamstrings. Hold 15 to 30 seconds and repeat with the other leg.

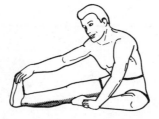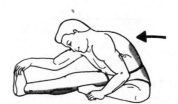

FIGURE 9.21

Stretching the Hamstrings

Bend your knees slightly and slowly lean forward from the waist until a stretch is felt in the hamstrings. Hold 15 to 30 seconds.

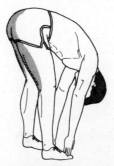

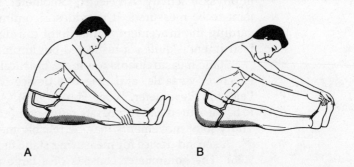

FIGURE 9.22

Stretching the Hamstrings
Extend both legs and lean forward. Pull back on the toes (B) to exert a stretch in the calves as well as the hamstrings. If you cannot reach your toes, reach as far forward as you can (A). Hold for 15 to 30 seconds.

A   B

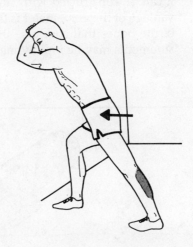

FIGURE 9.23

Stretching the Calf and Achilles Tendon
Assume the position shown above. Be sure that the heel of the extended leg remains in contact with the floor and that both feet are pointed straight ahead. Slowly move your hips forward until you feel a stretch in the calf of the extended leg. Hold 15 to 30 seconds and repeat with the other leg.

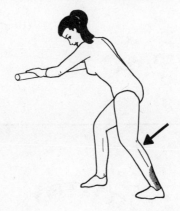

FIGURE 9.24

Stretching the Calf and Achilles Tendon
Bend the knee of the extended leg in this variation of FIGURE 9.23. This places the stretch upon the Achilles tendon. Hold 15 to 30 seconds and repeat with the other leg.

Assessing Flexibility

Flexibility may be assessed both statically and dynamically. Static measurements are easier to obtain and require less expertise but are less realistic than dynamic measures. Dynamic measures of flexibility are made while subjects are involved in physical activity. An electrogoniometer, such as the Elgon, is fastened to the joint to be measured. It provides a continuous stream of electrical signals regarding the movement of that joint during physical activity.[13] This measuring instrument is quite sophisticated but impractical for use with groups of people.

Static measurements are more practical although less functional. The most effective, versatile, and objective device for measuring static flexibility is the Leighton Flexometer.[14] (See Figure 9.25). A **Flexometer** is attached to the joint to be measured and records its range of motion from full flexion to full extension. Thirty joint movements may be reliably measured with this device.

A second device for measuring static flexibility is the goniometer (see Figure 9.26). The **goniometer** consists of a large protractor and two 15-inch straight edges. One of the edges is stationary and positioned at the zero line while the other rotates through 180 degrees. This instrument is not only inexpensive but it can be constructed with simple materials and a few tools. The major disadvantage of the goniometer is the subjective process of determining the long axes of the bones that comprise the joints, but the device is inexpensive and measurements may be rapidly made.

FIGURE 9.25

The Leighton Flexometer
(A) is the pointer, (B) the weight that keeps the pointer in a vertical position, and (C) the housing that rotates as the body part moves.

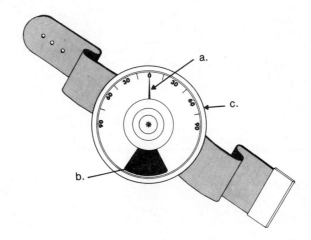

FIGURE 9.26

Large Goniometer

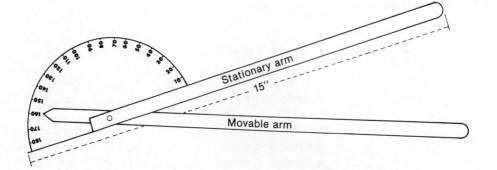

Field Tests

Field tests to measure flexibility may be employed in the absence of more so-phisticated devices. Three commonly used field tests include the sit-and-reach, back hyperextension, and shoulder flexion. The following paragraphs describe these three tests. After reading this material, you are encouraged to partake in the Self-Assessment on page 254 of this chapter to determine your flexibility standing.

The sit-and-reach test measures hip, low back, and hamstring flexibility. The testing device consists of a ruler attached to the top of a wooden box (Figure 9.27). The ruler extends 9 inches (23 centimeters) over the edge of the box facing the subject, who sits on the floor with both legs extended and both feet flat against the box. The subject places one hand on top of the other, and without bending the knees, slowly leans forward sliding the hands along the ruler as far as possible. The scores are read from the ruler, and the best of three trials is recorded. Bouncing is not permitted, and the knees must not bend at any time during this test.

The back hyperextension test measures the extensibility of the back muscles and spinal column. The subject lies in the prone position (face down) anchored by a partner who applies downward pressure on the back of the thighs (Figure 9.28). The subject arches his/her back while lifting the chest and chin as far as

FIGURE 9.27

The Sit-and-Reach Test

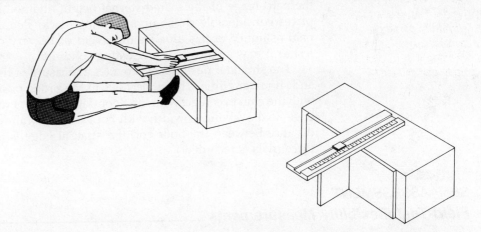

FIGURE 9.28

The Back Hyperextension Test
The scores are read from the ruler and the best of three trials is recorded. Bouncing is not permitted and the knees must not bend at any time during this test.

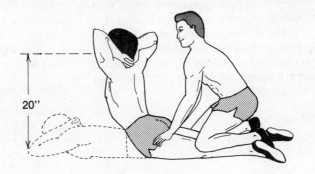

FIGURE 9.29

The Shoulder Flexion Test

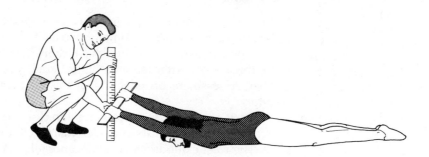

possible off the floor without using the arms. The distance between the floor and the sternal notch (the groove at the top of the breastbone) is measured and the best of three trials is recorded. Then the subject sits erectly against a wall and the distance between the floor and the sternal notch is measured in this position. This measurement helps compensate for differences in trunk length among subjects. The flexibility score may be determined by inserting both measures into the following formula:

$$\text{Back Hyperextension} = \frac{\text{hyperextension sternal height}}{\text{seated sternal height}}$$

Dividing the hyperextension sternal height by the sternal height seated yields the percentage of the seated sternal height attained by each subject. This test places considerable stress upon the low back. People who have experienced pain or injury to this area should avoid or be very careful in performing this test as it may aggravate a preexisting condition.

The shoulder flexion test provides a measure of the elasticity of the deltoids and shoulder girdle. The subject lies in the prone position, arms fully extended with the chin in contact with the floor (Figure 9.29). From this position, a straight edge held at shoulder width with both hands is raised as high as possible. The distance between the floor and the straight edge is measured and the best of three trials is recorded.

SELF-ASSESSMENT
Field Test Flexibility Measurements

It is important to maintain full range of motion throughout life. Loss of flexibility is caused by inactivity rather than aging. You may wish to quantify your current level of flexibility by performing each of the three field tests which were presented in this chapter. Be sure to warm up prior to doing each. Warming up should include light to moderate aerobic activities to heat the muscles, followed by gentle stretches of the muscles and joints to be tested.

Sit-and-Reach

Follow the procedure described on page 253 of this chapter, using a testing device similar to the one in Figure 9.27.

You do not need a testing box specifically designed for this measurement; a simple platform, ruler, and tape will work sufficiently. Record your three trials and compare the best effort to the standards found in Table 9.1.

Remember: Bouncing is not permitted, and the knees must not bend at any time during this test.

Back Hyperextension

Follow the procedure described on page 253 of this Chapter (Figure 9.28 gives a good visual demonstration of the exercise). However, because consistent norms are needed for the purpose of self-assessment against a population of peers, you will not use the hyperextension sternal height divided by seated sternal height formula. Rather, make three trials measuring the distance between the floor and the top of your chin, and compare your best effort to the standards found in Table 9.2.

Caution: People who have experienced pain or injury to the area should avoid this test, or, at very least, be extremely careful in exertion; this test could possibly aggravate a preexisting condition.

Shoulder Flexion

Follow the procedure described on page 000 of this chapter (see Figure 9.29 for a visual demonstration). Record three trials, and compare your best effort to the standards found in Table 9.3.

TABLE 9.1   Sit-and Reach Test Standards*

Men	Women	Classification
17.5 or above	18 or above	Excellent
15.75–17.4	16.5–17.9	Good
13.5–15.74	14.5–16.4	Average
10.5–13.4	12.25–14.4	Fair
Less than 10.5	Less than 12.25	Poor

*All scores are in inches. An individual's score is the best of three trials.

From R. R. Pate, *Norms for College Students: Health Related Physical Fitness Test*, American Alliance for Health, Physical Education, Recreation and Dance, 1985.

TABLE 9.2   Back Hyperextension Test Standards*

Men	Women	Classification
Above 21	Above 28	Excellent
18–21	25–28	Good
13–17	18–24	Average
9–12	12–17	Fair
Below 9	Below 12	Poor

*All scores are in inches. An individual's score is the best of three trials.

Adapted from B. Getchell, Physical Fitness A Way of Life, New York: John Wiley & Sons, 1983 and B. L. Johnson and J. K. Nelson, *Practical Measurements for Evaluation in Physical Education*, Burgess Publishing, 1986.

TABLE 9.3   Shoulder Flexion Test Standards*

Men	Women	Classification
26 or above	27 or above	Excellent
23–25	24–26	Good
18–22	19–23	Average
13–17	14–18	Fair
12 or below	13 or below	Poor

*All scores are in inches. An individual's score is the best of three trials.

Adapted from W. E. Prentice and C. A. Bucher, *Fitness for College and Life,* St. Louis: Times/Mirror Mosby College Publishing, 1988 and F. D. Rosato, *Fitness and Wellness: The Physical Connection*, St. Paul: West Publishing Co., 1986, 1st Edition.

POINTS TO PONDER

1. *Describe the relationship between flexibility and wellness.*
2. *Discuss the rationale for static stretching as a means of enhancing flexibility.*
3. *What are the major limitations of dynamic stretching?*
4. *Identify the principles that should be followed when employing static stretching.*
5. *Identify exercises which will stretch the hamstrings, low back, chest, shoulders, quadriceps, and achilles tendon.*
6. *What does the sit and reach test measure?*
7. *Define the myotatic reflex and describe its function.*

Chapter Highlights

Flexibility refers to the range of motion about a joint or series of joints. It is not a general ability; instead, it is specific to each joint. Flexibility may be improved with regular participation in activities that sensibly stretch the soft tissues—the muscles, tendons, ligaments, and connective tissue.

Flexibility training helps reduce low back problems, impedes loss of joint mobility, reduces the probability of joint injury, and enhances the quality of life by maintaining flexible movements into old age. The results of several studies support the notion that consistent participation in stretching exercises improves flexibility for young and old alike.

Static stretching is the preferred method. Dynamic or ballistic stretching may induce injury as a result of bobbing and bouncing movements. These rapid movements stimulate the stretch reflex and may stretch the muscles beyond their elastic limits. On the other hand, static stretching employs stretch positions that are achieved slowly and then held for 15 to 30 seconds. It is best to warm up the muscles with easy calisthenics prior to stretching.

Flexibility may be measured statically and dynamically. Dynamic measures of flexibility are more realistic with regard to suppleness during movement but these measures are difficult to attain. Therefore, static measures are more commonly used to assess flexibility. The Leighton Flexometer and the goniometer have been used with success. Field tests are also available to provide a measure of flexibility for specific joints.

References

1. H. A. deVries, *Physiology of Exercise*, Dubuque, Iowa: Wm. C. Brown Company Publishers, 1986.
2. B. Stamford, "Flexibility and Stretching," *The Physician and Sportsmedicine*, 12 (1984): 171.
3. C. L. Stanitski, "Low Back Pain in Young Athletes," *The Physician and Sportsmedicine*, 10 (1982): 77.
4. W. E. Prentice and C. A. Bucher, *Fitness for College and Life*, St. Louis: Times Mirror/Mosby College Publishing, 1988.
5. M. J. Adrian, "Flexibility in the Aging Adult," In *Exercise and Aging* E. L. Smith and R. C. Serfass (eds.), Hillside, N.J.: Enslow Publishers, 1981.
6. S. J. Hartley-O'Brien, "Six Mobilization Exercises for Active Range of Hip Flexion," *Research Quarterly for Exercise and Sport*, 51 (1980): 625.
7. G. W. Grey, "A Study of Flexibility in Selected Joints of Adult Males Ages 18–72," (University of Michigan: Doctoral Dissertation, 1955).

8. A. Jervey, "A Study of Flexibility of Selected Joints in Specified Groups of Adult Females," (University of Michigan: Doctoral Dissertation, 1961).

9. E. A. Chapman et al., "Joint Stiffness: Effects of Exercise on Young and Old Men," *Journal of Gerontology,* 27 (1972): 218.

10. K. Munns, "Effects of Exercise on the Range of Joint Motion in Elderly Subjects," in *Exercise and Aging* E. L. Smith and R. C. Serfass (eds.), Hillside, N.J.: Enslow Publishers, 1981.

11. M. Lesser, "The Effects of Rhythmic Exercise on the Range of Motion in Older Adults," *American Corrective Therapy Journal,* 32 (1978): 4.

12. E. T. Howley and B. D. Franks, *Health/Fitness Instructor's Handbook,* Champaign, Ill.: Human Kinetics Publishers, Inc., 1986.

13. P. V. Karpovich and W. E. Sinning, *Physiology of Muscular Activity,* Philadelphia: W. B. Saunders Co., 1971.

14. J. R. Leighton, "An Instrument and Technic for the Measurement of Range of Joint Motion," *Archives of Physical and Medical Rehabilitation,* 36 (1955): 571.

10

The Basics
of Nutrition

Chapter Outline

Mini Glossary

Amino Acids: the building blocks of proteins.

Carbohydrate: an organic compound composed of one or more sugars that are derived from plant sources.

Carbohydrate Loading: a method of overfilling the glycogen stores used by endurance athletes.

Crude fiber: the fiber that remains in food after it has been treated with harsh chemicals during laboratory analysis.

Dietary fiber: the fiber that remains after food is digested in the human body.

Disaccharide: a combination of two simple sugars.

Electrolyte: a substance capable of conducting an electrical current.

Fats: organic compounds that are composed of glycerol and fatty acids.

Fiber: the indigestible polysaccharides that are found in the stems, leaves, and seeds of plants.

Insoluble Fiber: include cellulose, lignin, and hemicellulose. Insoluable fibers add bulk to the contents of the intestine accelerating the passage of food remnants through the digestive tract. These reduce the risk of colon cancer as well as other diseases of the digestive tract.

Kilocalories: the amount of energy found in food, it is the quantity of heat needed to raise the temperature of one kilogram of water one degree centigrade.

Minerals: inorganic substances that exist freely in nature.

Monosaccharide: simple sugars such as table sugar, honey, molasses, etc.

Phospholipids: similar to a triglyceride except that one of the fatty acids is replaced by a phosphorous-containing acid.

Polysaccharides: the joining of three or more simple sugars to form starch and glycogen.

Protein: a food substance formed from amino acids.

Saturated fats: found primarily in animal flesh and dairy products. Chemically, it carries the maximum number of hydrogen atoms.

Soluble fiber: pectin, gums, and other substances that add bulk to the contents of the stomach. These lower blood cholesterol levels.

Sterol: one of the three major fats with a structure similar to cholesterol.

Triglycerides: consist of three fatty acids attached to a glycerol molecule.

Unsaturated fats: fatty acids in which one or more points is free of hydrogen atoms.

Vitamins: organic compounds found in food that are essential to normal metabolism.

Introduction

Carbohydrates, fats, protein, vitamins, minerals, and water are the basic nutrients which, when taken in proper amounts allow the body to perform its many functions. They provide fuel for muscle contraction, maintain and repair body tissues, regulate chemical reactions at the cellular level, conduct nerve impulses, and contribute to growth and reproduction. Carbohydrate, fat, and protein supply the calories in the diet.

Metabolism is the sum total of chemical reactions whereby the energy liberated from food is made available to the body. Two processes are involved: anabolism, in which substances are built into new tissues or stored in some form for later use; and catabolism, which involves the breakdown of complex materials to simpler ones for the release of energy for muscular contraction.

Catabolism occurs when food is combined with oxygen. This process, referred to as oxidation, transforms food materials into heat or mechanical energy. The energy value of food is expressed as a calorie. The term "calorie" will represent the large calorie (k-Cal), which is the unit that is commonly used to assign the caloric value to food.

Carbohydrates

Carbohydrates (CHO) are organic compounds composed of carbon, hydrogen, and oxygen that are arranged as monosaccharides or multiples of monosaccharides. Carbohydrates are found almost exclusively in plant sources. The only animal source containing an appreciable amount is milk.

Carbohydrates are classified as simple or complex. Simple carbohydrates consist of monosaccharides (glucose, fructose, and galactose) and disaccharides (sucrose, lactose, and maltose). **Monosaccharides** are single sugars (mono = one; saccharide = sugar); **disaccharides** consist of two sugars bonded together (di = two; saccharide = sugar). Glucose and fructose are the most commonly occurring single sugars in nature. Sucrose, lactose, and maltose consist of two single sugars bonded together. Table sugar (sucrose) is a combination of glucose and fructose. Lactose, a double sugar made from the bonding of galactose and glucose, is the major sugar found in milk.

The complex carbohydrates (**polysaccharides**) are made of many single sugars that are strung together to form starch and most of the fibers. Starch comes entirely from plant sources, the richest of which are seeds such as grains, peas, and beans. Legumes—butter beans, kidney beans, black-eyed peas, chick-peas (garbanzo beans), and soybeans—are about 40 percent starch by weight.[1] Root vegetables (yams), tubers (potatoes), and rice are examples of other sources of starch.

Most **fibers** are indigestible polysaccharides which are found in the stems, leaves, and seeds of plants. Human digestive enzymes are incapable of breaking the bonds that hold the units of fiber together, but bacteria in the digestive tract can dismantle a few of the fibers so that a small amount of absorbable energy is derived. Fiber is therefore not totally devoid of kilocalories (kcals) although their contribution to total body energy is negligible.[2]

The amount of energy found in food is measured in **kilocalories** which is the amount of heat needed to raise the temperature of a kilogram of water (about one quart) 1 degree centigrade. People simply refer to these as calories but this is technically incorrect. There are 1000 calories in one kilocalorie so the energy in food is measured in thousands of calories. All food energy values in this text refer to kilocalories.

The most common polysaccharide fibers are cellulose, hemicellulose, pectin, and gums. These are the "nonstarch polysaccharides in foods."[3] **Crude fiber** is the fiber that remains in food after it has been treated with harsh chemicals during laboratory analysis. **Dietary fiber** is the fiber that remains after food is digested in the human body. Dietary fiber is the type which is of interest here.

Table sugar, corn syrup, molasses, and honey are some examples of simple sugars. Americans, active and inactive, consume too much of these substances; approximately 60 to 80 pounds per person per year. Most of this is in the form of hidden sugar; that is, it is included in processed foods. Canned soups and vegetables, canned meats, cereal, dairy products, soft drinks, and many other items are laden with sugar. Simple sugars are called "empty calories" because they are rich in calories but provide little or no nutrition. Many authorities feel that the excessive consumption of simple sugars leads to obesity, diabetes, elevated cholesterol, heart disease, and dental caries.

Starches such as rice, potatoes, cereal grains, and unprocessed vegetables are some of the complex carbohydrates. These supply energy, vitamins, min-

One 6 oz potato contains 40 percent of the daily requirement of vitamin C. It is also high in fiber, niacin, and potassium. Many of the nutrients are located in or near the skin. It only contains 180 Kcals.

Toasting bread removes much of the moisture but none of the calories.

erals, fiber, and water. They are broken down through complex digestive processes to simple sugar for absorption by the body. One might conjecture that consuming simple sugars to begin with would save all of the intermediate steps needed to oxidize complex carbohydrates. The problem with this apparently logical position is that humans have not had enough time to adapt to the digestive demands of simple sugar. It's only in the last few decades that this category of food has become available. When consumed, it gets into the bloodstream rapidly and triggers an abnormal insulin response that causes large swings in blood sugar levels. On the other hand, the complex carbohydrates are broken down slowly, get into the blood stream slowly, and the insulin response is more precise.

Carbohydrates had received bad press until 10 to 15 years ago and many misconceptions about this most valuable source of nutrition still exist. Many uninformed dieters delete or severely reduce their consumption of such carbohydrates as bread, potatoes, rice, and other starches in the mistaken belief that these foods are primarily responsible for weight gain. Actually, these complex carbohydrates (starch and fiber) should be increased because they are filling, high in water content and nutrients, and low in calories. Simple or concentrated sugars such as table sugar, honey, molasses, and the like are the carbohydrates to avoid because they are calorie-dense while lacking in fiber and nutrients. The problem with the complex carbohydrates lies in how they are cooked and prepared for serving. Rich sauces, sour cream, margarine, and other fatty substances are heaped on potatoes, rice and pastas—doubling, tripling, or quadrupling their caloric value.

Diets that are low in carbohydrates promote lean tissue and water loss. Each gram of glycogen (the stored form of carbohydrate) is stored with three grams of water. If the glycogen stores are depleted and not replenished, the lost water is also not replaced. Diet vendors capitalize on this knowledge to effect quick but ineffective water weight loss. Low-carbohydrate diets can lead to dehydration. When dieters return to prediet eating patterns, glycogen and all of the water needed to store it are returned so that the dieter quickly regains some of the lost weight.

Complex carbohydrates are looked on favorably by the nutritional and medical community. They are low in fat and high in fiber, both of which can help protect against heart disease and certain types of cancer. Dietary fiber consists of a number of different substances which appear to affect the body in various ways. Fiber is classified as soluble or insoluble. **Soluble fiber** (pectin, gums, and other substances) comes from a wide variety of grains, fruits, and vegetables. Excellent sources include prunes, pears, oranges, apples, dry beans, cauliflower, zucchini, sweet potatoes, and oat and corn bran. Soluble fibers add bulk to the contents of the stomach. This slows stomach emptying, prolongs the sense of feeling full, and reduces the desire to eat for a longer period of time. It also slows the absorption of sugars from the small intestine so that the blood sugar level rises moderately resulting in a more precise insulin response. Regarding cardiovascular health, it is the soluble fibers that lower blood cholesterol levels.

Insoluble fibers include cellulose, lignin, and hemicellulose. The best sources of insoluble fibers are whole grain cereals and breads. Insoluble fibers add bulk to the contents of the intestine rather than the stomach. This accelerates the passage of food remnants through the digestive tract and decreases tissue exposure time to toxins and carcinogenic substances. Insoluble fibers reduce the likelihood of developing colon cancer. Also, some insoluble fibers attract water thus softening stools and preventing constipation, while others solidify watery stools helping to alleviate diarrhea. The improved motility of the digestive contents contributes to the health and tone of the intestinal muscles which increases their resistance to the formation of pouches which signifies the onset of diverticulitis. Diverticulitis is characterized by pouchlike formations in the intestinal wall which are subject to serious infection should they rupture.

Some Fiber Sources

The list below contains some of the common sources of dietary fiber. Dietary fiber is always an estimate rather than an exact value because of the variability inherent in food samples, and because no standardized test method has been developed for simulating the human digestive process. The estimates below are in grams (gm).

I. Grains (1 oz)	Dietary Fiber (gm)
Brown rice, cooked (½ cup)	2.4
Millet, cooked (½ cup)	1.8
Whole wheat bread (1 slice)	1.0
Spaghetti, cooked (½ cup)	0.8
White bread (1 slice)	0.6
White rice, cooked (½ cup)	0.1

II. Legumes (½ cup)	
Kidney beans	5.8
Pinto beans	5.3
Split peas	5.1
White beans	5.0
Lima beans	4.9

III. Vegetables (½ cup)	
Sweet potatoe (1 large)	4.2
Peas	4.1
Brussel sprouts	3.9
Corn	3.9
Potatoe, baked (1 med.)	3.8
Carrots (1 raw; ½ cup cooked)	2.3
Collards	2.2
Asparagus	2.1
Green beans	2.1
Broccoli	2.0
Spinach	2.0
Turnips	1.7
Mushrooms (raw)	0.9
Summer squash	0.7
Lettuce (raw)	0.3

IV. Fruits	
Blackberries (½ cup)	4.5
Prunes, dried (3)	3.7
Apples with skin (1)	2.6
Banana (1 medium)	2.0
Strawberries (¾ cup)	2.0
Grapefruit (½ med.)	1.7
Peach (1 med.)	1.6

IV. Fruits (continued)	Dietary Fiber (gm)
Cantaloupe (¼ small)	1.4
Raisins (2 tablespoons)	1.3
Orange (1 small)	1.2
Grapes (12)	0.5

Adapted from J. Anderson, *Plant Fiber in Foods*, Lexington, Ky: HFC Diabetes Research Foundation, Inc., 1986, and the *Nutrition Action Healthletter* (April, 1986).

The National Cancer Institute recommends a daily consumption of 20 to 35 grams of fiber. Ideally, this should come from a variety of foods representing both soluble and insoluble types of fiber. The average American consumes less than half of this amount. A diet high in fiber displaces some of the high-calorie foods that contain concentrated fats and sugar. The advantages of such a diet, from a health perspective, are quite obvious. However, adding fiber in large doses is not recommended because unaccustomed large amounts produce several side effects. Fiber must be added slowly in order to avoid bloating, flatulence, cramps, and diarrhea. Also, heavy fiber intake may interfere with the absorption of iron, copper, calcium, zinc, and magnesium. This possibility can be circumvented by eating a balanced diet in which the recommended amount of dietary fiber is not exceeded.[4]

Many authorities suggest that an increase in high-fiber foods would produce beneficial changes in the disease patterns in the United States. The Select Committee on Nutrition recommended that 55 to 60 percent of our total calories come from carbohydrates.[5]

When oxidized, carbohydrates yield approximately 4 calories per gram. Because the calories are oxygen-rich, they constitute our most efficient source of fuel. About 30 to 40 percent of the body's energy needs at rest are supplied by carbohydrates.[6] Mild to moderate exercise such as walking 4 mph, jogging 1.7 to 3.4 miles in 20 to 40 minutes, and cycling at 10 mph rely on carbohydrates to contribute up to 50 percent of the energy. More vigorous exercise relies principally on carbohydrates, while very intense exercise relies almost exclusively upon carbohydrates.

A mistaken notion centers around the ingestion of simple sugar such as candy bars for the purpose of obtaining quick energy for physical activity. Highly dense sugar-laden foods get into the blood stream rapidly. The body overreacts by secreting more insulin than is needed into the blood. This causes the blood sugar level to fall below normal values and reduces rather than enhances performance.[6] Foster and his associates found that exercise time to exhaustion was decreased by 19 percent when subjects were given simple sugar 30 to 45 minutes prior to exercise.[7] Conversely, **carbohydrate loading** enhances the storage of muscle glycogen and increases one's capacity for prolonged aerobic work. This text has attempted to develop a rationale for exercise as an important component of health and wellness. In this context, carbohydrate loading in the classic manner is unacceptable as a component of a healthy lifestyle. Classic carbohydrate loading requires a glycogen depletion phase consisting of a 20 mile run or its equivalent seven days prior to performance. This is followed by three days of a very low-carbohydrate, high-protein, high-fat diet. This is the type of unhealthy diet that Americans have been asked to avoid. This phase is followed by three days of a very high-carbohydrate diet. If you are an aspiring marathoner, forget the depletion phase when you load and go straight to an increase in carbohydrates of the complex variety. Loading is only beneficial for endurance events of marathon distance or beyond.[8]

Fats

Fats are energy dense organic compounds that yield approximately 9 calories per gram. They have a relatively low oxygen content when compared to carbohydrates and consequently are not as efficient as sources of fuel. It takes more than twice the amount of oxygen to liberate energy from fat than from carbohydrates. However, we store at least 50 times more energy in the form of fat than in carbohydrates.

Fats (lipids) consist of three major types: triglycerides, sterols, and phospholipids. The triglycerides are the most abundant type of fat, representing 95 percent of the fat that is eaten as well as that which is stored within the body. The **sterols** have a structure similar to cholesterol. The **phospholipids** are similar to a triglyceride except that one of the fatty acids is replaced by a phosphorous-containing acid. The **triglycerides** are composed of three fatty acids attached to a molecule of glycerol. Fatty acids are chains of carbon, oxygen, and hydrogen atoms which are classified as saturated or unsaturated based upon their chemical structure. A fatty acid is **saturated** when all of its carbons are occupied with hydrogen and **unsaturated** when some carbon sites in the chain are free of hydrogen.

Sources of saturated fats are butter, cheese, chocolate, coconuts and coconut oil, meats, milk, palm oil, and poultry. Saturated fats such as bacon grease, have a high melting point and solidify at room temperature. Unsaturated fats such as corn oil, have a lower melting point and remain liquid at room temperature. Monosaturated fats such as olive oil, also remain liquid at room temperature. Until a few years ago, nutritional research indicated that the monosaturates were neutral fats with no substantial role in certain disease processes. However, today the evidence strongly suggests that these fats are at least as good, or maybe better, than the polyunsaturates in lowering blood levels of cholesterol.[9] In fact, a diet where 40 percent of total calories consisted of fat, most of which was monosaturated, lowered cholesterol levels significantly better than a diet whose fat content was only 20 percent of the total calories.[10] The monosaturated fat diet reduced LDL cholesterol without reducing HDL cholesterol. The 20 percent fat diet significantly lowered HDL cholesterol. The American Heart Association (AHA) has recognized the emerging role of monosaturated fats in lowering cholesterol by recommending that they comprise one-third of the total intake of fat. Remember, the AHA also recommends lowering fat consumption to 30 percent of the total calories.

Monosaturated fatty acids, unlike saturated which has all its carbons occupied with hydrogen, contain one point in the carbon chain which is free of hydrogen. Sources of monosaturated fats include avocodos, cashew nuts, olives and olive oil, peanuts, peanut oil, and peanut butter. Polyunsaturated fatty acids have two or more points in the carbon chain which are free of hydrogen. Sources of polyunsaturated fats include almonds, corn oil, cottonseed oil, filbert nuts, fish, soft margarine, pecans, safflower oil, soybean oil, sunflower oil, and walnuts.

Polyunsaturated oils should be refrigerated to keep them from becoming rancid. They are vulnerable to spoilage when left to stand at room temperature because oxygen attacks those points in the chain that are unoccupied by hydrogen. To counteract spoilage the food industry adds hydrogen to some of the free bonds through the process of hydrogenation. The fat then loses its polyunsaturated characteristics as well as its health benefits.

The only pasta that contains cholesterol is egg noodles. One serving (1 cup cooked) has about 70 mg of cholesterol, nearly 25 percent of the daily recommended maximum.

Eating a fat-free diet is virtually impossible. Even vegetarian diets supply 5 to 10 percent of their calories from fat. Some fat in the diet is necessary for good health, however, the problem in the United States is that we consume too much fat. Some authorities contend that an optimal amount of fat in the diet is closer to 20 percent of the total calories as opposed to the AHAs suggested 30 percent. The human body can synthesize its fat requirements from carbohydrates, fats, and proteins with the exception of two fatty acids. Linoleic acid and linolenic acid are categorized as essential fatty acids because they cannot be manufactured in sufficient amounts within the body to meet physiological needs. Both are polyunsaturated fatty acids which can only be supplied through the diet. These fatty acids are widely distributed in plant and fish oils. Linoleic acid is an omega-6 fatty acid found mostly in plants while linolenic acid is an omega-3 fatty acid found in fish. The fatty acids in cold water fish are the most polyunsaturated of the fats.[11]

Fish Oil Effects are Not Fishy

New evidence is emerging which suggests that dietary intake of fish and fish oil may reduce the risk of heart attack. Dutch investigators studied hundreds of middle-aged males for 20 years and reported in the May edition of the 1985 *New England Journal of Medicine* that subjects who ate no fish were more than twice as likely to die of a heart attack as subjects who ate fish regularly.[12] At the same time American scientists reported that a diet rich in fish oils was more effective in reducing cholesterol in the blood than a diet rich in vegetable oils such as safflower and corn oil. The consumption of fish serves two purposes, (1) it replaces some of the saturated fat which would have normally been ingested, and (2) it seems to have intrinsic therapeutic value. Omega-3 fatty acids reduce the incidence of heart attack by lowering blood levels of cholesterol and, by inhibiting the process that forms blood clots. The blood platelets use arachidonic acid, which is formed from linoleic acid, to produce thromboxane A2. Thromboxane A2 initiates the clotting process by (1) stimulating the platelets to clump together, and (2) constricting blood vessels at the site of platelet aggregation. This is an important safety mechanism for controlling bleeding when the circulatory vessels are injured, but is a very hazardous process when initiated in the absence of bleeding.

The cells in the walls of blood vessels release prostacyclin which is a substance that dilates blood vessels and prevents platelet clumping. Fish oil acts by inhibiting the formation of arachidonic acid so that the prostacyclin effect dominates and decreases the tendency to form clots.

Atherosclerosis occurs because of damage to the cells lining the artery walls. Cell inflammation precedes the deposit of cholesterol. Fish oil maintains the integrity of the cell walls because it interferes with the process of inflammation and blocks the deposition of cholesterol. Omega-3 fatty acids also increase the amount of tissue plasminogen activator which dissolves clots that have previously formed in the coronary arteries. More than 70 studies have documented the effects of omega-3 fatty acids in reducing coronary risk as well as conferring other healthy benefits. For instance, these studies indicate that omega-3 fatty acids may enhance the body's natural defenses against the development of cancer, and they may reduce the inflammation associated with arthritis and asthma.

How much fish must be consumed to achieve all of this protection? Surprisingly, not a great deal. Authorities suggest that two to three fish meals per week will suffice. However, fish oil capsules and other fish supplements are ill advised at this point because: (1) the quantity of fish oil needed to produce these benefits is unknown, (2) the fish oils may contain toxins such as pesticides and other contaminants, (3) the fish oils are rich in vitamins A and D, which if taken in excess can cause vitamin toxicity, and (4) an excess of polyunsaturated oils can result in a vitamin E deficiency. Eating fish does not have the same deleterious effects. Also fish contains many other nutrients as well. Purified fish oils contain just oil and many calories.

Excellent sources of omega-3 fatty acids are: anchovies, herring, mackerel, sablefish, salmon, sardines, fresh tuna, and whitefish. Fish with moderately high omega-3 fatty acids include bass, bluefish, halibut, mullet, ocean perch, rainbow trout, rockfish, and smelt. Oysters are the only shellfish high in this important fatty acid.

Fat serves many vital functions. Fat is a significant energy source that provides up to 70 percent of the calories needed while the body is at rest. It is responsible for the storage, transport, and absorption of the fat soluble vitamins. Fat is an essential component of nerve fibers and cell walls and protects vital organs from physical trauma by acting as a shock absorber. Fat also acts as an insulator against the loss of body heat. Excessive amounts of dietary or stored fat are not required to support these functions.

Fat is the major supplier of energy during rest, mild exercise (below 60 percent of the aerobic capacity) and low-intensity exercise of long duration. Exercise for the purpose of weight loss should emphasize prolonged and consistent mild exercise. As exercise intensity increases, the percentage of energy derived from fat decreases.

Protein

Protein is one of the most misused and abused of the nutrients. It has been advertised as a high-energy food. In the Roman Empire, gladiators were fed large amounts of animal muscle tissue in the belief that this practice would build human muscle tissues. Many of today's body builders, weight lifters, and power lifters continue this practice. They consume enormous quantities of protein-rich foods and supplements in the belief that active people cannot obtain too much protein.

Protein is an essential nutrient that yields approximately 4 calories per gram but whose energy is liberated for the building and repair of body tissues; the formation of enzymes, hormones, antibodies and hemoglobin; the transportation of fats and other nutrients in the blood; the maintenance of acid-base balance in tissue fluids; and supplying energy for muscular work when there is a shortage of carbohydrates and fat.

Proteins are complex chemical structures containing carbon, oxygen, hydrogen, and nitrogen. These elements are combined into chains of different structures called **amino acids.** There is general agreement that the proteins of all living tissue consist of 20 different amino acids. Two other rare amino acids have been identified but are found in very few proteins. Eight of the amino acids are essential because they cannot be manufactured in the body; these can only be obtained through the diet.

Skinless turkey contains about 33 percent less fat than skinless chicken. Skinless dark turkey and chicken meat contains twice as much fat as skinless white meat, 20 percent more calories, and 10 percent less protein.

In order to build body tissues, all of the amino acids must be present simultaneously. This is analogous to building a house. Construction progresses unimpeded as long as all of the building materials are at the site, but if there isn't any mortar to lay the bricks, construction stops until it is supplied. Similarly, the building of body tissue progresses to completion when all of the amino acids (the body's building blocks) are present, but if one or more is missing construction stops at that point. Complete proteins, those containing all the amino acids, are found in meat, fish, poultry and dairy products. The proteins found in vegetables and cereal grains generally do not contain all of the amino acids but complementary foods from these two groups may be selected so that one supplies those amino acids missing in the other. See Table 10.1 for combinations of food which together provide complete proteins.

Legumes such as kidney and lima beans, black-eyed peas, garden peas, lentils, and soybeans are excellent sources of protein. Although their protein is not quite the caliber of that in meat they are rich in fiber, iron, and B-vitamins and they are low in fat.

Daily protein requirements vary according to our position in the life cycle. Infants require about 2.2 grams of protein per kilogram of body weight to support growth. Adolescents require 1.0 gram per kilogram and adults need 0.8 gram per kilogram. Table 10.2 summarizes the protein requirements by age.

TABLE 10.1   Complete Proteins from Vegetable Combinations

Categories of foods	Examples
Beans/wheat	Baked beans and brown bread
Beans/rice	Refried beans and rice
Dry peas/rye	Split pea soup and rye bread
Peanut butter/wheat	Peanut butter sandwich on wheat or whole grain bread
Cornmeal/beans	Cornbread and kidney beans
Legumes/rice	Black-eyed peas and rice
Beans/corn	Pinto beans and corn bread
Legumes/corn	Black-eyed peas and corn bread

Adapted from A. C. Grandjeans, *The Vegetarian Athlete,* 15 (1987): 191.

TABLE 10.2   Recommended Daily Allowance (RDA) for Protein

Age (yr)	RDA (grams/kilogram*)
0–½	2.2
½–1	2.0
1–3	1.8
4–10	1.1
11–14	1.0
15–18	0.9
19 and beyond	0.8

*Pregnancy increases the protein requirement by 30 grams per day and lactation increases the protein requirement by 20 grams per day.

The typical American diet contains more than adequate amounts of protein. There seems to be no advantage in consuming more than 15 percent of the total calories in the form of protein. Excessive intakes have altered the body composition of children[13] and enlarged the kidneys and livers of animals.[14] It can cause dehydration because extra water is needed to rid the body of unused or wasted nitrogen. This can be a significant problem for active people because they lose additional fluid in perspiration during a workout. Another problem associated with excessive protein intake is that it is usually accomplished by increasing the consumption of animal products which are also high in saturated fat. This may displace fiber in the diet possibly leading to constipation. In addition, these foods are expensive. Ingesting larger than normal amounts of protein does not enhance physical performance; but then, that is not protein's function.

Many people, competitors and noncompetitors alike, who are striving to develop strength and power have been taking amino acid supplements to build larger and more powerful muscles. Selected amino acids do not build larger muscles, only exercise can do that. However, these and other unfounded notions proliferate among uninformed participants who are constantly attempting to enhance performance with substances that might give them an edge beyond that achieved with training. William Evans, Chief of the Physiology Laboratory in the Human Nutrition Research Center on Aging at Tufts University stated that, "If you have an intestine, you don't need amino acid supplements. The intestine breaks down protein perfectly well. Furthermore, no research indicates that amino acid supplements improve strength, power, or muscle mass."[15]

Vegetarianism

Vegetarianism, with its biblical origins, is probably the oldest form of diet known. There are many reasons for pursuing such a style of eating from those that are health-related to those that are philosophical and cultural. Regardless of the reason, vegetarianism requires some basic nutritional knowledge in order to meet the recommended daily allowances for normal nutrition. The amount of knowledge required depends on the restrictiveness of the diet. This is reflected by the type of vegetarian diet that is practiced. Vegetarianism runs the gamet from strict adherence to plant foods to other less restrictive forms which allow animal products. The types of vegetarian diets are as follows:

1. Fruitarians: food choices consist of raw or dried fruit, nuts, honey, and vegetable oil.
2. Vegen: all plant food diet without animal foods, milk products, or eggs.
3. Lacto-vegetarian: vegetable diet plus milk and milk products.
4. Lacto-ovo-vegetarian: vegetable diet plus milk, milk products, and eggs.
5. Semivegetarian: vegetable diet plus some groups of animal products.
6. New Vegetarian: vegetable diet plus some groups of animal products. Emphasis is placed on foods that are organic, natural, and unprocessed or unrefined.

Active people who are strict vegetarians (vegens) many times have difficulty obtaining enough calories to meet their daily caloric expenditure.[16] Their diet consists of foods that are nutritionally dense, high in fiber, but low in calories. They may need to supplement with high-calorie foods such as nuts, seeds, legumes, and vegetable margarine. The problem with strict vegetarian diets is not only limited to low calorie intake. Vitamin B12 is found almost exclusively in animal products. Vitamin B12 supplements may be taken or the vegen may elect to use soybean milk fortified with

B12. Complete proteins may be obtained by matching appropriate foods as suggested in Table 10.1. The high-fiber content of vegetable diets interferes with the absorption of iron. Legumes are a good source of iron, however, the iron contained in these foods is less absorbable than that found in meats. Vegens can triple the absorption of iron from legumes by eating vitamin C rich foods at each meal.

There is no practical source of vitamin D in plant foods. Regular exposure to the sun should prevent a deficiency but vegetarians need to be aware of the positive relationship that exists between skin cancer and exposure to the sun's rays. It may be better to take a one-a-day vitamin/mineral supplement than to sun bathe. Calcium may be obtained from calcium-fortified soy milk, stone ground meal, legumes, almonds, sesame seeds, collards, mustard greens, and okra. The absorption of zinc is also inhibited by fiber.[17] Sources of zinc include legumes, soy products, nuts, and seeds.

Vegetarianism, as practiced by informed people, constitutes a very healthy style of eating. On the average, knowledgeable vegetarians are leaner, have lower cholesterol levels, and lower blood pressures than meat eaters. They also have lower rates of certain kinds of cancer, lower mortality from cardiovascular diseases, and greater longevity than their meat-eating counterparts.

POINTS TO PONDER

1. *Define anabolism, catabolism, and metabolism.*
2. *Define simple and complex carbohydrates and give some examples of each.*
3. *What are the major functions of soluble and insoluble dietary fiber?*
4. *How much fiber should people consume on a daily basis?*
5. *Name the major categories of fats and discuss the differences among them.*
6. *What are the essential fatty acids and identify both of them?*
7. *What are the health implications associated with the different categories of fats?*
8. *Discuss the role of fish oil as it relates to cardiovascular health.*
9. *Describe the daily protein requirements of children, adolescents, and adults.*
10. *What is a complete protein?*
11. *Identify and describe the different types of vegetarianism.*
12. *Discuss the advantages and disadvantages of following a vegetarian diet.*

Vitamins

One cup of broccoli or cauliflower contains more vitamin C than an orange. They are also high in fiber and, as with other "cruciferous vegetables," may protect against certain forms of cancer.

Vitamins are noncaloric organic compounds found in small quantities in most foods. All vitamins are either fat-soluble or water-soluble. The fat-soluble vitamins A, D, E, and K are stored in the liver and fatty tissues until they are needed. The water-soluble vitamins, C and the B complex group, are not stored for any appreciable length of time and must be replenished daily.

Vitamins function as coenzymes that promote the many chemical reactions that occur in the body around the clock. Vitamin deficiencies result in a variety of diseases; therefore, an adequate daily intake is necessary for optimal health. The recommended daily allowances (RDA) have been established for most of the vitamins. These amounts are needed to prevent the occurrence of diseases that are the result of vitamin deficiencies, but they do not represent optimal values. However, the RDA are based on the best available evidence. The recommended levels actually cover the nutritional needs of 98 to 99 percent of the American population.[18] However, an alarming trend—the practice of taking megadoses of vitamins in the mistaken belief that extremely large doses will prevent or cure anything—has surfaced in recent years. Manufacturers and advertisers have convinced the public that the American diet is so deficient in vitamins that supplementation is a necessity. Those who supplement heavily may experience vitamin toxicity, particularly from overindulgence in the fat-soluble group. When vitamins are taken in very large amounts they cease to function as vitamins and begin to act more like drugs. Also, large doses interfere or disrupt the action of other nutrients. See Tables 10.3 and 10.4 for problems associated with vitamin megadoses.

Are synthetic vitamins inferior to natural vitamins? Promoters of vitamin products that come from natural sources adamantly proclaim that this is correct, but see below for another viewpoint.

Synthetic versus Natural Vitamins

It should be repeated that the body's cells can't tell the difference between the synthesized vitamin and the "natural" vitamin, even though the marketers of "natural" vitamins would like you to believe otherwise. The word synthetic sometimes implies fake, as in a synthetic (fake) fur coat. To the chemist, however, to synthesize means to put together—and the product is not fake, it is identical to the real thing.

Vitamins sold as natural often have synthetics added anyway. For example, vitamin C pills made from rose hips would have to be as big as golf balls to contain significant amounts of the vitamin. The manufacturer therefore adds synthetic vitamin to the small amount of "natural" vitamin and sells the product for many times the original price.

As we said earlier, a cell picking up vitamins from the bloodstream can't tell the difference between the vitamins from pills and those from foods. However, the digestive tract often does respond to the vehicle in which nutrients arrive. For some reason, synthetic vitamin C seems to be better retained than "natural" vitamin C when both are supplied in pill form. But because the body evolved to utilize foods, not pills, we might guess that vitamin C would be retained even better if it came from foods. The lesson in this must be that it really is not natural to take any kind of pills.

Studies too numerous to mention in this text have shown that a deficiency in one or more water-soluble vitamins is inimical to physical performance. Work output deteriorates, fatigue occurs more rapidly, and there is a tendency toward muscular soreness as a result. Work output returns to normal when vitamin intake is restored, but above-normal amounts do not appear to promote further increases in work output, muscular strength, or resistance to fatigue.

The results of an excellent double-blind, crossover placebo study with 30 competitive male runners (average age 32 yr) were recently reported.[19] For three months, 15 of the subjects were given daily vitamin and mineral supplements while the other 15 received placebo pills. This was followed by a three-month "washout" period, that is, neither group received the true supplement. This was followed by a three-month crossover trial in which the original placebo group was switched to the vitamin and mineral supplement, and the original supplement group was switched to the placebo. This occurred without the

TABLE 10.3   Vitamin RDA, Sources, and Toxic Symptoms (Fat Soluable)

Vitamin (U.S. RDA)	Sources	Toxic Symptoms
Vitamin A (1000 RE)	Fortified milk and margarine, cream, cheese, butter, eggs, liver, spinach and other dark leafy greens, broccoli, apricots, peaches, cantaloupe, squash, carrots, sweet potatoes, and pumpkin.	Red blood cell breakage, nosebleeds, abdominal cramps, nausea, diarrhea, weight loss, blurred vision, irritability, loss of appetite, bone pain, dry skin, rashes, hair loss, cessation of menstruation, growth retardation.
Vitamin D (400 IU)	Self-synthesis with sunlight, fortified milk, fortified margarine, eggs, liver, fish.	Raised blood calcium, constipation, weight loss, irritability, weakness, nausea, kidney stones, mental and physical retardation.
Vitamin E (30 IU)	Vegetable oils, green and leafy vegetables, wheat germ, whole-grain products, butter, liver, egg yolk, milk fat, nuts, seeds.	Interference with anticlotting medication, general discomfort.
Vitamin K (no U.S. RDA)	Bacterial synthesis in digestive tract, liver, green leafy and cabbage-type vegetables, milk.	Interference with anticlotting medication, may cause jaundice.

knowledge of the subjects or the researchers who administered the supplements. The results indicated that vitamin and mineral supplementation did not significantly change performance. Unchanged were aerobic capacity, peak running speed on the treadmill, peak blood lactate concentrations, and there was no significant change in the time required to run 15 km (9.3 miles).

Active people get more vitamins in the diet than sedentary people because they consume more calories. If you are concerned about not getting enough vitamins in your diet but unwilling to make appropriate changes, then a one-a-day brand should do. More than this amount is unnecessary and costly.

Minerals

Minerals are inorganic substances that exist freely in nature. They are found in the earth's soil and water and they pervade some of its vegetation. Minerals maintain or regulate such physiological processes as muscle contraction, normal heart rhythm, body water supplies, acid-base balance of the blood, and nerve impulse conduction. Calcium, phosphorous, potassium, sulphur, sodium, chloride, and magnesium are the major minerals. These are classified as major

TABLE 10.4   Vitamin RDA, Sources, and Toxic Symptoms (Water Soluable)

Vitamin (U.S. RDA)	Sources	Toxic Symptoms
Thiamin B1 (1.5 mg)	Meat, pork, liver, fish, poultry, whole grain and enriched breads, cereals, pasta, nuts, legumes, wheat germ, oats.	Rapid pulse, weakness, headaches, insomnia, irritability.
Riboflavin B2 (1.7 mg)	Milk, dark-green vegetables, yogurt, cottage cheese, liver, meat, whole grain or enriched breads and cereals.	None reported, but an excess of any of the B vitamins could cause a deficiency of the others.
Niacin B3 (20 mg)	Meat, eggs, poultry, fish, milk, whole grain and enriched breads and cereals, nuts, legumes, peanuts, nutritional yeast, all protein foods.	Flushing, nausea, headaches, cramps, ulcer irritation, heartburn, abnormal liver function, low blood pressure.
Vitamin B6 (2.0 mg)	Meat, poultry, fish, shellfish, legumes, whole-grain products, green and leafy vegetables, bananas.	Depression, fatigue, irritability, headaches, numbness, damage to nerves, difficulty walking.
Folacin (Folic acid) (400g or Micrograms)	Green leafy vegetables, organ meats, legumes, seeds.	Diarrhea, insomnia, irritability, may mask a vitamin B12 deficiency.
Vitamin B12 (Cobalamin) (3g)	Animal products: meats, fish, poultry, shellfish, milk, cheese, eggs, nutritional yeast.	None reported.
Pantothenic acid (10 mg)	Widespread in foods.	Occasional diarrhea.
Biotin (300g)	Widespread in foods.	None reported.
Vitamin C (Ascorbic acid) (60 mg)	Citrus fruits, cabbage-type vegetables, tomatoes, potatoes, dark-green vegetables, peppers, lettuce, cantaloupe, strawberries, mangos, papayas.	Nausea, abdominal cramps, diarrhea, breakdown of red blood cells in persons with certain genetic disorders, deficiency symptoms may appear at first on withdrawal of high doses.

because they occur in the body in quantities greater than five grams. The trace minerals or micronutrients number a dozen or more. The distinction between the major and trace minerals is one of quantity rather than importance. Deficiencies of either can have serious consequences.

Sodium, potassium, and chloride are the primary minerals lost through perspiration. Sodium, the positive ion in sodium chloride (table salt), is one of the body's major **electrolytes** (ions that conduct electricity). Americans consume 6 to 18 grams of sodium daily but only one to three grams is recommended by the Food and Nutrition Board of the National Academy of Sciences.[20] Estimates vary regarding the origination of salt in the American diet. One estimate indicates that one-third comes from each of the following: processed foods, natural salt in foods, and the salt shaker. Another estimate indicates that as much as 75 percent of our salt intake comes from processed foods.[21]

Physically active people who sweat profusely for prolonged periods of time may require some salt replacement. Symptoms of salt depletion include nausea, weakness, loss of appetite, and muscle cramps. A general rule regarding salt replacement concerns the amount of liquid that one must drink in a day to replace that which is lost because of sweating. Each extra quart of water above four quarts should be accompanied by a gram of salt.[14] However, conscious salt replacement should not occur indiscriminately since most Americans consume too much. Physically active people attain more than the normal amount through their diets because of their extra food consumption.

Sodium is found in the fluid outside of the cells while potassium is found within cellular fluid. The temporary exchange of sodium and potassium across the cell's membrane permits the transmission of neural impulses and the contraction of muscles. Low potassium levels interfere with muscle cell nutrition and lead to muscle weakness and fatigue. Potassium is essential for the maintenance of the heart beat. Starvation and very low-calorie diets for prolonged periods may produce sudden death from heart failure as potassium storage drops to critically low levels. Vomiting, diarrhea, and diuretics (medication to rid the body of excess water) reduce potassium levels. Chronic physical activity that produces heavy sweating may gradually diminish the potassium levels. Potassium should be replaced daily and this can be easily accomplished because it is contained in most foods. It is particularly abundant in oranges, grapefruit, bananas, dates, nuts, fresh vegetables, meat, and fish.

As with vitamins, mineral intake may also be abused. Excess amount of both major and trace minerals produce a variety of symptoms (see Tables 10.5 and 10.6).

Water

People may survive for a month or more without food but a few days without water will result in death. All body processes and chemical reactions take place in a liquid medium, therefore it is imperative to be fully hydrated and to make a special effort to replace water when it is lost. Under normal conditions adults drink 1.2 to 1.4 liters of fluid each day. More is needed when the weather is hot and humid or when one is physically active regardless of weather conditions.

Approximately 40 to 60 percent of the body's weight consists of water. A sizeable amount is stored in the muscles and some is stored in fat. By virtue of his larger muscle mass, the average male stores more water than the average female. Sixty-two percent of the total amount of water is found in the intracellular compartment (water which is within the cells), while the remaining 38 percent is extracellular (water in the blood, lymph system, spinal cord fluid, saliva, etc.).

TABLE 10.5   RDA, Sources, and Toxic Symptoms (Major Minerals)

Minerals (U.S. RDA)	Selected Sources	Toxic Symptoms
Calcium, Phosphorus (1000 mg)	Calcium: milk and milk products, small fish (with bones), tofu, greens, legumes. Phosphorus: all animal tissues.	Excess calcium is excreted except in hormonal imbalance states. Excess phosphorus can create relative deficiency of calcium.
Magnesium (400 mg)	Nuts, legumes, whole grains, dark green vegetables, seafoods, chocolate, cocoa.	Not known.
Sodium (no U.S. RDA)	Salt, soy sauce, moderate quantities in whole (unprocessed) foods, large amounts in processed foods.	Hypertension.
Chloride (no U.S. RDA)	Salt, soy sauce, moderate quantities in whole (unprocessed) foods, large amounts in processed foods.	Normally harmless (the gas chlorine is a poison but evaporates from water), disturbed acid-base balance, vomiting.
Potassium (no U.S. RDA)	All whole foods: meats, milk, fruits, vegetables, grains, legumes.	Causes muscular weakness, triggers vomiting, if given into a vein, can stop the heart.
Sulfur (no U.S. RDA)	All protein-containing foods.	Would occur only if sulfur amino acids were eaten in excess; this (in animals) depresses growth.

Water level in the body is maintained primarily by drinking fluids, but solid foods also contribute to water replenishment. Many foods—fruits, vegetables and meats—contain large amounts of water. Even seemingly dry foods such as bread contain some water. Solid foods add water in another way—they contribute metabolic water, which is one of the by-products of their breakdown to energy sources.

Most water loss occurs through urination, while small quantities are lost in the feces and in exhaled air from the lungs. Insensible perspiration (that which is not visible) accounts for a considerable amount of water loss. Exercise and hot humid weather increase sweating, so more water must be consumed during these times. Exercise in hot weather and water replacement guidelines were discussed in Chapter 6.

Guidelines for Healthy Eating

The following dietary guidelines will enable you to evaluate your current eating habits. These guidelines differ from dieting per se in that they provide a sensible

TABLE 10.6   RDA, Sources, and Toxic Symptoms (Trace Minerals)

Minerals (U.S. RDA)	Selected Sources	Toxic Symptoms
Iodine (150 g)	Iodized salt, seafood.	Very high intakes depress thyroid activity.
Iron (18 mg)	Red meats, fish, poultry, shellfish, eggs, legumes, dried fruits.	Iron overload: infections, liver injury.
Zinc (15 mg)	Protein containing foods: meats, fish, poultry, grains, vegetables.	Fever, nausea, vomiting, diarrhea.
Copper (2 mg)	Meats, drinking water.	Unknown except as part of a rare hereditary disease (Wilson's disease).
Fluoride (no U.S. RDA)	Drinking water (if naturally fluoride containing or fluoridated), tea, seafood.	Fluorosis: discoloration of teeth.
Selenium (no U.S. RDA)	Seafood, meat, grains.	Digestive system disorders.
Chromium (no U.S. RDA)	Meats, unrefined foods, fats, vegetable oils.	Unknown as a nutrition disorder. Occupational exposures damage skin and kidneys.
Molybdenum, Manganese (no U.S. RDA)	Molybdenum: legumes, cereals, organ meats. Manganese: widely distributed in foods.	Molybdenum: enzyme inhibition. Manganese: poisoning, nervous system disorders.
Cobalt (no U.S. RDA)	Meats, milk, and milk products.	Unknown as a nutritional disorder.

approach to healthy, low-calorie eating that can be maintained for life rather than for a few weeks or months.

Fig bars have double the fiber and less than half the fat calories of other cookies, but they are high in sugar and total calories.

1. Eat more fresh fruit, vegetables (some should be consumed raw), and cereal grains. These are low in calories, high in fiber, and filling. Fresh fruit contains natural sugar and may satisfy your craving for sweets. Canned fruit is acceptable if it is packed in its own juice rather than in syrup. Olives, avocados, and coconuts are the exceptions in that the first two are high in fat while the latter is high in saturated fat, so reduce consumption of these foods.

2. Gradually increase consumption of food high in soluble and insoluble fiber for the reasons previously discussed in this chapter.

3. Many dieters abstain from eating bread. This is a mistake because it is chewy, nutritious, filling, and relatively low in calories. Acceptable breads include sourdough, French, Italian, pita, and whole grain.

   Don't load bread down with butter, margarine, jellies, jams, creamed cheese, peanut butter and the like because these substances can double or triple the number of calories in a slice of bread. If you must use these toppings the key is to spread them lightly.

Rice, macaroni, pastas, and potatoes are excellent low-calorie foods provided they, too, are not loaded down with such goodies as butter, margarine, sour cream, and rich sauces.

4. Increase your consumption of fish particularly those that are rich in omega-3 fatty acids.

5. Eat more poultry; it is high in protein and low in fat. Skin a chicken before cooking it because 50 percent of its fat is located in and directly beneath the skin. Turkey skin is usually too tough to be eaten.

   Avoid or only occasionally eat domesticated duck and goose because these are high in fat. Wild duck and geese are more acceptable. Quail and dove are low in fat.

6. Reduce consumption of red meat (beef and pork) and select the leaner cuts. Leaner cuts are cheaper, and are healthier for the wallet as well as the body. Round steak is relatively cheap and approximately 80 percent water, with the remainder consisting of muscle tissue and fat. With all of the visible fat trimmed prior to cooking, round steak becomes a weight watcher's delight. Beef fillets are tender because they are marbled with fat.

   Bacon and sausage are high in fat, salt, and nitrates and should be consumed sparingly. Hot dogs and lunch meats (cold cuts) are usually high in fat and salt. However, there are some lunch meats that are 97 percent fat-free. Also, hot dogs made from chicken or turkey have less fat than those made from beef but they still have substantial calories which come from their fat content. Salt in lunch meats and hot dogs has yet to be reduced. Organ meats such as liver and kidneys are nutritious but are high in cholesterol. Brains are especially high in cholesterol. All of these foods are to be avoided or eaten sparingly. Cholesterol is a primary risk factor for heart disease and salt is associated with an increase in blood pressure, which is another of the primary risk factors.

7. Dairy products are important sources of nutrition but many of these products are high in fat and saturated fat. Therefore, emphasize low fat dairy foods such as skim milk and cheeses and other foods made from skim milk. Skim milk has all of the nutrition of whole milk without the fat; therefore, it is lower in calories.

   As a general rule, no more than three eggs should be eaten per week because they are very high in cholesterol. However, all of the cholesterol is found in the yolk. The egg whites instead are actually a good source of protein.

8. Choose margarines, liquid oil shortenings, salad dressings, and mayonnaise made from unsaturated oils. Oil from corn, cottonseed, safflower, sunflower, canola, and olive are good examples. Read the labels, however, because if these oils are hydrogenated by the manufacturer (a process which converts unsaturated oil into the more harmful saturated oil), any advantage to be gained by using them is lost.

   Saturated fats come from animal sources and too much of these in the diet can be harmful as they become part of the artery-clogging process. Unsaturated fats are preferred because these are not implicated in the causation of heart disease, in fact, they may help to reduce the cholesterol level in the blood. However, fat, whether saturated or unsaturated, is rich in calories. Fats yield 9 Kcals per gram as opposed to the 4 Kcal yield

The 3½ percent fat in whole milk supplies 50 percent of the calories. Fat supplies 30 percent of the calories in 2 percent milk; 18 percent of the calories in 1 percent milk; and 2 percent of the calories in skim milk.

per gram from protein and carbohydrate. The key to consuming fat is to reduce the intake of fat to 30 percent of the total calories. Of the total intake of fat calories, saturated fat should not be more than one-third of the fat calories.

9. Go easy on seeds and nuts, particularly if they are salted, because of the relationship between high salt intake and high blood pressure. These snacks are also very high in fat and total calories. However, nuts are a good source of many nutrients. Two whole walnuts or 10 large peanuts contain 5 grams of fat or the equivalent of 45 Kcals of fat. This is the caloric equivalent of a teaspoon of butter or margarine.

10. Avoid other high-calorie snacks—those rich in sugar and/or fat such as candy, cookies, cakes, pies, ice cream, honey, molasses, syrup, and commercially fried food such as potato chips and other deep-fried snacks.

11. Limit your intake of cola drinks. Also limit your daily intake of coffee and tea. These beverages contain caffeine, a strong stimulant which affects the central nervous system. The effect reaches a peak one to four hours after it is consumed. While caffeine is not addictive, it is habit forming. It has produced arrhythmias (irregular heart beats) and should be avoided by those who are subject to these irregularites. Table 10.7 illustrates some of the sources of caffeine.

Expresso coffee is roasted for a longer period of time than the popular American coffees and as a result has less caffeine.

12. Drink alcohol moderately or not at all. Alcohol is second only to fat in caloric density and these are essentially empty calories containing very few nutrients. Beer and wine contain some nutrients but the majority of their calories come from alcohol. Hard liquors have no nutrients and all of their calories come from alcohol.

Alcohol is a mood-modifying depressant drug that has profound effects upon the brain and central nervous system. Reaction time slows down and judgment is impaired under its influence. Most important, do not drink and drive.

13. Reduce your consumption of processed foods. Canned vegetables and soups, as well as frozen and canned entrees are generally high in sugar and salt. Read labels on cans and boxes and you will find these two additives in most processed foods. They are relatively cheap sources of adding flavor while catering to Americans' acquired taste for these substances.

Processed foods are also high in fat—most likely in saturated fat—and therefore higher in calories than their unprocessed or raw counterparts.

14. Patronize fast food restaurants less frequently. These places serve food that is generally high in fat and salt. For instance, pizza is a very nutritious food but it is extremely high in salt. Chicken is usually low in fat and calories but the preparation techniques in fast food places increase the caloric value so that it is at least equal to and often greater than a large hamburger. Check the Kcals, fat, and sodium content of foods in the Fast Foods Listing in Appendix A. Fast foods are not necessarily junk foods, but should be carefully chosen and should not be eaten regularly.

TABLE 10.7 Selected Sources of Caffeine

Beverages	Serving Size (oz)	Caffeine (mg)
Coffee, drip	5	110–150
Coffee, perk	5	60–125
Coffee, instant	5	40–105
Tea, 5-minute steep	5	2–5
Tea, 3-minute steep	5	40–100
Coca-Cola	12	45
Hot cocoa	5	2–10
Coffee, decaffeinated	5	2–5

Foods	Serving Size	Caffeine (mg)
Milk chocolate	1 oz	1–15
Bittersweet chocolate	1 oz	5–35
Chocolate cake	1 slice	20–30

Over-the-Counter Drugs	Dose	Caffeine (mg)
Anacin, Empirin, or Midol	2	64
Excedrin	2	130
NoDoz	2	200
Aqua-Ban (diuretic)	2	200
Dexatrim (weight control aid)	1	200

The caloric content of foods can be altered by the way they are prepared. The following are some methods of reducing, or at least not increasing, the caloric value of food.

1. Do not fry foods. The process of frying, whether with saturated or unsaturated oil, adds many calories. For instance, if you bake or boil one potato and fry another of equal size, the fried potato will be calorically enhanced by as much as 150 percent while the other preparations will add no calories. Potatoes that are fried absorb significant amounts of the high-calorie oil in which they are cooked. Even fried foods that have been well-drained retain much of the fat in which they were fried. Actually, potatoes are 80 percent water and are low-calorie items that are nutritious and filling.

2. Roast, bake, broil, boil, grill, and stew rather than fry. If you roast meat in an oven, it should be placed on a rack so that the drippings will fall into a pan below. Prepared in this manner, the meat will not soak in fatty gravy. If you wish to use this gravy, place it in a refrigerator for cooling. The fat will solidify on top and can easily be removed.

   You can reduce the fat content of soups and stews in the same way. After the fat is removed, they can be reheated and served.

SELF-ASSESSMENT

Nutrition Inventory

Directions

We have presented what you should be doing nutritionally, and now you will have the opportunity to examine your eating patterns in the assessment quiz presented in Table 10.8. Answer each of the questions as accurately as possible. Note the number of "yes" answers at the end of each section, and then transfer these figures into the appropriate blank in Table 10.9. This will show you how well or how poor you are doing in each area of nutrition. Finally, total the section scores for an overall score and compare it to the key given in Table 10.9. If your score is in the "poor" or "fair" category, it is time to start making some changes in your nutritional patterns.

TABLE 10.8 Nutrition Quiz

Section 1 *Do I:*	*Response*	
1. Limit consumption of meat, fish, poultry or egg servings to once or twice a day?	yes	no
2. Eat red meats (beef, ham, lamb, or pork) three times or less per week?	yes	no
3. Remove all visible fat from meat prior to cooking?	yes	no
4. Limit consumption of eggs to three or four per week including those cooked in other foods?	yes	no
5. Occasionally have meatless days by substituting legumes and nuts for protein?	yes	no
6. Usually broil, bake, roast, or boil meat, fish, or poultry and abstain from frying?	yes	no

Total "Yes" Answers _____

Section 2 *Do I:*	*Response*	
1. Have two or more cups of milk or the equivalent in milk products daily?	yes	no
2. Drink or use low fat or skim milk (2% or less butterfat)?	yes	no
3. Limit ice cream or ice milk to twice per week or less?	yes	no
4. Generally consume less than 3 tsp. of margarine or butter per day?	yes	no

Total "Yes" Answers _____

Section 3 *Do I:*	*Response*	
1. Usually consume at least one-half cup of citrus fruit or juice (oranges, grapefruit, etc.) daily?	yes	no
2. Have at least one serving of dark green or deep orange vegetables daily?	yes	no
3. Eat fresh fruit and vegetables daily?	yes	no
4. Cook vegetables without fat, such as bacon drippings or ham hock?	yes	no
5. Eat fresh fruit for desert more often than cakes, cookies, and other pastries?	yes	no

Total "Yes" Answers _____

TABLE 10.8   Continued

Section 4 Do I:	Response	
1. Usually eat whole grain breads?	yes	no
2. Usually eat whole grain cereals which are good sources of fiber?	yes	no
3. Eat cereals which have no sugar or are low in sugar?	yes	no
4. Substitute brown rice for white rice?	yes	no
5. Consume at least 4 servings of bread or cereal grain products each day?	yes	no

Total "Yes" Answers _____

Section 5 Do I:	Response	
1. Remain within 5 to 10 lbs. of your optimal weight for your height?	yes	no
2. Drink less than 1½ oz. of alcohol (one to two drinks) per day?	yes	no
3. Abstain from adding salt to food after it is served and do you prefer foods that are lightly salted or not salted at all?	yes	no
4. Try to avoid foods high in refined sugar?	yes	no
5. Always eat a breakfast of at least cereal and milk, egg and toast, or other protein carbohydrate combination with fruit or fruit juice?	yes	no

Total "Yes" Answers _____

TABLE 10.9   Nutrition Quiz Score Evaluation

Section	Excellent	Good	Fair	Poor	Score
1. Meat/meat alternate choices	5–6	4	3	2–0	_____
2. Dairy choices	4	3	2	1–0	_____
3. Fruit/vegetable choices	5	4	3	2–0	_____
4. Grain choice	5	4	3	2–0	_____
5. Potpourri	5	4	3	2–0	_____

Total Score _____

Key: Excellent   24–25
Good   19–23
Fair   14–18
Poor   13 or less

Adapted from M. A. Boyle and E. N. Whitney, *Personal Nutrition* (St. Paul: West Publishing Co., 1989.)

POINTS TO PONDER

1. *Name the fat and water-soluble vitamins.*
2. *Discuss the validity of this statement: Natural vitamins are more effective in promoting and maintaining good health than the synthetic vitamins.*
3. *Discuss the potential harmful effects of taking megadoses of vitamins.*
4. *Identify some foods and beverages which contain caffeine.*
5. *What affect does caffeine have upon the body?*
6. *Is caffeine addictive?*
7. *Identify the major nutritional drawbacks associated with the consumption of fast foods.*

Chapter Highlights

Carbohydrates are organic compounds composed of one or more sugars derived from plant sources. Complex carbohydrates are the body's preferred source of fuel. The consumption of simple sugars should be reduced significantly or avoided because they are calorie-dense and nutrient-poor. Carbohydrates are the major source of fuel for intense exercise.

Americans are advised to consume 20 to 35 grams of fiber from a wide variety of foods. Fiber should be increased gradually to the recommended amount. The type of fiber that is consumed should be split evenly (approximately) between the soluble and insoluble fibers because each contributes to good health in unique ways.

Fats are energy-dense organic compounds that yield approximately 9 calories per gram. Saturated fats are found in animal flesh and dairy products; unsaturated fats are found in plants. Americans consume too much fat and should lower the total by substantially reducing saturated fats. Monosaturated and polyunsaturated fats should make up two-thirds of the fat intake. Each has the capacity to lower the level of blood cholesterol. Two to three fish meals per week provides enough omega-3 fatty acids to provide significant protection from cardiovascular disease. Fat is a major supplier of energy during rest and mild exercise.

Protein is required for building and repairing body tissues. It is made of 20 amino acids, eight of which are essential and must be supplied by the diet. Protein is not a major supplier of energy for physical work except under conditions of very low or starvation levels of food intake.

Vitamins are noncaloric organic compounds found in small quantities in most foods. They are either fat-soluble (Vitamins A, D, E, and K) or water-soluble (Vitamins B and C). They are coenzymes that promote many chemical reactions. Minerals are inorganic substances that exist freely in nature. Sodium, potassium, and chloride are the primary minerals lost through perspiration. Sodium and potassium are involved as electrolytes for the contraction of muscles. Vitamin and mineral supplementation may be abused. There is no evidence to indicate that megadoses of these substances enhance health, however, there is considerable evidence that large doses are harmful.

Humans may survive for weeks without food, but only a few days without water. All bodily processes and all chemical reactions take place in a liquid medium; therefore, the maintenance of adequate body fluids is imperative.

References

1. M. A. Boyle and E. N. Whitney, *Personal Nutrition*, St. Paul: West Publishing Co., 1989.
2. W. D. Holloway et al., "Digestion of Certain Fractions of Dietary Fiber in Humans," *The American Journal of Clinical Nutrition*, 31 (1978): 927.
3. D. A. T. Southgate, "The Relation Between Composition and Properties of Dietary Fiber and Physiological Effects," in *Dietary Fiber: Basic and Clinical Aspects*, G. V. Vahouny and D. Kritchevsky (eds.), New York: Plenum Press, 1986.
4. E. N. Whitney and E. M. N. Hamilton, *Understanding Nutrition*, St. Paul: West Publishing Co., 1987.
5. Select Committee on Nutrition and Human Needs, Dietary Goals for the United States (Washington, D.C.: U.S. Government Printing Office, 1977).
6. M. H. Williams, *Nutrition for Fitness and Sport*, Dubuque, Iowa: Wm. C. Brown Co., Publishers, 1983.
7. C. Foster et al., "Effects of Prexercise Feedings on Endurance Performance," *Medicine in Science and Sports*, 11 (1979): 1.
8. D. L. Costill, *Inside Running: Basics of Sports Physiology*, Indianapolis, IN: Benchmark Press, Inc., 1986.
9. "Saturation Point," *Tufts University Diet and Nutrition Letter*, 4 (Dec., 1986): 2.
10. "Is Olive Oil Right?" *Tufts University Diet and Nutrition Letter*, 4, (May, 1986): 1.
11. L. Lamb (ed.), "Current Thinking About Fish Oil," The Health Letter, 32, (Sept. 9, 1988): 1.
12. D. Kromhout et al., "The Inverse Relation Between Fish Consumption and 20-Year Mortality from Coronary Heart Disease," *New England Journal of Medicine*, 312, (1985): 1205.
13. "Infections and Undernutrition," *Nutrition Reviews*, 40, (1982): 119.
14. J. Klug, "Overeating Possible Cause of Renal Disease," *Internal Medicine News*, (Dec. 1982): 1.
15. L. E. Koszuta, "Experts Speak Out on Fitness and Nutrition," *The Physician and Sportsmedicine*, 16, (1988): 42.
16. A. C. Grandjean, "The Vegetarian Athlete," *The Physician and Sportsmedicine*, 15, (1987): 191.
17. J. H. Freeland-Graves et al., "Zinc Status of Vegetarians," *Journal of the American Dietetic Association*, 77, (1980): 655.
18. E. N. Whitney et al., *Understanding Normal and Clinical Nutrition*, St. Paul: West Publishing Co., 1987.
19. L. M. Weight et al., "Vitamin and Mineral Supplementation: Effect on the Running Performance of Trained Athletes," *American Journal of Clinical Nutrition*, 47, (1988): 192.
20. USDA and USDHHS, Nutrition and Your Health: Dietary Guidelines for Americans. (1985).
21. T. Ratto, "The Great Salt Controversy," *Medical Self-care Magazine*, 69, (May/June 1986): 35.

11

The Reduction Equation:
Exercise + Sensible Eating
= Weight Control

Chapter Contents _____

Mini Glossary

Adipose Tissue: fat cells.

Amenorrhea: Failure to menstruate.

Android Obesity: male pattern of fat deposition in the abdominal region.

Anorexia Nervosa: A psychological and emotional disorder characterized by excessive underweight.

Basal Metabolic Rate (BMR): The energy required to sustain life while in the rested and fasted state.

Body Composition: The percentage of lean versus fat tissue in the body.

Bulimarexia Nervosa: An eating disorder characterized by episodes of secretive binge eating followed by purging.

Gynoid Obesity: Female pattern of fat deposition in the thighs and gluteal areas.

Hydrostatic Weighing: A method for determining specific gravity and percent body fat by underwater weighing.

Resting Metabolic Rate (RMR): The conditions for measuring BMR are difficult to achieve and when they are approximated the term resting metabolic rate is used. It is an approximation of the energy required to sustain life while in the resting state.

Skinfold Measurement: A method for determining percent body fat by measuring a pinch of skin at selected sites with a skinfold caliper.

Thermogenic Effect of Food (TEF): The energy required to digest and absorb food.

Very-Low Calorie Diet: Diets which contain 800 kcals per day or less.

Weight Cycling: Repeated cycles of weight loss followed by weight gain.

Introduction

The effects of diet and exercise on weight reduction and weight maintenance are covered in this chapter. It begins with the definition of body composition, lean body mass, essential and storage fat. Overweight and obesity, which are not synonomous, are discussed and their differences are delineated. The connection between wellness and the maintenance of optimal body composition is established.

Exercise is an important component for reducing body weight (specifically fat weight) while sparing or enhancing muscle tissue. Exercise uses calories, stimulates metabolism, and brings appetite in line with energy expenditure. On the other hand, dieting without exercise produces diminishing returns because metabolism slows down as caloric needs decrease. After a few weeks of dieting the body goes into a survival mode and adapts to the reduced caloric intake. The diet becomes less effective and continued weight loss is more difficult to accomplish. Eventually the diet will end, some or all of the old eating patterns will be reestablished, and the lost weight will be regained. If dieting becomes cyclical, each attempt at losing weight will take longer, but the lost weight will be regained quicker and the likelihood that additional weight will be gained increases. Very-low calorie diets should be avoided. Without supplementation it is impossible to receive the required nutrients and the effect of low caloric intake on metabolism is devastating.

Anorexia nervosa and bulimia, two different eating disorders or appetite disorders, with some common characteristics are discussed.

Finally two methods for assessing body composition are presented. These are accompanied by a method for determining optimal body weight based upon the body composition measurement.

Body Composition Defined

When considered in its simplest form, **body composition** refers to the amount of fat versus lean tissue in the body. Lean tissue includes all tissue exclusive of fat; that is, muscles, bones, organs, fluid, and so on. Fat includes essential as well as storage fat. Essential fat, which is found in the bone marrow, organs, muscles, intestines, and the central nervous system, is indispensable to normal physiological functioning. The amount of essential fat in the male body is equal to approximately 3 percent of the total body weight. The amount of essential fat in the female body is equal to about 12 percent of the total body weight. The disparity in the amount of essential fat between the sexes is probably because of sex-specific essential fat stored in the females' breasts, pelvic area, and thighs. Essential fat constitutes a lower limit beyond which fat loss is undesirable and unhealthy because normal physiological and biological functioning may be impaired.

Storage fat is found in adipose tissue. For most Americans this represents a substantial energy reserve. **Adipose tissue** is found subcutaneously (under the skin) and around the organs, where it acts as a buffer against physical trauma. It is desirable to reduce storage fat for health and aesthetic reasons. Reasonable goals for total body fat (essential plus storage fat) differ for both sexes. Excellent values for males and females are 12 and 18 percent respectively. Females who become excessively lean (below 12 to 14 percent fat), such as long-distance runners and ballerinas, often experience menstrual dysfunction. Irregular menses (menstrual cycle), oligomenorrhea (infrequent menses) and **amenorrhea** (no menses), are frequent problems for exercising women who reduce their total body weight and/or fat excessively. Loss of body weight and fat are among several factors associated with menstrual dysfunction. Emotional stress, inadequate nutrition, hypothyroidism, and pituitary tumors are some other factors related to the onset of menstrual problems.[1] Anorexia nervosa, which is most prevalent among middle-class white females between the ages of 11 and 24, is a form of self-starvation that produces amenorrhea.[2] Although these young people often lose 25 to 60 percent of their normal weight, they tend to perceive themselves as being "fat." Some have literally starved themselves to death. Parallels have been drawn between anorectics and highly trained, very lean male and female athletes. A paradox exists in that females who exercise heavily strengthen their bodies but those who develop "athletic amenorrhea" lose calcium from their bones, especially those of the vertebrae.[3] Bone responds to exercise by acquiring more calcium and growing stronger, but highly intense exercise carried out on a regular basis tends to weaken the bones. "By lowering hormone levels, regular heavy exercise leads to loss of calcium from bones and thus weakens them. Which bones are affected, and in what way, depends on the type and intensity of exercise."[3] The menstrual cycle returns to normal when exercise is reduced and weight is gained.[4,5] Bone mineral content loss is probably reversible and returns to normal values as well, but this has not been clearly established.[4]

Excessive leanness has been implicated in the death of 14 young and middle-aged marathon runners. A common element shared by these runners was a very restricted diet coupled with vigorous exercise.

Lean Runners and Fatal Heart Irregularities

Many dedicated runners are quite thin. Others run to avoid obesity. Being too thin for whatever reason or accomplished by whatever means can be a health hazard. That is particularly true when the thinness is accomplished by unwise dietary restrictions. Dr. Thomas Bassler has commented further on marathon runners he has studied who evidently died from fatal heart irregularities (*J Amer Med Assoc 252:* 1984, 483). In 12 of the 14 of his cases who had autopsies, the marathon runners had little or no evidence of any fatty-cholesterol changes in their coronary arteries, or narrowing of these arteries. It is unlikely that coronary artery disease played any part in their deaths. The two men who did not have an autopsy had normal electrocardiograms and no reason to suspect that they had coronary artery disease. None smoked but according to Bassler they were lean to the point of being "almost cachectic." As a group they were young with an average age of 44 and a range from 18 to 61 years of age.

A review of their dietary habits revealed marked weight loss in some men. Eleven of these men had severely restricted their diet. Bassler thinks the explanation for their deaths was a fatal heart irregularity and proposes to call these nutritional arrhythmia. He warns against diets that are overly restrictive for runners. He singles out the "compulsive, cachectic vegetarian athlete," recommending that he be encouraged to eat a balanced diet.

To this should be added that any activity that uses lots of calories requires increased nutritional support. Some exercise physiologists consider exercise a means of "controlled starvation" because of its use of energy and they analyze its effects in weight reduction in that manner. In any case, with the known facts about excessive dieting, improper dieting and leanness from exercise, it is apparent that being too lean can be a hazard. Leanness itself is probably not a hazard if the diet still provides enough calories and enough nutrients, including important minerals such as potassium. The diet must provide enough energy to not utilize the body's essential protein. There is some evidence that when body protein is utilized that it is extracted from nonmuscular sources first, such as the liver. Studies of fasting deaths have also suggested that there is a critical level of body fat. Admittedly this is far below the level of fat most individuals have, but in the exercise zealot or the starvation victim the critical level can be reached.

"Lean Runners and Fatal Heart Irregularities," *The Health Letter*, vol: 24, no. 5, (Sept. 14, 1984) 1. Health Letter, copyright 1985. Used by permission.

According to psychiatrist Alayne Yates, "obligatory" runners—those who are compelled to run regardless of injury or circumstance—have the following characteristics in common with anorectic women: "inhibition of anger, extraordinarily high self-expectations, tolerance of physical discomfort, denial of potentially serious debility, and a tendency toward depression."[6] One of the problems associated with this study was the comparison of male obligatory runners to anorectic females. A more decisive study was directed by Jonathan Chang.[6] He identified, by questionnaire, 43 obligatory runners (22 men and 21 women). He then selected 24 consecutive anorectic subjects who were diagnosed with criteria developed by the American Psychiatric Association. All subjects completed the Minnesota Multiphasic Personality Inventory. After analyzing the data, Chang concluded that there was, "no connection between obligatory runners and anorectic women. The only similarities were superficial."

Development of Adiposity

Overweight and obesity have complex physiological and psychological causes but the principles involved in weight loss are very simple. Energy cannot be destroyed; it is either used for work or converted into another form for storage. Individuals are in equilibrium when the calories consumed equal the calories used. Weight maintenance is lost when the equation is unbalanced in either direction. If the calories consumed exceed those that are used, the excess is converted into fat and stored. If the calories used exceed those that are consumed, weight will be lost because a portion of the stored fat must be mobilized to supply the extra need for fuel.

Scientifically, the principle is beautifully uncomplicated. We have made the process complex by inventing hundreds of ways to achieve weight loss painlessly and rapidly. Unfortunately, most of these methods are fruitless; some are actually dangerous and usually benefit only those who invent and promote them. The preferred course of action is to prevent obesity from occurring rather than treating it after the fact. From this standpoint, it might be useful to know some basics about the development of adipose cells. As with other organs, adipose tissue (fat cells) normally grows by increasing in number (hyperplasia) or size (hypertrophy). Fat cell number and size vary from one body part to another.

Fat cells enlarge significantly during the initial six months of postnatal (after birth) life and by the end of the first year are similar in size to those of adolescents.[7] It appears that fat-cell size remains fairly stable from one year of age to puberty, but fat-cell number increases progressively during this time. During puberty, males and females experience substantial increases in both fat-cell size and number. However, there are gender differences in the deposition of subcutaneous fat. Males distribute fat primarily in the upper half of the body and females deposit it in the lower half of the body. Further, the percentage of fat reaches peak values during early adolescence for males and then declines during the remainder of adolescent growth, while females show a continuous increase in the percentage of fat from the onset of puberty through age 18.[8]

Excess fat storage is the result of hypertrophy and/or hyperplasia of adipose cells. Obese children beyond two years of age have a greater number of fat cells than children of normal weight.[8] Not long ago, it was hypothesized that the number of adipose cells was fixed soon after birth.[9] This controversial theory no longer appears to be credible.[10] Some researchers have suggested that overfeeding in infancy promotes the formation of excess fat cells, and further, that overfeeding predisposes affected children to later obesity. Current evidence indicates that obesity later in life is unaffected by overfeeding in early life, and conversely, underfeeding in early life does not prevent or preclude the development of obesity or adipose cell number later in life.[11] The consequences of early feeding patterns on later obesity are not clear. An interesting sidelight is that breast feeding, compared to bottle feeding, seems to deter adiposity but only in early childhood.[12,13]

Food deprivation during various stages of pregnancy has produced some intriguing results. Young men whose mothers experienced famine during the first and second trimesters of pregnancy had a higher than normal incidence of obesity. But food deprivation during the last trimester resulted in a significantly reduced incidence of obesity.[14] Neonatal (newborn) adiposity appears to be influenced by maternal fatness. Both obese and diabetic mothers have babies that are fatter and heavier at birth than babies of normal weight mothers.[15] However, the evidence suggests that neonatal adiposity does not predict obesity in childhood.[16] However, children who are obese have only a one-in-four chance of becoming normal weight adults and if the extra pounds are not removed by adolescence, the chances decrease to one in twenty-eight.[17] Based upon this evidence, the prevention of adult obesity should begin with efforts to prevent childhood obesity.

Body Composition and the Wellness Connection

The majority of Americans of all ages and both sexes can avoid obesity. It is a matter of choice, effort or lack of it, awareness of the hazards of obesity, and a commitment to do something about it. High-level wellness cannot be attained by the obese because the quality of their lives is diminished and the hazards of obesity are well known. These have been articulately and forcefully reinforced by the 14-member panel of authorities that was very explicit regarding the hazards of obesity and overweight.

The National Institutes of Health (NIH) convened a panel of experts to develop a consensus statement regarding the health implications of obesity. While this was a formidable task, and while segments of the study were criticized, the fact remains that for the majority of people the higher their weight escalates the greater the risk of developing health problems. The panel cited the strong association between obesity and high blood pressure, Type II diabetes, and high blood cholesterol levels.[18] Obese women are more likely to die from cancer of the uterus, breast, ovaries, and gallbladder than normal weight women. Obese men are more likely to die from cancer of the colon, prostate, and rectum. The relationship between obesity and cardiovascular disease is well established but now it appears that the distribution of fat is as important as the amount of storage fat. Males tend to deposit fat in the abdominal region **(android obesity)** while females tend to deposit fat in the thighs and gluteal areas **(gynoid obesity).** The masculine pattern of obesity is associated with the development of diabetes, hypertension, heart disease, and death independent of the total degree of obesity.[19,20,21] Even 15 extra pounds of android obesity presents a risk for either sex.

Moderate obesity increases mortality by 42 percent independent of gender; morbid obesity increases the mortality of males by 79 percent and females by 61 percent.[22] As a result of its effect on longevity and its high positive association with severe chronic disease, obesity should be regarded as a serious medical and psychological problem. The following points regarding obesity support these findings.

1. Regional differences exist between the sexes with regard to fat cell distribution in both obese and nonobese subjects.
2. Moderate obesity is caused primarily by fat-cell size increases followed subsequently by an increase in fat-cell number.

3. Men and women with male abdominal type obesity are more susceptible to several catastrophic disease processes.
4. Even limited abdominal obesity should be considered a risk for cardiovascular disease.
5. Obesity is a serious disease.

In addition to these health hazards, the obese suffer from economic and social discrimination, poor body image, and a depressed self-concept. A survey of 1500 executives revealed that body weight was inversely related to earning power. Only 10 percent of the executives in the upper income bracket were more than ten pounds overweight, while 40 percent of those in the lower bracket were more than ten pounds overweight.[23] Excessive weight seems to be hazardous to purse and wallet. Fat people are victims of discrimination because our culture is "slim" oriented. We have become enamored with the thin silhouette. Advertisements cater to the young and the slim. Clothing is made for thin people and modeled by thin people. The latest Gallup Poll indicated that we are in the midst of a second fitness revolution.[24] The first fitness movement was led by white middle and upper class males. It began in the 1960s, when deaths caused by cardiovascular disease were at their peak. The primary motivation for exercise during this time was the enhancement of health. The second movement is characterized by a tremendous influx of women participants, it crosses socioeconomic lines, and, while health enhancement still is the major motivator, many participants are seeking optimum development of their potential as human beings. Health enhancement remains the predominant reason for participating in fitness activities but Americans are "not just pursuing exercise for its own sake, for the thinner look or a faster running time. Instead they're lured onward by the belief that exercise transforms their lives and helps them become the best humans they can be." Exercise is viewed as a tool for building a new self. The obese and overweight are the antithesis of this emerging spirit, thus establishing a climate for further discrimination. Fat people pay higher insurance premiums, obese children are ridiculed by their slim peers, and armed forces personnel are drummed out of service if they gain weight beyond an acceptable level. Female subjects (ages 18 to 68) enrolled in a weight loss program had distorted perceptions of their body image.[25] All 68 subjects saw themselves as being significantly more obese than they actually were. The error of estimate was even larger among those women who eventually dropped out of the program. As the women lost weight over 16 weeks, their estimates became more realistic and self-concept was positively affected. The inverse relationship between obesity and self-concept may be reversed with successful weight loss. Forty-five obese males successfully lost weight through exercise and nutritional counseling and their scores on the Tennessee Self-Concept Scale improved significantly.[26]

Fortunately obesity is reversible and so too are many of the risks with which it is associated. The preferred course of action would be to prevent obesity from occurring rather than trying to deal with it after the fact. This requires knowledgeable management of dietary and exercise habits both by individuals and their parents. Parents should teach and practice sound nutritional and exercise habits so that their children can proceed normally through periods in life when they are particularly vulnerable to fat cell proliferation.

Exercise plays a significant role in weight loss, weight maintenance, and the prevention of weight gain. The many benefits of exercise are well-documented.

The Effects of Exercise On Body Composition _____

Exercise Burns Calories

A persistent misconception is that aerobic exercises do not burn enough calories to make the effort worthwhile. Misinterpretation of caloric expenditure tables has contributed substantially to this misunderstanding. The tables show, for example, that to lose one pound one must walk 35 miles, or chop wood for seven and one-half hours, or cycle for eleven hours, or play basketball for eight and one-half hours. The tables are essentially correct for 150 lb people. In weight-bearing activities (walking, jogging, aerobic dance, rope jumping, to name a few), calories are consumed according to body weight. Larger people burn more, smaller people burn less. Table 11.1 provides an estimate of the caloric cost of selected activities on a per-minute basis according to body weight. This is a more realistic method of assessment. Simply multiply your body weight by the calories per minute per pound column and then multiply this value by the number of minutes spent participating in the activity.

The caloric expenditure charts have spawned other misconceptions. First, the energy expenditures refer to fat tissue (there are 3500 calories in a pound of fat) and not to a pound of weight as measured with a bathroom scale. Scale

TABLE 11.1   Estimated Caloric Cost of Selected Activities

Activity	Cal/Min/Lb*	Activity	Cal/Min/Lb*
Aerobic dance (vigorous)	.062	Jogging (5 MPH)	.060
Basketball (vigorous, full court)	.097	Laundry (taking out and hanging)	.027
Bathing, dressing, undressing	.021	Mopping floors	.024
Bed-making (and stripping)	.031	Peeling potatoes	.019
Bicycling (13 MPH)	.071	Piano playing	.018
Canoeing (flat water, 4 MPH)	.045	Rowing (vigorous)	.097
Chopping wood	.049	Running (8 MPH)	.104
Cleaning windows	.024	Sawing wood (crosscut saw)	.058
Cross-country skiing (8 MPH)	.104	Shining shoes	.017
Gardening: Digging	.062	Shoveling snow	.052
Hedging	.034	Snowshoeing (2.5 MPH)	.060
Raking	.024	Soccer (vigorous)	.097
Weeding	.038	Swimming (55 yd/min)	.088
Golf (twosome carrying clubs)	.045	Table tennis (skilled)	.045
Handball (skilled, singles)	.078	Tennis (beginner)	.032
Horseback riding (trot)	.052	Walking (4.5 MPH)	.048
Ironing	.029	Writing while seated	.013

*Multiply cals/min/lb by your body weight in pounds and then multiply that product by the number of minutes spent in the activity.

From *Physical Fitness for Practically Everybody: The Consumers Union Report on Exercise*, Mount Vernon, N.Y.: The Consumers Union of the U.S., 1983.

Young and middle-aged regular exercisers were compared for percentage of body fat. Result: body fat percent was linked to the number of hours of aerobic workout, not to age. Keeping fit means you don't have to settle for a slow decline into flabbiness.
–USDA Human Nutrition Research Center/Tufts University

weight includes the loss of liquid and muscle as well as fat, while providing no clues to the relative losses of each. The scale is a poor criterion with which to judge the success of weight loss. Second, these charts fail to fully account for the calories burned during recovery from exercise. The body does not turn off like a water tap when the workout is over. Instead, metabolism remains elevated for a period of time commensurate with the type, intensity and duration of exercise performed. It may extend for a few minutes following light exercise to as long as 24 hours following exhaustive exercise. The point is that the extra calories burned during the recovery period alone may result in a significant weight loss in a year's time. Third, one does not have to walk 35 miles in a single exercise session. The cumulative effect of exercise is what counts and this concept seems to be misunderstood by the general public. The calories expended in exercise today add to those which were expended yesterday and both will add to those expended tomorrow, and so on. Walking one extra mile per day will lead to the loss of one pound of fat in approximately 35 days for an average size male. This is a modest weight loss but it does add up to 10.5 pounds in a year. Two extra miles a day result in a 21 pound weight loss. This is a worthy accomplishment, particularly when one considers that excess weight accumulates slowly; we do not wake up one morning suddenly fat. We may perceive that it happened that way but the truth is that weight gain is insidious, taking months or years to occur. When we finally face the fact that the weight gained is beyond our acceptable limit, then we resolve to remove the excess as rapidly as possible. Impatient Americans, accustomed to instant tea, instant mashed potatoes, and instant rice also want instant weight loss and instant fitness. The laws of physiology and common sense dictate that this strategy is unsound and destined to fail. Success is dependent upon effort, time, and patience.

Physical activity is the most effective way to rid the body of calories but it is not the only way that the body uses calories. The process of digesting and absorbing food requires energy and represents another source of using calories. The energy for these processes, known as the **thermogenic effect** of food (TEF), is supplied by some of the food which is eaten.[27] Research interest in TEF has resurfaced as investigators attempt to piece-out the influence of various factors involved in energy storage and utilization. Metabolism may be elevated for as long as several hours following a meal. What would happen to metabolism if aerobic exercise were combined with the TEF effect since both individually boost metabolism? Some authorities suggest that mild exercise, such as walking, be performed shortly after ingesting a meal because such activities potentiate the TEF.[28] This concept is attractive. From a weight loss perspective, it is certainly much better than taking a nap after a meal. However, there is substantial individual variation in TEF so its effectiveness in weight management has yet to be elucidated. As a result of this uncertainty, we will concentrate on the effect of calories expended from physical activity.

Aerobic exercise contributes significantly to weight loss. According to the American College of Sports Medicine, aerobic exercises that use 300 to 500 calories per bout promote favorable changes in body composition. Use Table 11.1 to determine the number of minutes you must participate in your favorite activities to burn the recommended number of calories. The obese person will expend more calories in the initial stage of the exercise program. The caloric expenditure will decline as body weight is lost but the participant will compensate by exercising longer and harder as fitness improves.

Exercise and Appetite: Eat More, Weigh Less

To the uninitiated, the title of this section must seem at least paradoxical if not impossible. How can one eat more and weigh less? It sounds like a bit of alchemy or a get-rich-quick sales pitch. But wouldn't it be nice to "have your cake and eat it too"—without gaining weight? This is especially intriguing since it is known that Americans are eating less and getting fatter. Since weight gain and loss are a combination of calories consumed and calories expended, it is obvious that the reduction in caloric consumption has been accompanied by a greater reduction in calories expended. This explains our continued weight gain.

The results of animal and human studies during the last 35 years have been equivocal and confusing regarding the effect of exercise on appetite. The data have shown that exercise may decrease, increase, or have no effect upon food intake.

Just a few short years ago, the scientific community adopted the position that one hour of mild to moderate exercise would exert an anorexigenic effect (reduction in appetite).[29] The theory was that food intake would decrease during the early days of exercise as one was making the transition from inactivity to moderate exercise and persist until the level of exercise increased to above moderate levels. At this point the appetite would increase to be in balance with energy expenditure. Other researchers tested these assumptions but were unable to produce similar results. Exercise did not seem to suppress the appetite except temporarily immediately after exercise. Most studies indicated that people either continued to eat the same amount or increased their food intake when they began exercising and were allowed to eat freely. The food intake and energy expenditure of military cadets was carefully monitored for 14 days.[30] Their food intake was depressed during exercise days and increased during the off-days. The researchers concluded that moderate exercise undertaken regularly tends to be accompanied by a slight increase in food intake. Blair and his associates reported that both male and female joggers consumed more calories than sedentary controls.[31] Wood investigated the effect of a year of jogging on previously sedentary middle-aged males.[32] The subjects were encouraged not to reduce their food intake or to attempt to lose weight during the course of the study. At the end of one year the men who ran the most miles lost the most fat. The more miles the men ran the more they increased their food intake, and the more fat the men lost, the more they increased their food intake. There was a positive relationship between miles run and food intake but negative relationships between miles run and fat lost and food intake and fat loss. Obese and nonobese young males participated in one hour per day of vigorous exercise for 18 weeks.[33] The researcher did not provide the caloric cost of this activity but the fact that it was classified as vigorous indicates an energy expenditure of approximately 400 to 600 calories. The subjects' food intake did not keep pace; there was a slight 100 to 200 calorie increase. The subjects lost both weight and body fat while gaining muscle mass.

Two studies at St. Luke's Hospital in New York showed that the effect of exercise on the appetite is regulated to some extent by the degree of obesity at the start of the program.[34] Fifty-seven days of moderate treadmill exercise resulted in a 15 pound weight loss by obese female subjects. Their caloric intake during exercise compared to the preexercise period was essentially unchanged. This study was repeated with women who were close to "ideal weight" according to insurance company charts; the results were very different. Moderate treadmill exercise produced an immediate surge in appetite and these women maintained their "ideal body" weight.

Zuti and Golding investigated the relationship between exercise, diet, and weight loss.[35] They analyzed the effects of three different strategies upon the quantity and quality of weight loss. Each strategy was designed to elicit a loss of one pound per week. The subjects were overweight women 25 to 45 years of age. A summary of the results of the study appears in Table 11.2.

The "Diet only" group reduced food intake by 500 calories per day and did not exercise. The "Exercise only" group did not diet; instead, they increased their physical activity by 500 calories per day. The "Diet and exercise" group reduced their caloric intake by 250 calories per day while increasing their caloric expenditure by the same amount. The aim of all three strategies was to lose one pound per week (500 cals/day × 7 days = 3500 cals) and this objective was essentially accomplished. But the significant outcome of this study was that 21 percent of the total loss experienced by the "Diet only" group was in the form of lean tissue. This occurred despite a nutritionally sound diet of modest calorie restriction. The other two groups lost fat (the true goal of weight loss programs) and gained rather than lost lean tissue.

Following the Zuti and Golding approach, investigators recently examined the effect of dieting and weight training on body composition. The subjects were 40 obese females whose average age was 33 years.[36] The subjects were randomly assigned to one of four groups: (1) a control group who did not diet or exercise, (2) a diet only group, (3) an exercise only group, and (4) a diet plus exercise group. The exercise program consisted of supervised weight training and the diet was designed so that each individual would lose two pounds per week. The diet group also received a protein supplement. Measurements taken at the end of the study showed that two groups, the exercise only, and the exercise plus diet significantly increased their lean body weight and their strength. The researchers concluded that exercise and diet acted independently during weight loss. Weight training affected those variables associated with muscle components while dieting affected those variables associated with fat components. This study reinforces the need for including both sensible exercise and dietary modifications in a weight loss program.

Muscle atrophies and metabolism slows with diet only strategies. All muscles are affected adversely including those of the heart and the more severe the diet the greater the loss. Data which illustrated this effect was presented at the 1987 Scientific Session of the American Heart Association convention. Twenty-one obese women ages 18 to 40 were put on diets of 800 to 1000 kcals per day (low-

Most Americans gain 15 to 25 pounds between the ages of 25 and 50—even when their eating habits haven't changed. Reason is that people become less active with time which results in a need for fewer calories.
—Tufts University Diet and Nutrition Letter

TABLE 11.2 Average Weight Lost by Groups

Weight Loss Strategy	Fat Tissue Loss (lb)	Lean Tissue Change (lb)	Total Weight Loss (lb)
Diet only	−9.3	−2.4	−11.7
Exercise only	−12.6	+2.0	−10.6
Diet and exercise	−13.0	+1.0	−12.0

calorie diet) or 1300 to 1600 kcals per day (moderate-calorie diet).[37] Some of the subjects remained sedentary, some did aerobic exercise and others combined aerobic exercise with circuit weight training. All of the women lost weight during the 12 weeks of the study. Those on the low-calorie diet lost 26 pounds while those on the moderate-calorie diet lost 15 pounds. Echocardiographic assessments showed that all of the low-calorie subjects experienced a reduction in left ventricular mass (the heart chamber that pumps blood to all tissues of the body) but the loss was greater in the nonexercising group. Exercising subjects on the moderate-calorie diet had an increase in left ventricular size. It seems that the harmful effects of very low-calorie diets cannot be offset entirely even with exercise, but heart muscle increased when exercise was combined with moderate calorie restriction.

Weight loss attempts in the U.S. have emphasized dietary restriction with continued sedentary living. This combination has led to consistent failure. Weight loss with this method is temporary and the majority of these weight watchers lose and gain weight many times during their lives. The eating patterns established during the diet period are short-lived. "Dieting actually makes the fat person even more unlike the slim person; he or she is simply a fat person reluctantly eating less, and the transformation into a true slim person has not occurred. It is not at all surprising, then, that the 'eat less' approach to weight loss and permanent weight control has not worked."[38] Each failure stimulates a rebound effect. The dieter regains the lost weight plus a few more pounds and each new attempt at weight loss produces more frustration and requires a more stringent diet. This pattern known as **weight cycling** results in weight loss which comes primarily from muscle mass, while the weight which is regained is mostly in the form of fat.[39]

Exercise Stimulates Metabolism

Approximately 65 to 70 percent of the energy liberated from food is expended to maintain the essential functions of the body.[40] The energy to accomplish these functions is the **basal metabolic rate (BMR).** This "basal" measurement is made while the subject is rested, fasted, and in a thermally neutral environment. Because these conditions are often difficult to achieve, it is more appropriate to substitute the term resting metabolic rate (RMR) to indicate that ideal conditions have been approximated. The **resting metabolic rate (RMR)** refers to the amount of energy required to sustain life while in the resting state. The RMR is measured in calories and pertains to the energy required to maintain body temperature and cellular metabolism. It is affected by age, sex, secretions from endocrine glands, nutritional status, sleep, fever, climate, body surface area, and muscle tissue. Principally because of less muscle tissue, the RMRs of females is 5 to 10 percent lower than males and 15 percent lower than that of very muscular males. Males who are overweight primarily because of heavy musculature have higher RMRs, higher TEF, and respond more readily to exercise/diet approaches to weight loss then overweight men whose excess weight is primarily fat.[27] The energy needed to sustain the RMR constitutes a significant amount of the total number of daily calories expended by the average adult. Then from a weight management perspective, it is advantageous to preserve and/or enhance the RMR and to do nothing to reduce it. Exercise fits the bill very nicely.

In the past, the decline in RMR was presumed to be a natural aspect of aging. But age per se has relatively little effect. It seems that the acquired changes accompanying aging are primarily responsible for the decline in RMR. deVries stated that "it has been shown that the loss in human muscle tissue with age can entirely account for the downward trend in basal metabolism."[41] Muscle tissue uses more energy than fat during rest and/or physical activity. Authorities estimate that we lose 3 to 5 percent of our active protoplasm (mostly muscle tissue) each decade after 25 years of age. This loss is directly attributed to physical inactivity as we age and results in the all-too-common negative changes that are seen in body composition.

Physical activity is the key to weight management because it uses calories and accelerates metabolism. It also prevents or attenuates the weight loss plateau that the majority of dieters experience. This plateau represents a period of time when weight loss decelerates substantially or stops temporarily.[42,43]

Researchers measured the food intake and energy expenditure of a group of three-month-old infants. The measurements were repeated when they were one year old.[44] Infants who were overweight by their first birthday were expending 21 percent less energy than normal weight infants even though the two groups did not differ in food intake. It is difficult to control and distinguish between genetics (all overweight infants in this study had overweight mothers) and environmental influences in studies such as these, however, the researchers strongly suggest that encouraging physical activity may be more effective than food restriction in preventing obesity in vulnerable infants. Low energy expenditure is also a major contributor to obesity in adults.[27,45,46,47,48]

Young and middle-aged subjects who were within plus or minus 5 percent of their ideal weight as determined by height, weight, and frame size charts illustrated the body composition changes that occur with age. Although both groups were within the ideal range for weight, the middle-aged subjects had twice as much body fat as the young subjects. These data show quite well that lost muscle weight that is replaced by a gain in fat weight produces negative changes in body composition even in the absence of weight gain. Fat is less dense than muscle so it occupies more room in the body; hence the change in the configuration of the body. Table 11.3 illustrates some of the changes in body composition that occur as Americans age. The examples are hypothetical but they are based upon fact.

TABLE 11.3   Effects of Physical Inactivity on Body Composition

Subject	Body Weight at age 20 (lb)	Body Weight at age 60 (lb)	Activity Level	Lean Tissue*	Fat	Body Composition
1	150	150	Inactive	Lost 12–20%	Gain	Changed
2	150	135	Inactive	Lost 12–20%	No Gain	Changed
3	150	165	Inactive	Lost 12–20%	Gain	Changed
4	150	150	Active	No Loss	No Gain	Unchanged

*The lean tissue values in the table apply to males, but the same trend is evident to a lesser degree in females because they have less lean tissue to lose.

Subject 1 typifies the inactive person who maintains his body weight while aging but experiences a change in body composition. The bathroom scale provides no clues regarding the change but the mirror and fit of his clothes do. He must hold a tight reign on appetite because his resting caloric requirements have diminished. Subject 2 is inactive and chooses to lose weight with age to keep from becoming fatter—rare in our society. He loses one-quarter to one-half a pound per year after age 30. This individual has lost muscle tissue but has reduced his body weight. His body composition has changed as a result—he is smaller all over. Because of the decline in metabolism from the loss of muscle, along with a lower body weight which diminishes the caloric cost of any weight-bearing movement, this individual must eat progressively less as the years pass to prevent a gain in fat tissue. Hunger would be a constant companion with this strategy. Subject 3 is probably most representative of the typical American who gains both fat and weight with age. Subject 4 is physically active throughout life. There is little muscle loss and no gain in fat weight. Many examples of this modern-day phenomenon continue to jog, cycle, swim, and so on. Programs that build and maintain muscle tissue preserve the RMR and perpetuate a youthful body composition.

Best Time to Exercise

Is there a best time of the day to exercise? Anytime it fits into your busy schedule may be the best time. However, those individuals whose major goal is weight loss might find that there are better times during the day for exercise. The two times most often suggested are before breakfast and prior to the evening meal.

Runners participated in a 30-minute run after a 12 hour fast (before breakfast) and after a 3 to 4 hour fast (after lunch). They used the same number of kcals with each run but two-thirds of the kcals used before breakfast came from fat while only half of the kcals after lunch came from fat. The reason for the difference in the percentage of fuel used is probably because of the low circulating level of insulin in the morning. Breakfast ends a natural fast which occurs while we sleep. Blood levels of insulin rise after a meal and decrease during a fast. Insulin suppresses the release of free fatty acids from adipose tissue and encourages the body to use carbohydrates. Conversely, low levels of blood insulin stimulate the body to burn fat as fuel. Since the goal of weight loss is to lose excess fat, it may not be a bad idea to exercise at a time when fat utilization is preferred by the body.

Exercise before the evening meal may simultaneously accomplish two goals. First, it may alleviate the stress that has built-up during the day. Second, exercise which is intense enough to increase body temperature will temporarily suppress the appetite. Ostensibly, if supper is eaten during this time, we will eat less because we are not quite as hungry. If your goal is weight loss, you might give some consideration to these approaches.

POINTS TO PONDER

1. *Define the terms body composition, overweight, and obesity.*
2. *Differentiate between essential and storage fat and describe the influence of gender on each.*
3. *Discuss the development of adipose tissue.*

4. *Can a nonsmoking obese individual with normal cholesterol and blood pressure be considered in a state of high-level wellness? Defend your answer.*

5. *Why should exercise be an integral part of a weight-loss program? How would you convince a dieter who is reluctant to exercise?*

6. *What evidence can you cite to support the notion that exercise increases metabolism over the long term.*

The Effects of Diet on Body Composition

Metabolism is adversely affected by calorie restriction. In its quest for homeostasis (the tendency to maintain a constancy of internal conditions) the body adapts to the reduced calorie intake by lowering the metabolic rate. This effort to economize in response to less food intake is a survival mechanism that protects people during lean times. Because the body learns to get by with less, the difference between calories eaten and calories needed narrows. This defense mechanism makes it possible for prisoners of war to survive internment in concentration camps. This same defense mechanism is operative in individuals who voluntarily reduce their food intake with the same result: a drop in RMR. As the RMR decreases, so too does the effectiveness of dieting. Regular vigorous exercise has the opposite effect: it accelerates the metabolic processes and increases body temperature during and after physical activity. The RMR may remain elevated for some time after exercise and probably contributes to more calories used as a result than had been previously thought. Under exercise conditions, the body is spending rather than hoarding.

Some of the most popular of today's diets were evaluated in *The Walking Magazine.* This information is presented in Table 11.4.

Dieting reduces basal heat production. In one study, the basal heat of dieting obese subjects dropped to 91 percent of prediet levels in two weeks on a 500-calorie-per-day diet.[49] After the initial two weeks they switched to 20 to 30 minutes of exercise at 60 percent of their aerobic capacity. Basal heat production increased to normal values in three to four days and continued to increase for the next two weeks to a value equal to 107 percent of the prediet level. Meanwhile, the basal heat production of sedentary controls on a 500-calorie-per-day diet for the four weeks dropped to 81 percent of their prediet levels. This drop in heat production or energy expenditure partially explains why the actual weight lost by dieting is often less than the predicted weight loss.

More restrictive diets produce greater losses of lean tissue. Fasting or starvation results in substantial losses of lean tissue. The brain and central nervous system require glucose (sugar) as their only source of fuel. Glucose is produced from the breakdown of dietary carbohydrates, but fasting or starvation means zero nutrient intake. Under these circumstances, the body's protein from muscles, liver, and other organs is converted to glucose for the brain and central nervous system. Ninety percent of the body's glucose is formed in this manner and the other 10 percent comes from glycerol (fat). The conversion of protein to glucose is a wasteful process because only half of the amino acids (the structure of protein) are used, while the other half must be removed. Ninety-five percent of all fat cannot be converted to glucose. The body adapts to fat as a major

TABLE 11.4   The Walking Magazine's Guide To 1989's Most Popular Diets

Type	Description	Weight Loss	Health Drawbacks	Pros/Cons
Balanced (available in book stores) ■ Weight Watchers Quick Success Program (Weight Watchers International) ■ Jane Fonda's New Workout & Weight Loss Program ■ I Don't Eat (But I Can't Lose Weight) ■ Complete University Medical Diet ■ Jane Brody's Nutrition Book ■ Fit or Fat Target Diet ■ Popcorn Plus Diet ■ Getting Thin ■ Setpoint Diet ■ Nautilus Diet	Recommends 1,000 or more calories/day. At least 50% carbohydrate, less than 30% fat, 15% to 20% protein. Variety of foods from four basic food groups. (Regular exercise and lifestyle changes.)	1 to 2 lb./week. Promotes permanent loss of fat, especially if combined with regular exercise.	None (no side effects in healthy people). Diet includes an adequate amount of food in all the major food groups. No specialized medical supervision necessary in healthy people.	Provides variety and good nutrition. Combined with exercise, diet can be used as a basis of lifelong weight control. No vitamin supplementation necessary. Weight lost is fat, not muscle.
High Carbohydrate ■ Bloomingdale's Eat Healthy Diet ■ Pritikin Permanent Weight Loss Manual	Calorie level varies. Encourages increasing carbohydrate intake to more than 60% of diet. Can severely restrict protein and fat intake. Some advocate exercise and positive lifestyle changes.	Gradual or rapid, depending on calorie intake.	May be too low in protein and require vitamin and mineral supplements.	If protein level and calorie intake are adequate, high-carbohydrate diets are safe and effective. However, they may be so restrictive that they can be hard to stick to.
Formula/Rx (available through a physician or hospital-run program) ■ HMR (Health Management Resources) ■ Medifast ■ Optifast	Suggests only 800 calories or less/day. Requires dieters to forgo food for about 12 weeks and eat only a protein supplement. After initial fast, food is gradually reintroduced. May encourage exercise and lifestyle changes.	Very rapid, 3 to 4 lb./week. Protein supplements claimed to reduce loss of muscle tissue. Unknown: whether dieters keep weight off.	Can produce severe metabolic disturbances, heart beat irregularities, hair loss, dehydration, kidney problems and sense of feeling cold. Vitamins and mineral supplements required.	Expensive. Cost can run as high as $500 per month. Only for obese people (20% or more overweight), to off-set a weight-related health problem, or who have failed on other diets. Requires close medical supervision.
Formula/OTC (over the counter) ■ Nutrament ■ Slender ■ Slim Fast	May advocate less than 1,000 calories/day. Replaces one or more meals with a low-calorie shake or food bar that contains some combination of protein, carbohydrates, fats, vitamins, minerals.	Can be rapid, 3 or more lb./week if daily calorie level falls below 1,000. May promote water and muscle loss. Weight often regained.	May be low in protein, carbohydrates, vitamins or minerals. Can be dangerous if used for sole source of nutrition.	Teaches reliance on patented products, not on sound, lifelong eating habits.
Low Carbohydrate/High Protein ■ Dr. Atkins' Diet Revolution ■ Complete Scarsdale Medical Diet ■ Doctor's Quick Weight Loss Diet (Stillman, "water diet") ■ 35-Plus Diet for Women	Calorie level varies. Severely restricts carbohydrates, such as bread, cereals, grains, starchy vegetables.	Rapid, 3 or more lb./week. Promotes loss of water and muscle tissue. Weight usually regained.	Usually unbalanced. May be very high in saturated fat and cholesterol. Can cause fatigue, headaches, nausea, dehydration and dizziness.	Does not promote good eating habits. Nutritional claims are unsound.
Very Low Calorie ■ Diet Principal ■ Rotation Diet	Suggests less than 1,000 calories/day for part of diet or for its entirety. Based on low-fat, high-carbohydrate foods.	Rapid, 3 or more lb./week. Initial loss is water and muscle, not fat. Weight usually regained.	May be unbalanced and require vitamin and mineral supplements.	Usually does not teach long-term good eating habits.
Food Combination ■ Beverly Hills Diet ■ Fit for Life ■ Rice Diet Report	Usually less than 1,000 calories/day. Often makes false claims that specific foods or combinations burn fat; suggests eating one type of food, to exclusion of others.	Can be rapid, depending on calorie intake. Weight generally regained.	Unbalanced. May be dangerously low in protein; often deficient in vitamins and minerals. Can result in dizziness, diarrhea, gas, hair loss, brittle nails and loss of vital muscle tissue.	Based on unsound nutritional guidelines. Weight is lost because of reduction in calories, not magic food formula; can be dangerous. May be extremely restrictive and monotonous.

Reprinted with permission from The Walking Magazine, June 1989, © 1989, Raben Publishing Co., 711 Boylston St., Boston, MA 02116.

supplier of fuel by converting fatty acids to ketone bodies. Ketone bodies are organic acids that disturb the acid-base balance of the blood. They are the product of the incomplete breakdown of fat when carbohydrates are not available. The brain and central nervous system partially adapt and receive 50 percent of their fuel from ketones. The other 50 percent continues to come from the breakdown of the body's protein. Consequently, the RMR decreases significantly during the time of deprivation as the body attempts to conserve its lean tissue and fat stores. As the protein-containing organs progressively shrink, they perform less and less metabolic work and reduce the body's energy needs. The slowed-down metabolic engine results in less fat loss while body weight continues to fall rapidly. Concurrently, ketone bodies accumulate in the blood because they are produced in quantities that outstrip the body's ability to use or excrete them. The increase in blood acid level is potentially dangerous. Starvation should be avoided except for the extremely obese and then only under hospitalized medical supervision.

Very-low calorie diets (800 kcals/day or less), including those which have been promoted as having a "protein sparing effect," have often been associated with medical complications if they are followed long enough to produce substantial weight loss. The consequences of these diets include cardiac arrhythmias and sudden death.[50] These diets produce distinctive EKG (electrocardiogram) patterns that depict abnormal rhythm disturbances which are probably caused by protein depletion of the myocardium and/or cell membrane instability from rapid weight loss.[5] In addition to these risks, crash dieting typically results in a return to prediet weight when the diet ends. Repeated weight loss and recovery (weight cycling) predispose dieters to lower resting metabolic rates.[51] Cycle dieters lose muscle and gain fat in its place. Rats who were cycled took 21 days to lose a specified amount of weight and 46 days to regain it during the first cycle.[39] The second cycle took twice as long (40 days) to lose the same amount of weight but it was regained three times faster (14 days). Evidence emerging from human studies is showing a similar effect to weight cycling.

Most humans who diet and have lost and regained weight more than once are cycle dieters. Dieting without exercise has not worked for the majority of people. If you are thinking of losing weight, do it right the first time because cycling makes it more difficult each succeeding time.[51] Losing weight correctly requires sensible eating and sensible exercise for a lifetime. Here are some points to bear in mind.

1. Cycle dieting enhances the body's efficiency in converting food to fuel. As a result, fewer calories supply more of the energy and the calories saved are converted to fat.
2. Cycling may increase the activity of lipoprotein lipase, a fat-storing enzyme, which increases the body's ability to store fat.
3. Repeated dieting may alter the number and/or the size of fat cells.
4. Women may possibly react more negatively to the effects of dieting than men because a certain amount of fat is necessary to maintain fertility.
5. Repeat dieters tend to add weight in the masculine pattern increasing the risk for several chronic diseases.

Based upon these observations repeat dieting is inimical to both health and successful weight loss.

Just how successful are weight loss programs that rely solely upon manipulation of dietary intake? The statistics are dismal. The U.S. Department of Public Health has estimated that only 5 percent of all dieters are successful in reducing to a target weight and maintaining the loss for one year.[52] Further, only 2 percent are successful in achieving permanent weight loss; 98 out of 100 people who employ diet-only strategies fail to achieve permanent weight loss.

A widely held assumption is that the obese eat substantially more than thin people. The evidence indicates that they eat the same or less than normal-weight individuals. Obese girls who were observed during summer camp ate less and were less active than normal-weight girls. Similar results were obtained from observations of boys at summer camp. Studies of obese adults have shown that the inception of their weight gain could be traced back to a time when a decrease in physical activity, rather than an increase in appetite, occurred. This pattern is evident through observation of people who are attempting to fit into and establish a career after college. The attention and time devoted to physical activity decreases but their appetites do not. Six to twelve months after graduation they are 5 to 15 pounds heavier.

Exercise and the Underweight

The focus thus far has been on weight loss rather than weight gain, but the purposeful gain of weight represents a real problem for the underweight. What constitutes underweight? This question has not been satisfactorily answered. Actuarial statistics indicate that those who are significantly below the average in body weight have a higher expected mortality rate. Marked underweight may be indicative of underlying disease and is as much of a risk for early death as obesity.

Being underweight may pose as much of a cosmetic problem for an affected individual as obesity is for an obese individual. An effective weight gain program should include regular resistance exercise in conjunction with three well-balanced meals plus a couple of nutritious, between-meal snacks. Nuts, cheese, dried fruit, and fruit juice make excellent snacks. In addition, there are some commercial drinks that can be used for the purpose of increasing caloric consumption. Protein supplementation is unnecessary and can be harmful if taken in excessive amounts. Despite Herculean efforts, many underweight people find it to be more difficult to gain a pound than it is for the obese to lose one. Very lean people should not attempt to gain weight by increasing the fat content of their diet. This is an unhealthy eating pattern for anyone regardless of their body weight.

The amount and type of weight gain should be closely monitored. It is desirable to gain muscle tissue without increasing fat stores. Overeating without exercise will not accomplish this objective and it will not enhance physical appearance.

Some people are obsessed with becoming and remaining thin. **Anorexia nervosa** and **bulimarexia nervosa** are two eating disorders reflective of the preoccupation with thinness.[53] Although they share some common characteristics, anorexia and bulimia are different eating disorders. The major commonality between the two is an intense fear of becoming overweight. The anorexic accomplishes this primarily through starvation while the bulimic gorges and then purges by vomiting or by using laxatives and diuretics.[54] Bulimics seldom starve to the point of emaciation, in fact, they are often moderately overweight.[2] This eating disorder is characterized by episodes of secretive binge eating, menstrual irregularities, swollen glands, frequent weight fluctuation, and the inability to stop eating voluntarily. Bulimia is not caused by anorexia nervosa and many bulimics do not become anorexic, but many anorexics are bulimic.

Anorexia: Voluntary Starvation Amidst Plenty

Anorexia Nervosa is a psychological disorder characterized by a voluntary refusal to eat. It is the relentless pursuit of thinness. According to the American Psychological Association true anorexia involves weight loss of at least 25 percent of original weight, amenorrhea, distorted perception of body image, intense fear of becoming obese in spite of persistent weight loss, refusal to maintain normal body weight, and no identifiable physical illness to account for the weight loss.

Anorexia usually occurs in the mid to late teens to middle and upper class females. Evidence indicates that there are nine or ten anorexic females for every affected male but the disease is becoming more common in males.

Several theories have been advanced as possible causes of anorexia but none has been proven. Some researchers believe that underlying psychological problems such as the inability to deal with stress, fear of puberty, and the inability to separate from parents are the primary causes. Others believe that the cultural pressure to maintain a slim appearance is the primary cause.

About half of the anorexics are bulimic, that is they go on eating binges which are immediately followed by such purging tactics as self-induced vomiting, use of laxatives, diuretics, ipecac, and excessive amounts of exercise. These techniques combine to wreak havoc upon an already fragile fluid and mineral balance. Two to three percent of the anorexics suffer fatal heart irregularities from such practices.

Anorexics exhibit a characteristic set of signs and symptoms. The most obvious of these is a significant weight loss. Other signs include amenorrhea, social withdrawal, personality change, obsession with food and dieting, compulsive exercise, an overlying sense of unhappiness, slowed heart rate, the appearance of a layer of soft hair on the skin and a constant feeling of being cold even in a warm environment.

Treatment includes some restoration of the lost weight in order to make the mind more receptive to psychotherapy. The preferred method is to establish a contract for weight gain with the anorexic. If this technique fails then intravenous or tube feeding in a hospital may be necessary. When the body weight recovers to a nonlife-threatening level, then psychotherapy is initiated to discover the underlying causes. Several approaches such as group therapy, family therapy, and behavior modification may be employed to attempt a cure. A cure occurs when the individual is no longer obsessed with weight.

How thin is too thin? There are no hard and fast answers. The height-weight charts provide some clues. Individuals who are well below average for their height and frame size are underweight. They may be undermuscled or underfat or both. A better criterion concerns the percentage of total weight composed of fat. Healthy males who have more than five percent body fat are not endangering those biological functions that require fat. However, such males may not be satisfied with their very slim physical appearance. Females should not reduce their fat stores to levels that disturb the menses. For college-age women, seventeen to eighteen percent body fat presents a slim, trim appearance with enough fat for the reproductive system to function in a normal manner.

Assessment of Body Composition _____

The assessment of body composition has presented some problems. The only direct method available involves the separation of lean from fat tissue in cadavers. Only a few cadavers have been dissected in this manner because of the difficulty in obtaining them, the amount of time and effort required by the process, and the limited usefulness of the ensuing data. Such problems have stimulated scientists to develop indirect methods of analysis. These techniques provide an estimate of body composition; because they are estimates, some degree of error is associated with each. Two of the indirect measures, skinfold measurements and hydrostatic weighing, will be discussed.

If you can remain objective, standing naked before a full-length mirror will provide the answer to the basic question, "Am I fat?" This method does not yield the percentage of your weight in the form of fat, so it does not serve as a good guide to the amount of weight that must be lost. The pinch-an-inch tests provide a bit more information but still leaves much to be desired.

Skinfold Measurements

Skinfold measurements are based upon the assumption that 50 percent of the body's fat lies beneath the surface of the skin, that it can be separated from muscle tissue, and that it can be accurately and reliably measured. The thumb and index finger are used to pinch the loose skin over the site to be measured. This pinch, consisting of a double layer of skin plus subcutaneous fat, comprises the skinfold which is measured with a special caliper. The most accurate calipers maintain a constant jaw pressure of 10 grams per square millimeter of surface area. The Lange and Harpenden calipers meet these criteria and have been two of the most popular devices for measuring skinfolds. In recent years, several inexpensive calipers have emerged that are relatively accurate when used by well-trained technicians. These range in price from $10 to $30 while the Lange and Harpenden are in the $200 to $220 range.

The technique for taking skinfold measurements is not complicated but in order to become proficient one must practice measuring the different sites for all ages and both sexes. Standardize the method by observing the following suggestions:

1. Mark each site according to the directions given in Figures 11.1 through 11.5.
2. Take two measurements at each site unless there is a difference of more than 1 mm between the two; if there is, take a third measurement and average the two closest readings.
3. The calipers should be applied about one-quarter to one-half of an inch below the fingers. This allows the calipers rather than the fingers to compress the skinfold.
4. The calipers should maintain contact with the skinfold for two to five seconds in order for the reading to stabilize.

Use Tables 11.5 and 11.6 to convert millimeters of skinfold thickness to percent body fat. Table 11.5 uses the sum of chest, abdominal, and thigh skinfolds by age to estimate percent body fat for males. Table 11.6 uses the sum of triceps, supraillium and thigh skinfolds by age to estimate percent body fat for females.

FIGURE 11.1

Triceps Skinfold
Take a vertical fold on the midline of the upper arm over the triceps, halfway between the acromion and olecranon processes (tip of the shoulder to the tip of the elbow). The arm should be extended and relaxed when the measurement is taken. All skinfold measurements should be taken on the right side.

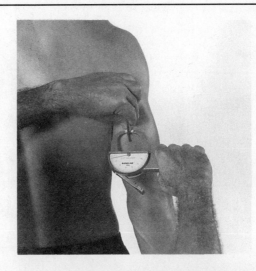

FIGURE 11.2

Suprailium Skinfold
Take a diagonal fold above the crest of the ilium directly below the mid-axilla (armpit).

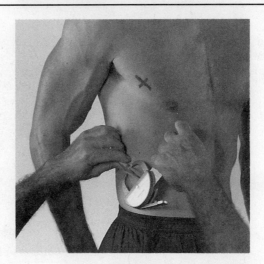

FIGURE 11.3

Thigh Skinfold
Take a vertical fold on the front of the thigh midway between the hip and the knee joint. The midpoint should be marked while the subject is seated.

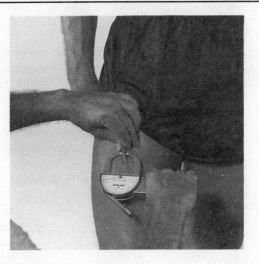

Chest Skinfold
Take a diagonal fold one-half of the distance between the anterior axillary line and the nipple.

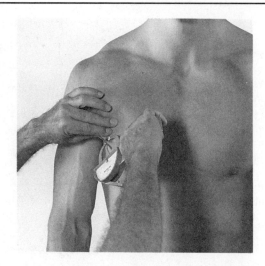

Abdominal Skinfold
Take a vertical fold about one inch from the navel.

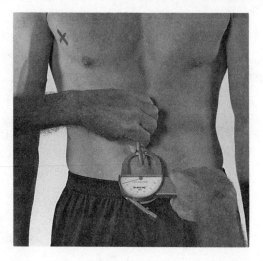

Hydrostatic Weighing

Hydrostatic weighing, as the name implies, involves the weighing of subjects while they are completely submerged. It is a more accurate measure than the skinfold technique provided that the subject is capable of a maximal exhalation of air from the lungs and can remain submerged and still for 6 to 10 seconds. Accuracy is enhanced still further if the technician has the equipment to measure residual air (the amount of air remaining in the lungs following a maximal expiration). Without such equipment, residual air can be estimated from a table of constants which have been developed for age and sex.

The equipment for hydrostatic weighing includes an autopsy scale calibrated in grams with a capacity of approximately 8 kilograms. This is suspended over the shallow end of a swimming pool or tank at least three feet deep. A light-weight seat is attached to the scale. The subject is suspended chin-deep in the

TABLE 11.6   Percent Fat Estimate for Women: Sum of Triceps, Suprailium, and Thigh Skinfolds

Sum of Skinfolds (mm)	Age to Last Year								
	Under 22	23–27	28–32	33–37	38–42	43–47	48–52	53–57	Over 57
23–25	9.7	9.9	10.2	10.4	10.7	10.9	11.2	11.4	11.7
26–28	11.0	11.2	11.5	11.7	12.0	12.3	12.5	12.7	13.0
29–31	12.3	12.5	12.8	13.0	13.3	13.5	13.8	14.0	14.3
32–34	13.6	13.8	14.0	14.3	14.5	14.8	15.0	15.3	15.5
35–37	14.8	15.0	15.3	15.5	15.8	16.0	16.3	16.5	16.8
38–40	16.0	16.3	16.5	16.7	17.0	17.2	17.5	17.7	18.0
41–43	17.2	17.4	17.7	17.9	18.2	18.4	18.7	18.9	19.2
44–46	18.3	18.6	18.8	19.1	19.3	19.6	19.8	20.1	20.3
47–49	19.5	19.7	20.0	20.2	20.5	20.7	21.0	21.2	21.5
50–52	20.6	20.8	21.1	21.3	21.6	21.8	22.1	22.3	22.6
53–55	21.7	21.9	22.1	22.4	22.6	22.9	23.1	23.4	23.6
56–58	22.7	23.0	23.2	23.4	23.7	23.9	24.2	24.4	24.7
59–61	23.7	24.0	24.2	24.5	24.7	25.0	25.2	25.5	25.7
62–64	24.7	25.0	25.2	25.5	25.7	26.0	26.7	26.4	26.7
65–67	25.7	25.9	26.2	26.4	26.7	26.9	27.2	27.4	27.7
68–70	26.6	26.9	27.1	27.4	27.6	27.9	28.1	28.4	28.6
71–73	27.5	27.8	28.0	28.3	28.5	28.8	29.0	29.3	29.5
74–76	28.4	28.7	28.9	29.2	29.4	29.7	29.9	30.2	30.4
77–79	29.3	29.5	29.8	30.0	30.3	30.5	30.8	31.0	31.3
80–82	30.1	30.4	30.6	30.9	31.1	31.4	31.6	31.9	32.1
83–85	30.9	31.2	31.4	31.7	31.9	32.2	32.4	32.7	32.9
86–88	31.7	32.0	32.2	32.5	32.7	32.9	33.2	33.4	33.7
89–91	32.5	32.7	33.0	33.2	33.5	33.7	33.9	34.2	34.4
92–94	33.2	33.4	33.7	33.9	34.2	34.4	34.7	34.9	35.2
95–97	33.9	34.1	34.4	34.6	34.9	35.1	35.4	35.6	35.9
98–100	34.6	34.8	35.1	35.3	35.5	35.8	36.0	36.3	36.5
101–103	35.3	35.4	35.7	35.9	36.2	36.4	36.7	36.9	37.2
104–106	35.8	36.1	36.3	36.6	36.8	37.1	37.3	37.5	37.8
107–109	36.4	36.7	36.9	37.1	37.4	37.6	37.9	38.1	38.4
110–112	37.0	37.2	37.5	37.7	38.0	38.2	38.5	38.7	38.9
113–115	37.5	37.8	38.0	38.2	38.5	38.7	39.0	39.2	39.5
116–118	38.0	38.3	38.5	38.8	39.0	39.3	39.5	39.7	40.0
119–121	38.5	38.7	39.0	39.2	39.5	39.7	40.0	40.2	40.5
122–124	39.0	39.2	39.4	39.7	39.9	40.2	40.4	40.7	40.9
125–127	39.4	39.6	39.9	40.1	40.4	40.6	40.9	41.1	41.4
128–130	39.8	40.0	40.3	40.5	40.8	41.0	41.3	41.5	41.8

From A. S. Jackson and M. L. Pollock, "Practical Assessment of Body Composition," *The Physician and Sportsmedicine,* 13, no. 5, (May 1985):86.

water, exhales completely, and bends forward from the waist until entirely submerged. This position is maintained for 6 to 10 seconds—enough time for the scale's pointer to stabilize. Five to ten trials are needed and the three heaviest readings are averaged. The individual's net underwater weight is calculated by subtracting the weight of the seat and its supporting structure, plus a weight belt if needed, from the gross underwater weight. The typical underwater weighing apparatus appears in Figure 11.6.

FIGURE 11.6

Underwater Weighing Apparatus
a.) Subject in the ready position for underwater weighing. b.) Subject in the process of being weighed.

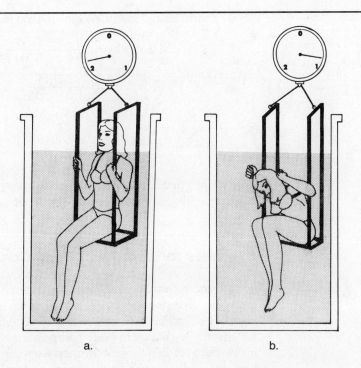

a.   b.

Desirable Body Weight

Desirable body weight may be determined easily when percent body fat has been ascertained. For example, a 20-year-old male who weighs 160 pounds has a measured body fat of 20.5 percent. Reducing his fat weight to 15 percent of his total weight would place him in an acceptable category for his age and sex. How much weight should he lose to accomplish this objective? The calculations are as follows:

1. Find Fat Weight (FW) in pounds

$$\text{FW (lb)} = \frac{\text{Body Weight (BW)} \times \text{Percent Fat}}{100}$$

$$= \frac{160 \times 20.5}{100}$$

$$= \frac{3285.12}{100}$$

$$= 32.85 \text{ lb}$$

2. Find Lean Weight (LW) in pounds

$$\text{LW (lb)} = \text{BW (lb)} - \text{FW (lb)}$$

$$= 160 - 32.85$$

$$= 127.15 \text{ lb}$$

3. Find Desired Body Weight (DBW) in pounds

$$
\begin{aligned}
\text{DBW (lb)} &= \frac{\text{LW}}{1.0 - \% \text{ fat desired}} \\
&= \frac{127.15}{1.0 - .15} \\
&= \frac{127.15}{.85} \\
&= 147.2 \text{ lb}
\end{aligned}
$$

This subject needs to reduce his body weight from 160 pounds to 147.2 pounds to achieve his goal of 15 percent body fat.

Exercises for Improving Body Composition

Body composition may be improved by increasing muscle tissue and decreasing fat tissue. Exercise represents the only viable way to accomplish both of these objectives. Aerobic activities that use 300 to 500 calories per workout are suitable for effecting a change in body composition. This can be accomplished by choosing one or a combination of the many aerobic activities available, such as walking, jogging, cycling, swimming, rowing, aerobic dance, and many more. Court games such as handball, racquetball, squash, and badminton may change body composition if played vigorously. This requires a fair degree of skill on the part of participants and entails singles competition against compatible opposition. Anaerobic activities such as weight training and calisthenics also have the capacity to improve body composition. Chapter 12 discusses these and other activities in greater detail and analyzes their contributions to the components of physical fitness.

The potential to change body composition through exercise has led to attempts to change only selected sites. Spot reduction implies that one can reduce the fat content of a particular body part by doing specific exercises related to that part. Sit-ups and leg-lifts have been commonly used to reduce abdominal fat and waist girth while leaving the remainder of the body unchanged. The attractiveness of this concept has led an unsuspecting public to believe that with a little effort we can sculpt our bodies to suit our fancies.

Spot reduction is a myth promoted by charlatans or unknowledgeable people who have a gimmick, gadget, or system to sell which is supposedly designed to achieve reductions in localized areas of the body. The truth is that the buyer will probably reduce nothing but the contents of ones wallet or purse. Localized exercise produces muscle tone and strength but it does not reduce the amount of fat at a given site. It may tighten up localized areas resulting in a difference in girth. For example, sit-ups done over a long period of time will strengthen and tighten the abdominal area. The stronger abdominal musculature helps to hold back the viscera and in this respect may reduce waist girth, but fat content remains unchanged. In order to reduce fat stored in the abdominal region, or in the back of the arm, or in the buttocks, the person must expend more calories than those that are consumed. This way, fat is lost from everywhere in the body, including the site in question. If spot reduction were a reality, people with fat faces could chew gum every day and eventually become people with thin faces. It just doesn't work.

The Weight Equation: Input Minus Output

To provide you with some insight into your eating and exercise habits and their effect upon weight and body composition, you should engage in the following process.

Input

Dietary Recall

First, complete a three-day dietary recall for two week days and one weekend day. Table 11.7 provides the format for a practical recording log for this experiment, and Table 11.8 gives a sample entry including a food item and all contributing condiments. During the three-day period which starts with breakfast on the first day and concludes at midnight of the third day, record all foods and beverages that are consumed except water and diet drinks (which are essentially acaloric). During this period, try to eat as you normally do. Be as accurate and as honest as possible—this is the only way that you can get a clear picture of your nutritional habits. This record should include all meals and all snacks, solid and liquid.

When this data has been collected, move to the Selected Foods List found in Appendix B. This list consists of some of the common foods eaten by Americans (although it is by no means all-inclusive). The foods and beverages are broken down into approximate caloric value as well as the amount of proteins, fats, and carbohydrates they contain. Insert these values for the foods and beverages that you have recorded and total the number of kcals consumed per day for the three days. For some food items you may need to consult the Fast Foods List found in Appendix A. (Note that this list does not include entries for carbohydrates or protein).

Output

Resting Metabolic Rate

Next, calculate your Resting Metabolic Rate (RMR). Use the factor 1.0 kcals per kilogram of body weight per hour for males (1 kcal/kg/hr), and 0.9 kcals per kilogram of body weight per hour for females (0.9 kcals/kg/hr). (The lb/kg conversion is 2.2 lb per 1 kg.) Using an example of a 160 lb male, the calculations are:

1. Change body weight in pounds to kilograms:

$$160 \text{ lbs} \div 2.2 \text{ kg} = 72.7 \text{ kg}$$

2. Multiply weight in kilograms by the RMR factor:

$$72.7 \text{ kg} \times 1 \text{ kcal/kg/hr} = 72.7 \text{ kcals/hr}$$

3. Multiply kcals/hr × 24 hours:

$$72.7 \text{ kcals/hr} \times 24 \text{ hrs} = 1744.8 \text{ kcals/day}$$

4. The RMR is 1744.8 kcals/day

Daily Activity Caloric Expenditure

Next, you need to approximate the number of kcals expended in daily activities as estimated by the amount of muscular movement you do during the course of a day. This is a rough approximation but you should be in the ball park if you follow the guidelines below and select the category that fits you best.

1. *Sedentary.* Student; desk job; etc; mostly sitting in your occupation and leisure time. Add 40 to 50 percent of the RMR.
2. *Light Activity.* Teacher; assembly line worker; walk two miles regularly. Add 55 to 65 percent of the RMR.
3. *Moderate Activity.* Waitress; waiter; aerobic exercise at about 75 percent of max heart rate. Add 65 to 70 percent of the RMR.
4. *Heavy Activity.* Construction worker; aerobic exercise above 75 percent of max. heart rate. Add 75 to 100 percent of RMR.

Input Minus Output

Add the approximate number of calories expended in voluntary physical activity to the RMR, and then compare this value to the average number of kcals consumed during the three-day dietary recall period. If you are in weight maintenance, the two values should be similar. If you are gaining or losing weight, this should be reflected in the direction of the difference between the two values.

The dietary recall will let you know the types of food that you are eating, the total number of kcals consumed, and how many kcals are derived from fats, carbohydrates, and proteins. If you are attempting to lose weight, the dietary recall may target some trouble spots by pointing out those foods which are contributing more than their share of kcals. Your strategy would be to cut back on these while at the same time increasing your physical activity level.

TABLE 11.7   Dietary Recall Sample Log

Time	Food /Beverage	Amount	kcals	Carbo-hydrates	Protein	Fat

TABLE 11.8   Example Entry for Dietary Recall Log

Time	Food/Beverage	Amount	kcals	Carbo-hydrates	Protein	Fat
12:20 A.M.	Hamburger	¼ lb.	327	0	36	7
	Bun	1	120	21	3	2
	Cheese (swiss)	1 slice	105	1	8	8
	Tomatoes	2 slices	10	1.5	trace	trace
	Lettuce	1 leaf	5	1	trace	trace
	Mayonnaise	1 tsp.	100	trace	trace	11

Each of the condiments and food accompanyments (bun, cheese, etc.) contain calories and contribute to the total number of kcals in the quarter-pound hamburger, so each is listed separately. You should also record the amount of carbohydrates, fats, and protein. Remember that carbohydrates and protein yield 4 kcals/gram, and fat yields 9 kcals/gram. This will show you where the calories are coming from.

You should slowly work up to burning 300 to 500 kcals per exercise session and participate 4 to 5 times per week. Refer to Table 11.1 and select several activities which are of interest and determine the number of minutes required to expend 300 to 500 kcals for your weight. If you have been sedentary, start slowly by expending 100 kcals per exercise session. As your level of fitness improves, increase the duration of exercise and the number of kcals used until you reach the desired level. Consider the fact that it is not necessary to burn all of the calories in one exercise session; you can split up the calories used by exercising several times per day.

Recall that we calculated desirable body weight for a 20 year old male subject (see page 309). His body weight was 160 lbs and his body fat was 20.5 percent. He needed to lose 12.8 lbs to achieve his desirable body weight. We will continue to use this subject as our example:

1. Let us assume that the subject's 3-day dietary recall indicates that he is consuming 2600 kcals/day.
2. His RMR, as calculated from the RMR example, is 1744.8 kcals/day.
3. Determine the kcals expended in daily activities. This 20-year-old is essentially sedentary both occupationally and in his leisure time, so we will multiply the RMR by 45 percent and then add this value back to the RMR.

   $1744.8 \times .45 = 785.2$ kcals burned in daily activities

4. Add the RMR kcals to the kcals burned for daily activities to get the total energy expenditure for one day.

   $1744.8 + 785.2 = 2530$ total kcals/day

5. Compare dietary recall kcals consumed to daily kcals expended.

Dietary recall:	2600 kcals
Daily expenditure:	2530 kcals
	70 kcals/day

6. This subject is consuming 70 kcals/day more than he needs. Bear in mind that a difference this small can be due to the error inherent in our method for determining RMR. This method yields an approximate value only. A second source of error involves the accuracy with which the dietary recall was handled. A third source of error involves the accuracy with which he compared the foods eaten to the values in the Selected Foods List. A fourth source of error involves how normally he ate during the recording time for the dietary recall. If our subject is in reality slowly gaining weight, however, the consumption of 70 extra kcals per day may be an accurate reflection of what is truly occurring. Seventy extra kcals per day would result in an insidious seven pound weight gain in a year.

Be careful and precise, then, and this process of calculating intake and output can provide you with the necessary information to successfully assess where you are, and should help you to determine what your course of action should be.

POINTS TO PONDER

1. *What physical problems are associated with very-low calorie diets?*
2. *Define weight cycling and discuss the reasons for its ineffectiveness as a weight management technique.*
3. *How should those who are underweight gain weight in a healthy manner?*
4. *Define anorexia nervosa and bulimarexia nervosa.*
5. *How do these two eating disorders differ; what do they share in common?*
6. *Discuss the steps which should be followed for assessing body composition with skinfold calipers.*
7. *What is hydrostatic weighing? Give a brief description of the technique.*
8. *A female weighs 155 pounds and is 32 percent fat. She would like to get down to 22 percent body fat. How much weight should she lose to achieve this goal?*

Chapter Highlights _____

Body composition refers to the amount of fat versus lean tissue in the body. Lean tissue consists of muscles, bones, organs, fluids; in short, any tissue that is not fat. Fat may be classified as essential or stored. Essential fat is necessary for many physiological functions, while stored fat is an energy reserve found in adipose tissue. Essential fat is sex-linked; females require more than males. Excessive leanness among females is associated with menstrual dysfunction.

Overweight is rampant in America. "Overweight" is a nebulous term in that it provides no clues to the composition of weight. Obesity refers to more than normal amounts of body fat; 20 percent or more for males, 30 percent or more for females. Both the number and the size of fat cells may be increased. Weight control is more difficult for those who have developed more than the usual number of fat cells.

Obesity is a health hazard that contributes to a variety of disorders and diseases and leads to premature death. In addition, the obese suffer from economic and social discrimination, poor body image, and depressed self-concept. Obesity is reversible! Suitable exercise and sensible changes in one's eating patterns, both of which can be sustained for a lifetime, are the appropriate course of action.

Exercise burns calories during the workout and in the recovery period that follows. Appetite may be suppressed for an hour or two following exercise but then it returns to normal. Sedentary people who begin an exercise program either continue to eat the same amount or slightly increase their food intake. Obese people generally do not eat more than slim people; they often eat less. Their obesity is not caused by overeating but rather to lack of exercise.

Exercise stimulates metabolism by maintaining and/or building muscle tissue while decreasing fat tissue. Males have higher resting metabolic rates (RMR) than females, primarily because of their extra muscle tissue. Dieting without exercise lowers the RMR because of lean tissue loss. Dieting-only strategies have failed miserably in producing permanent weight loss.

Marked underweight is a risk for early death because it may be a symptom of underlying disease. A healthy underweight individual may gain weight through muscle-building exercises coupled with an increase in caloric intake. Anorexia nervosa is a psychological condition of extreme underweight that requires professional treatment.

Body composition can be assessed through a number of indirect methods. Skinfold measures with a reliable caliper are reasonably accurate in skilled hands provided that the group being measured is similar to the reference group from which the standard measurements were taken. Hydrostatic weighing is probably more accurate than skinfold measurements, but it is not without its own problems.

Aerobic exercises that burn 300 to 500 calories per session can change body composition for the better primarily by reducing the amount of body fat. Anaerobic exercises such as weight training and calisthenics also affect body composition by building muscle tissue. Combining both types of activities is very effective.

References

1. M. M. Shangold, "Athletic Amenorrhea," *Clinical Obstetrics and Gynecology*, 28, (1985): 664.

2. S. C. Lipnickey, "Beyond Dieting: A Preventive Perspective on Eating Disorders," in *Health 89/90*, Guilford, Conn: The Dushkin Publishing Group, Inc., 1989.

3. "Athletic Amenorrhea and Bone Density," *The Harvard Medical School Health Letter*, 10, (December 1984): 5.

4. B. L. Drinkwater et al., "Bone Mineral Density After Resumption of Menses in Amenorrheic Athletes," *Journal of The American Medical Association*, 256, (1986): 380.

5. F. Munnings, "Exercise and Estrogen in Women's Health: Getting a Clearer Picture," *The Physician and Sportsmedicine*, 16, (1988): 152.

6. F. Caldwell, "Runners vs. Anorectics—No Contest," *The Physician and Sportsmedicine*, 12, (1984): 21.

7. C. M. Poissonnet et al., "Growth and Development of Adipose Tissue," *The Journal of Pediatrics*, 113, (1988): 1.

8. J. L. Knittle et al., "The Growth of Adipose Tissue in Children and Adolescents," *Journal of Clinical Investigation*, 63, (1979): 239.

9. A. F. Roche, "The Adipocyte Number Hypothesis," *Child Development*, 52, (1981): 31.

10. A. Hager et al., "Body Fat and Adipose Tissue Cellularity in Infants: A Longitudinal Study," *Metabolism*, 26, (1977): 607.

11. F. X. Hausberger and J. E. Volz, "Feeding in Infancy, Adipose Tissue Cellularity and Obesity," *Physiology and Behavior*, 33, (1984): 81.

12. M. S. Kramer et al., "Infant Determinants of Childhood Weight and Adiposity," *Journal of Pediatrics*, 107, (1985): 104.

13. W. S. Agras et al., "Does a Vigorous Feeding Style Influence Early Development of Adiposity," *Journal of Pediatrics*, 110, (1987): 799.

14. G. P. Ravelli et al., "Obesity in Young Men After Famine Exposure in Utero and Early Infancy," *New England Journal of Medicine*, 295, (1976): 349.

15. R. Kliegman et al., "Intrauterine Growth and Postnatal Fasting Metabolism in Infants of Obese Mothers," *Journal of Pediatrics*, 104, (1984): 601.

16. R. I. Berkowitz et al., "Physical Activity and Adiposity: A Longitudinal Study From Birth to Childhood," *Journal of Pediatrics*, 106, (1985): 734.

17. R. I. Berkowitz, "Physical Activity, Eating Style, and Obesity in Children: A Review," *Behavioral Medicine Update*, (Reprint).

18. "First, Understand What Causes Weight Gain," *Tufts University Diet and Nutrition Letter*, 3, (January 1986): 3.

19. M. Krotkiewski et al., "Impact of Obesity on Metabolism in Men and Women," *Journal of Clinical Investigation*, 72, (1983): 1150.

20. S. K. Fried and J. G. Krall, "Sex Differences in Regional Distribution of Fat Cell Size and Lipoprotein Lipase Activity in Morbidly Obese Patients," *International Journal of Obesity*, 11, (1987): 129.

21. C. D. Besten et al., "Resting Metabolic Rate and Diet-Induced Thermogenesis in Abdominal and Gluteal-Femoral Obese Women Before and After Weight Reduction," *American Journal of Clinical Nutrition*, 47, (1988): 840.

22. R. J. Meyers et al., "Accuracy of Self-Reports of Food Intake in Obese and Normal-Weight Individuals: Effects of Obesity on Self-Reports of Dietary Intake in Adult Females," *American Journal of Clinical Nutrition*, 48, (1988): 1248.

23. F. Rosato, *Jogging for Health and Fitness*, Englewood, Colorado: Morton Publishing Company, 1988.

24. T. G. Harris and J. Gurin, "Look Who's Getting It All Together," *American Health*, 42, (1985).

25. J. K. Collins et al., "Body Percept Change in Obese Females After Weight Reduction Therapy," *Journal of Clinical Psychology*, 39, (1983): 507.

26. M. A. Short et al., "Effects of Physical Conditioning on Self-Concept of Adult Obese Males," *Physical Therapy*, 64, (1984): 194.

27. C. Pierre, "Maximizing Metabolism: Can Calorie Burning Be Increased?" *Environmental Nutrition*, 12, (February 1989): 1.

28. A. R. Tagliaferro et al., "Effects of Exercise Training on the Thermic Effect of Food and Body Fatness of Adult Women," *Psychology and Behavior*, 38, (1986): 703.

29. J. Mayer et al., "Relation Between Caloric Intake, Body Weight, and Physical Work: Studies in an Industrial Male Population in West Bengal," *American Journal of Clinical Nutrition*, 4, (1956): 169.

30. O. G. Edholm et al., "The Food Intake and Individual Expenditure of Individual Men," *British Journal of Nutrition*, 9, (1955): 286.

31. S. N. Blair et al., "Comparison of Nutrient Intake in Middle-Aged Men and Women Runners and Controls," *Medicine and Science in Sports and Exercise*, 13, (1981): 310.

32. P. D. Wood et al., "Increased Exercise Level and Plasma Lipoprotein Concentrations: A One-Year, Randomized, Controlled Study in Sedentary Middle-Aged Men," *Metabolism*, 32, (1983): 31.

33. J. A. Dempsey, "Anthropometrical Observations on Obese and Nonobese Young Men Undergoing a Program of Vigorous Physical Exercise," *Research Quarterly*, 35, (1964): 275.

34. P. Wood, *California Diet and Exercise Program*, Mountain View, Calif: Anderson World Books, Inc., 1983.

35. B. Zuti and L. Golding, "Comparing Diet and Exercise As Weight Reduction Tools," *The Physician and Sportsmedicine*, 4, (1976): 49.

36. D. L. Ballor et al., "Resistance Weight Training During Caloric Restriction Enhances Lean Body Weight Maintenance," *American Journal of Clinical Nutrition*, 47, (1988): 19.

37. L. Lamb (ed.) "Exercise Protects Heart During Dieting," *The Health Letter*, 31, (February 12, 1988): 3.

38. P. Wood, "The Science of Successful Weight Loss" *Food and Fatness*, 1, (March 1984): 3.

39. "Dieting-Induced Obesity: A Hidden Hazard of Weight Cycling," *Environmental Nutrition*, 10, (February 1987) Reprint.

40. O. E. Owen et al., "A Reappraisal of Caloric Requirements in Healthy Women," *The American Journal of Clinical Nutrition*, 44, (1986): 1.

41. H. A. de Vries, "Physical Fitness Guidelines for Older Adults," *President's Council on Physical Fitness and Sports Newsletter*, Washington, D.C.: March, 1980.

42. M. Chinnici, "Picking The Perfect Diet," *The Walking Magazine*, 4, (May/June 1989): 40.

43. A. J. Siegel, "New Insights About Obesity and Exercise," *Your Patient and Fitness*, 2, (Jan/Feb 1989): 12.

44. S. B. Roberts et al., "Energy Expenditure and Intake in Infants Born to Lean and Overweight Mothers," *New England Journal of Medicine*, 318, (1988): 461.

45. A. Tremblay et al., "The Effect of Exercise-Training on Resting Metabolic Rate in Lean and Moderately Obese Individuals," *International Journal of Obesity*, 10, (1986): 511.

46. J. O. Hill et al., "Effects of Exercise and Food Restriction on Body Composition and Metabolic Rate in Obese Women," *American Journal of Clinical Nutrition*, 46, (1987): 622.

47. C. P. Donahoe et al., "Metabolic Consequences of Dieting and Exercise in The Treatment of Obesity," *Journal of Consulting and Clinical Psychology*, 52, (1984): 827.

48. E. Ravussin et al., "Reduced Rate of Energy Expenditure as a Risk Factor for Body-Weight Gain," *New England Journal of Medicine*, 318, (1988): 467.

49. C. Shultz et al., "Effects of Severe Caloric Restriction and Moderate Exercise on Basal Metabolic Rate and Hormonal Status in Adult Humans," *Federal Proceedings*, 39, (1980): 783.

50. A. J. Moss, "Caution: Very-Low Calorie Diets Can Be Deadly," *Annals of Internal Medicine*, 102, (1985): 121.

51. S. N. Steen et al., "Metabolic Effects of Repeated Weight Loss and Regain in Adolescent Wrestlers," *Journal of the American Medical Association*, 260, (1988): 47.

52. "You Can Lose Weight and Keep It Off," *Tufts University Diet and Nutrition Letter*, 7, (March 1989): 1.

53. J. M. Isner et al., "Anorexia Nervosa and Sudden Death," *Annals of Internal Medicine*, 102, (1985): 49.

54. A. E. Andersen, *American Anorexia/Bulimia Association Newsletter*, 9, (1986): 9.

12

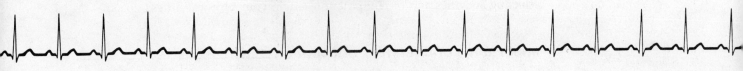

Fitness for Life

Introduction

Your knowledge and understanding of how to achieve wellness through physical fitness should be considerably enhanced by the time you have reached this point in the text. This chapter will focus on selected physical activities which contribute in varying ways to the development and maintenance of physical fitness. Also, equipment that promotes active or passive exercise will be discussed with regard to their contributions to physical fitness. This information should be helpful in selecting activities and/or equipment to attain your physical fitness goals.

Importance of Lifetime Participation

Exercise will provide lasting benefits if it is programmed as an integral part of one's lifestyle. The results of exercise are short-lived; that is, the benefits begin to wane 48 to 72 hours after the last workout. The development and maintenance of physical fitness depends upon consistent participation that adheres to the principles of intensity, frequency, duration, progression, and overload. Sporadic exercise does not promote physical fitness nor does it contribute to health. In fact, a recent study discussed in Chapter 3 indicated that infrequent participation increases the risk for a heart attack during exercise.[1] Those who exercise regularly and vigorously have a slightly elevated risk of heart attack during exercise but the long-term compensatory health advantages clearly outweigh the minimal risks. Some selected health benefits of exercise that have received support through research and anecdotal evidence appear in Table 12.1.

The feeling of well-being achieved by an increase in one's energy level is a bonus to the health benefits listed in Table 12.1. People who exercise regularly feel good! They consistently report feeling younger and more relaxed; they sleep better, feel better, have more energy, and even report less flu, colds, and other infections.

TABLE 12.1   A Summary of Selected Health-Related Benefits Associated with Regular Exercise

Regular Exercise:

I. Reduces the risk of cardiovascular disease
   1. Increases HDL-C
   2. Decreases LDL-C
   3. Favorably changes the ratios between total cholesterol and HDL-C, and between LDL-C and HDL-C
   4. Decreases triglyceride levels
   5. Promotes relaxation; relieves stress and tension
   6. Decreases body fat and favorably changes body composition
   7. Reduces blood pressure especially if it is high.
   8. Blood platelets are less sticky
   9. Less cardiac arrhythmias
   10. Increases myocardial efficiency
       a. lowers resting heart rate
       b. increases stroke volume
   11. Increase oxygen-carrying capacity of the blood

TABLE 12.1 Continued

Regular Exercise:

II. Helps control diabetes
   1. Cells are less resistant to insulin
   2. Reduces body fat

III. Develops stronger bones that are less susceptible to injury

IV. Promotes joint stability by
   1. Increasing muscular strength
   2. Increasing strength of the ligaments, tendons, cartilage, and connective tissue

V. Contributes to fewer low back problems

VI. Acts as a stimulus for other lifestyle changes

VII. Improves self-concept

Lifetime participation in physical activity may motivate the exerciser to follow a general program of health habits—such as adhering to a low fat diet, eliminating smoking, moderating alcohol, and regularly monitoring the blood pressure. It seems scientifically sound to encourage everyone to exercise and achieve high levels of physical fitness. Though the benefits of exercise "may not all be caused by exercise per se, it seems a good way to help accomplish a number of worthwhile goals toward better cardiovascular health."[2]

Business and industry have adopted multifaceted illness-prevention programs in order to reduce employee health care costs. The incidence of injury and the number of absences because of illness seem to decrease with participation in illness-prevention programs. Establishing a cause-and-effect relationship between these programs and the changes that occur is now being attempted.

Industry Invests in Sweat

Wellness programs featuring physical fitness, smoking cessation, blood pressure detection and control, nutritional counseling, and substance abuse education, are finally beginning to catch on in business and industry. These programs appeal to management because they are cost-effective; that is, the dollars spent on prevention are considerably less than the cost of after-the-fact medical care. In other words, its cheaper to keep employees healthy than to pay their sick bills. The following data exemplify the effectiveness of physical fitness programs in the workplace.

- A recent survey by Robert Half International Inc. of New York indicated that executives in the $30,000 to $55,000 salary range who participated in one or more sports earned an average of $3,120 more than their inactive colleagues.
- Exercising employees of Canada Life were compared to nonexercising employees of North American Life Assurance Co. The exercising group increased their productivity by 2.7 percent, reduced absenteeism by 22 percent, and the annual worker turnover was reduced by 16 percent. Health care costs were lowered by the equivalent of half-a-day spent in the hospital and three physician visits per worker. This translated to a conservative $7.50 savings per worker-year; this was much more than the cost of establishing and maintaining the physical fitness program.
- A study of 3200 Tenneco employees showed that those who exercised regularly received higher job performance ratings and more merit pay than sedentary employees.

- More than half of the NASA employees who began regular exercise improved their energy level and their job performance rating.
- New York State employees who participated in a five-year exercise program reduced their risk of heart disease and were absent less often from work.
- In one year, New York Telephone Co. realized an estimated savings of $14.3 million as a result of decreased medical and hospital care costs and reduced absenteeism due to physical fitness programs.

Many corporations are reducing the number of management positions in order to trim expenses and streamline the chain of command. Physically fit personnel will have a better chance of retaining their jobs as well as a better opportunity to advance up the corporate ladder than their sedentary coworkers.

Company physical fitness programs have contributed to less worker turnover. In addition, they are attractive "perks" that corporations employ to recruit qualified personnel. The message is becoming eminently clear—physical fitness pays off for the employers and employees.

Rating Selected Exercises and Sports

Kenneth Cooper probably did the most extensive work on rating exercises and sports. He developed a point system by which many physical activities can be compared on the basis of their contribution to cardiorespiratory or aerobic endurance. The point system is more accurate for some activities than for others. The rhythmic and continuous activities such as walking, jogging, cycling, swimming, rope jumping, and so on, are easier to quantify because the pace or tempo can be controlled. Therefore, values obtained for these activities by age and body weight are more accurate than those that have been developed for nonrhythmic sports such as racquetball, handball, badminton, tennis, soccer, and so forth. Many of these sports have the potential for developing and maintaining fitness. Meeting the proper intensity, frequency, and duration is more difficult with sports than for the rhythmic fitness activities. In sports, overload is applied by playing for a longer duration or more frequently. Intensity is difficult to manipulate since it is dependent upon skill level. As skill improves one can step up in competition and attain a better workout. Progression is connected to skill level. It cannot be planned in a manner similar to the rhythmic and continuous activities. However, sport participation adds a challenging, competitive, and fun element to one's fitness adventures. To get the most from sports, one should have a reasonable amount of skill, play against equally skilled opposition, be motivated to do one's best, and be physically fit prior to participation.

A number of years ago, the President's Council on Physical Fitness and Sport (PCPFS) enlisted the aid of seven experts to evaluate 14 popular physical activities for their contribution to physical fitness and general well-being. A summary of these ratings appears in Table 12.2. These activities remain popular and the ratings are equally valid today as when they were originally conceived.

Rhythmic and Continuous Activities

If these exercises and activities are to contribute to the development and maintenance of physical fitness they must meet the requirements established for intensity, frequency, duration, progression, and overload.

TABLE 12.2   Rating 14 Sports and Exercises*

Benefits	Activity						
	Jogging	Bicycling	Swimming	Skating (Ice or Roller)	Handball/ Squash	Skiing— Nordic	Skiing— Alpine
Physical Fitness							
Cardiorespiratory endurance (stamina)	21	19	21	18	19	19	16
Muscular endurance	20	18	20	17	18	19	18
Muscular strength	17	16	14	15	15	15	15
Flexibility	9	9	15	13	16	14	14
Balance	17	18	12	20	17	16	21
General Well-Being							
Weight control	21	20	15	17	19	17	15
Muscle definition	14	15	14	14	11	12	14
Digestion	13	12	13	11	13	12	9
Sleep	16	15	16	15	12	15	12
Total	148	142	140	140	140	139	134

*The ratings are on a scale of 0–3, thus a rating of 21 is the maximum score that can be achieved (a score of 3 by all seven panelists). Ratings were made on the following basis: Frequency = 4 times per week minimum; duration = 30 to 60 minutes per session.

TABLE 12.2   Continued

Benefits	Activity						
	Basketball	Tennis	Calisthenics	Walking	Golf**	Softball	Bowling
Physical Fitness							
Cardiorespiratory endurance (stamina)	19	16	10	13	8	6	5
Muscular endurance	17	16	13	14	8	8	5
Muscular strength	15	14	16	11	9	7	5
Flexibility	13	14	19	7	9	9	7
Balance	16	16	15	8	8	7	6
General Well-Being							
Weight control	19	16	12	13	6	7	5
Muscle definition	13	13	18	11	6	5	5
Digestion	10	12	11	11	7	8	7
Sleep	12	11	12	14	6	7	6
Total	134	128	126	102	66	64	51

**Golf rating was made on the basis of using a golf cart or caddy. If you walk the course and carry your clubs the values improve.

From C. C. Conrad, "How Different Sports Rate in Promoting Physical Fitness," *Medical Times* (reprint), May 1976, p. 4. Used by permission.

Aerobic Dancing. Aerobic dancing is usually performed in a group under the leadership of an instructor (see Fig. 12.1). Programs and routines differ, with some emphasizing aerobic exercise while others emphasize flexibility and/or muscular strength and endurance. This lack of standardization makes comparisons between programs difficult. Also two participants in the same class may differ regarding the quality of the workout, that is, one may perform enthusiastically with boundless energy while another performs languidly.

The American College of Sports Medicine has just recently developed guidelines and procedures for certifying aerobic dance instructors. This will be very helpful in producing quality programs. Here are some points to clarify before signing up for an aerobic dance class.

1. Has the instructor had classes in human anatomy, exercise physiology, kinesiology, first aid, and CPR (cardiorespiratory resuscitation)?
2. Does the instructor screen prospective students for medical problems or require a medical exam for entrance into the program?
3. Is the class small enough to be supervised effectively?
4. Is the major portion of class time devoted to aerobic activity? Does the instructor emphasize monitoring the intensity of the workout by heart rate and perceived exertion? Is this done several times during the class period?
5. Does class begin with a sufficient warm up and end with a cool down period?
6. Is the aerobic component continuous and long enough to produce a training effect?

FIGURE 12.1

Aerobic Dance Class

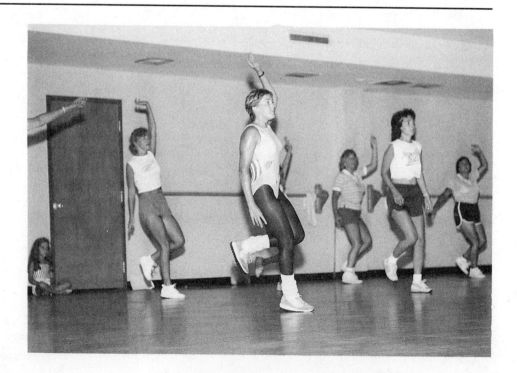

Most aerobic dance injuries are caused by overuse. Moderating the frequency and duration of participation and individualizing programs could reduce the number of injuries that occur.
—Yoshiteru Mutoh

Properly performed, aerobic dance has the potential to train the cardiorespiratory system, but performed too often on nonresiliant surfaces with inappropriate footwear, it can substantially increase the likelihood of injury.[3,4,5] Instructors in these studies incurred more injuries than their students because they performed more often. Most injuries occurred below the knee, with shin splints being the most common. Inactive people should approach aerobic dancing cautiously. Even though they are urged by instructors to proceed at their own pace, the tendency to keep up with the group is quite strong among many beginners. This can lead to soreness, pain, or injury. Those who expect to perform at the level of the class from the outset should enter the program already fit. If not, be patient and proceed slowly. You will quickly reach the level of the group.

Aerobic dancing is one of the few fitness activities which has the potential for developing all of the components of physical fitness. A knowledgeable instructor can structure the class to accomplish this desirable objective.

Another alternative is to begin by participating in low-impact aerobics. In this activity, one foot is in contact with the floor at all times. Target heart rates are achieved by combining leg movements and vigorous arm movements. These classes are excellent for sedentary people, the overweight, the elderly, and those who have lower extremity joint problems.

Cross-Country Skiing. A comparison of the world's elite athletes reveals that the cross-country skiers rank first in terms of cardiorespiratory endurance. Cross-country skiing exercises many muscle groups. Pulling with the poles develops the muscles of the arms, shoulders, back, and chest; while the gliding leg movements develop the leg muscles. Vigorous contractions of all of these muscle groups together enhance the cardiorespiratory system. Cross-country skiing significantly contributes to all of the components of fitness.

Availability and access to snow is the major limiting factor associated with cross-country skiing. A major advantage is that almost anyone can learn the fundamentals of this activity in a very short period of time so that joy in participation occurs early. This activity combines skiing and hiking.[6] The gear required for cross-country skiing costs only a fraction of downhill skiing gear and its not necessary to travel to a high-priced skiing resort to participate. Actually, one can cross-country ski in a local park or meadow.

Participants of cross-country skiing burn 600 to 900 kcals per hour depending on their skill level and the terrain. World class skiers burn more than 1000 kcals per hour. Needless to say, it is excellent for weight management provided that the frequency and duration are appropriate. Cross-country skiing should be supplemented by a daily program of stretching exercises.

Cycling. Outdoor cycling is a weight bearing but very efficient form of locomotion. The PCPFS panel rated it as the second best activity for developing physical fitness. Pedaling at approximately 15 mph is required in order to achieve a training effect, but this and all other aerobic activities are monitored best with exercise heart rate and perceived exertion. It is sometimes difficult to maintain the heart rate in the appropriate zone. Hills require hard work on the up side (the heart rate may exceed the target) but the temptation to coast on the down side is great. The result may be large heart rate swings.

Outdoor cycling is an excellent fitness activity for all age groups and is particularly good for the overweight and those with leg and joint problems. Weather is one of the limiting factors to outdoor cycling; cold, snow, ice, and rain are not conducive to riding a bike. Traffic presents the greatest hazard to the cyclist. Cyclists should wear protective equipment. A helmet, gloves, elbow and knee pads, and reflectors should be worn on all outdoor rides.

Stationary cycling is a nonweight-bearing activity allowing one to exercise indoors in a controlled environment against a resistance that maintains the heart rate in the proper zone (see Fig. 12.2). This is an excellent activity for the obese and the elderly because the hazards associated with falling and negotiating a bike in traffic are eliminated. Stationary cycling is a superb exercise but, for many, a boring one. To alleviate the boredom of going nowhere, a reading stand can be mounted on the handlebars or you may watch a favorite television program.

Pedalling efficiency occurs by adjusting the height of the seat to accommodate a slightly bent knee in the downstroke. This allows the cyclist to exert maximum force through a relatively full range of motion and applies to both outdoor and stationary cycling.

Cycling does not contribute to upper body strength or total body flexibility, thus it should be accompanied by daily stretching and resistance exercises three times per week. But cycling is excellent for the cardiorespiratory system. While

FIGURE 12.2

Exercising on a Stationary Bike

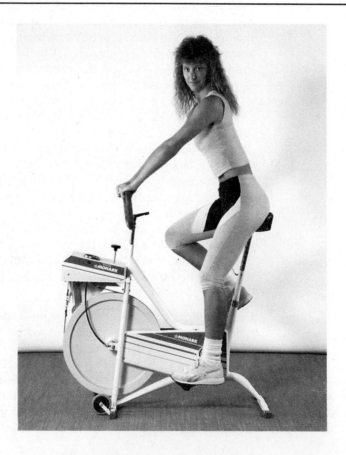

there is considerable risk associated with outdoor cycling, stationary cycling is a very safe activity resulting in very few injuries.

Jogging. According to the PCPFS panel, jogging is the best physical fitness activity of the 14 evaluated. Jogging is a most efficient and economic way to develop aerobic fitness (see Fig. 12.3). It is economical in terms of the amount of time needed to produce improvement and the monetary expense needed to get started. The only expense involves the purchase of a good pair of well-fitting jogging shoes; the remainder of the outfit can be improvised from clothing you already possess. There are some general guidelines for the purchase of jogging shoes.

Shoes made especially for jogging have some common characteristics. The heel should be about one-half inch higher than the sole and it should be well padded. The sole should consist of two separate layers with the outer layer made of a durable rubberized compound for traction and longevity. The inner layer should be thick and pliable and made of shock absorbing material. It is desirable for the heel and sole to flare out so the impact with the ground can be distributed over a wide area. This is critical because the jogger's foot hits the ground 600 to 750 times per mile, with each foot strike absorbing a force equivalent to three times the body weight.

Flexibility, another characteristic of a good shoe, can be determined by grasping the heel in one hand and the toe in the other and bending it. If it does not bend easily, it is too stiff and inflexible for jogging.

Proper fit is another important factor. The shoes should be one-half inch longer than the longest toe and the toe box should allow enough room for the

FIGURE 12.3

Jogging
This is an especially enjoyable activity when conducted with friends.

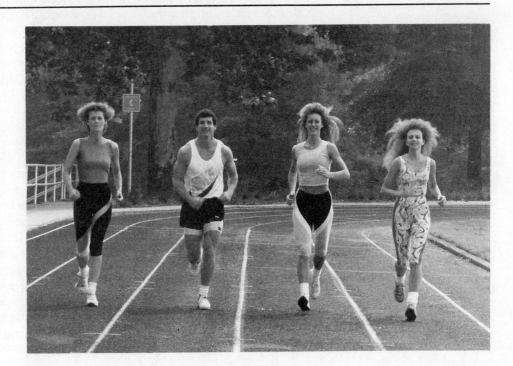

toes to spread. The toe box should be high enough not to pinch down on the toes. The heel of the foot should fit snugly in the padded heel of the shoe for maximum support and minimum friction. The shoe should have a good, firm arch support.

It is best to jog on level grassy or artificial surfaces such as those found on some running tracks and football fields. The sidewalks and streets are the worst surfaces for jogging and should be especially avoided by beginners. Joggers periodically can run on hard surfaces after the muscles, tendons, ligaments and cartilage have been conditioned. Orthopedic physicians unanimously agree that even long-time joggers cannot consistently use these surfaces with impunity. Eventually, stress injuries will occur. Powell reviewed the literature regarding the incidence of jogging-related injuries and found that a linear relationship existed between the frequency of injury and weekly mileage.[7] The knee joint seems to be most vulnerable.[8]

Although rated the number one fitness activity, jogging is not a total conditioner. It does not contribute to upper body strength or flexibility. In fact, it contributes to inflexibility of the lower back, hamstrings, and calf muscles. A daily stretching program is important for joggers.

Rope Jumping. The results of a study of the effect of rope jumping on the cardiorespiratory endurance that appeared in a popular magazine, helped to promote this aerobic activity.[9] The study indicated that 10 minutes of rope jumping trained the cardiorespiratory system as well as 30 minutes of jogging. It is easy to see why rope jumping dramatically increased in popularity. It sounded too good to be true, and it was. A faulty research design led to an equally faulty conclusion. Since that study, investigations featuring better research protocols showed that rope jumping takes as much time as jogging to produce similar effects.[10] An interesting and somewhat ironic fact is that a previous record holder for endurance rope jumping (he jumped continuously for six hours and turned approximately 59,000 revolutions of the rope) jogged 90 to 100 miles per week preparing for his assault on the record book. During this time, he jumped for 10 minutes per day and for two hours once every two weeks.[11]

The energy requirement of rope jumping, though substantial, is lower than jogging for the same heart rate.[10,12] This is probably because of the fact that jogging uses more muscles than rope jumping, especially when jumpers become highly skilled and efficient. Because of the high-heart rates elicited by rope jumping, it is too strenuous for sedentary people. Conversely, it is probably not strenuous enough for very fit people.

Rope jumping is a very inexpensive fitness activity that can be performed both indoors and outdoors (see Fig. 12.4). It is best to jump upon a resilient surface such as a plywood platform. This can easily be constructed with a three to four foot square of one-inch thick plywood framed with 2 × 4s. Indoor/outdoor carpet is also a good surface for jumping. The rope should be heavy enough to twirl easily and it should be attached to a set of swivel handles. If you want to try rope jumping before investing in a good rope, you can cut a length of clothesline and tie a knot in both ends. The proper length of a jump rope can be determined by holding both ends of the rope (where they join the handles) against one shoulder and let the loop hang down toward the floor. If the loop falls between the ankle bone and the floor, the rope is the proper length.

Landing on the toes while jogging is functionally incorrect. The entire biomechanical sequence designed to dissipate the force of landing breaks down if heelstrike is avoided.
—Kurt Jepson

Landing on the toes is a functional necessity when jumping rope. Landing on the heels would result in poor impact absorption.
—Kurt Jepson

FIGURE 12.4

Rope Jumping
Note that the elbows are
close to the body and the
subject jumps on the balls
of his feet.

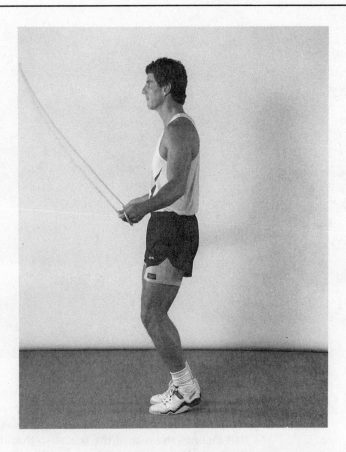

Rope jumping does not contribute to flexibility or muscular strength and should be supplemented by activities that promote both of these components of fitness.

Rowing. Rowing is an excellent cardiorespiratory and muscular conditioner that exercises many muscle groups. It was not evaluated by the PCPFS panel, however, competitive rowers rank among the best of the world's endurance athletes and they are muscularly fit as well. Rowing provides a good cardiovascular workout without the trauma on the legs and feet that occurs during jogging and court games, and it also confers an upper body workout at the same time.

This exercise, for the average person, is performed on a stationary rowing machine rather than in a boat or a racing scull (see Fig. 12.5). This is advantageous because the exercise can be performed at one's home and the resistance of the oars can be set to elicit the desired heart rate. Many people find stationary rowing boring, but according to the June 1984 *Sporting Goods Dealer*, the sale of rowing machines increased by 179 percent from 1982 to 1983. The cost of rowing machines runs from $150 for department store rowers to $3000 for sophisticated computerized ergometers which calculate speed, distance covered and kcals expended during the workout. The average person needs a durable lightweight model that is easily stored and costs about $350 to $400. The rower should sit

Rowing on a Stationary Rower

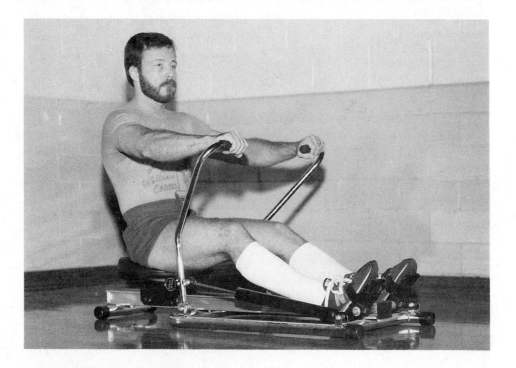

solidly on the floor without wobbling or jumping as you row. The seat and oars should move smoothly without binding. An option to consider is an attachment that inclines the rear of the frame so that the resistance can be increased during the leg extension phase of the stroke.

One caution regarding rowing as a form of exercise: it involves vigorous arm work and isometric gripping of the oars. This may raise the blood pressure to unacceptably high levels for hypertensives and those with cardiovascular disease.

Rowing is excellent for aerobic and muscular conditioning and contributes to flexibility if participants stroke through a full range of motion.

Swimming. Swimming is an excellent aerobic and muscular activity that employs continuous motion of the arms and legs against the resistance of the water. Swimming laps for 30 to 45 minutes constitutes a very good workout. Three months of swim training significantly improved the cardiovascular function of middle-age (age 30 to 48) people.[13] Most subjects began by swimming one lap. They progressed to one mile within three to four weeks and were up to two miles by the end of the three-month study. Although swimmers have a slightly lower exercise capacity than cross-country skiers and runners, swimming is still a good aerobic conditioner.

To receive a training effect, one must swim continuously for at least 30 minutes. Easy paddling and floating do not contribute to fitness. In recognition of the growing number of people who are swimming for fitness, many pool directors are designating times and lanes for lap swimming. To make their workout more interesting, many swimmers alternate swimming strokes every other lap. This also results in the use of some different muscles while utilizing in different ways those muscles which are common to several strokes.

The major advantage of swimming is that participants do not experience the physical trauma to muscles and joints that is associated with weight-bearing activities. It is particularly good for people who are prone to injury, have varicose veins, are obese or asthmatic, or who are rehabilitating an injury.

The disadvantages of swimming for fitness are that a pool must be available and one must know how to swim. According to the PCPFS panel, swimming contributes to all of the components of fitness, but least to muscular strength.

Water aerobics is an activity that is gaining in popularity (see Fig. 12.6). It is not swimming, but features various movements and exercises performed against the resistance of the water. Exercises performed in this manner may produce a better aerobic workout than swimming laps and it certainly reduces the orthopedic demands of exercise because of the buoyancy of the body in water. Water offers resistance to movement which is universal and three dimensional. Regardless of the angle of movement, water will resist it. This is impossible to duplicate with land based exercise. Theoretically, every voluntary muscle can be exercised in the water.

Walking is a natural form of locomotion that may be a lead-in to more vigorous exercise or it can be the means to develop and maintain physical fitness. The many forms of walking may be placed along a continuum from regular or natural gaited walking on one end to race walking on the other. Some of the different types of walking that appear somewhere between the two extremes of the continuum are pace, power, aerobic, fitness, health, rhythmic, and walking with weights. Actually some of these different forms of walking are really not so different from each other. The type of walking which is selected depends on several factors, one of which should include the major objective for participation.

FIGURE 12.6

Water Aerobics

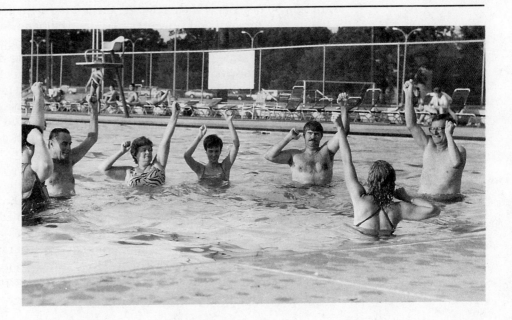

Natural gaited walking is an excellent exercise for those who are deconditioned, overweight, elderly, have medical limitations, or for any one whose sole objective is to exercise for health enhancement. When participants are able to walk three miles in 45 minutes without undue fatigue, they are ready for more vigorous exercise if they so choose. Walking with weights, race walking, and other forms of speed walking are excellent forms of activity for those who wish to attain a higher level of physical fitness than can be achieved with natural gaited walking.

Walking with weights as a physical conditioner has been examined by a number of investigators.[14,15,16] Light hand-held weights increase the energy expenditure of walking if the arms are swung vigorously. Hand-held weights that are carried passively (without vigorous arm swinging) do not appreciably increase the energy expenditure above that of walking without weights. Carrying weights in a backpack or vest is not quite as good as swinging hand-held weights because weights carried in this manner are not actively involved in loading the muscles. Vigorous swinging of the arms with or without hand-held weights seems to be the stimulus which increases the energy demand. As you recall, the more muscles that are vigorously involved in exercise the greater the oxygen demand. Ankle weights increase the energy expenditure of walking but less than hand-held weights for the same speed.[17] Walking on hilly terrain increases the energy cost to a level comparable to that of carrying hand-held weights.[16] In a two-phased study, fast walking without weights elevated heart rates to the exercise training zone.[18] Phase one involved untrained middle-aged men and women who walked at an intensity level which was sufficient to raise the heart rate into the target zone. Phase two, involved ten highly trained men who were instructed to achieve and maintain their target heart rate during a 30-minute walk. These subjects were able to reach and maintain the target heart rate for an average of 25 minutes which indicated that even highly fit individuals can reach their target and receive a training effect from fast walking.

Fast walking can be very enjoyable and challenging when a few basics are mastered. It is a heel-toe activity which is aided by rapidly pumping arms that are bent 90 degrees at the elbow. As the left leg steps forward, the right arm is swung in a forward and upward direction. The hand, which is loosely closed, should reach ear-height and then it is vigorously returned to the starting position following the same plane. As the right arm is coming down the right leg and left arm are moving forward. These repeated contralateral, well coordinated movements, result in a rapid turnover of the limbs and increases walking speed. The hands should not go above the height of the ear because this will slow arm turnover and consequently leg speed. The arms should not be pumped across the body because this creates rotational motion which detracts from horizontal momentum.

Adding weights while walking burns extra calories but it adds some risk as well. Isometric gripping of hand-held weights causes the systolic blood pressure to rise. Vigorous swinging of the arms stresses the shoulder and elbow joints and may cause damage in those who are unaccustomed to such forces. Ankle weights may change the foot strike enough to lead to groin injuries. Weights may also contribute to muscle soreness and may discourage some deconditioned people from continuing the program. These problems may be circumvented by starting slowly, increasing speed, and adding weights progressively over a pe-

Getting the most out of walking requires some attention to technique, a few reasonable goals, and a little self-assurance that walking for fitness is not only fun but can also be your ticket to a lifetime of good health.
—The Walking Magazine

FIGURE 12.7

Fitness Walking

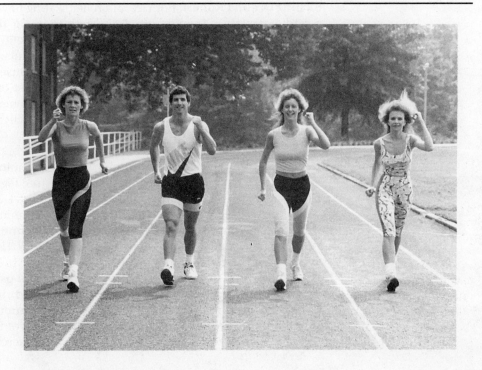

riod of time. Hand-held weights should not be tightly squeezed and the use of ankle weights should be discouraged.

Walking is a practical and convenient form of exercise which can be undertaken almost anywhere and at any time (see Fig. 12.7). The physical trauma to the lower half of the body is less than that of running and most of the court games. The impact is only one-third to one-half that of running. The force occurs more centrally on the heel when walking whereas the load is accepted on the outside border when running. Does this mean that a special shoe is needed for walking?[19] The experts are not in complete agreement on this topic. Those who do not support the notion that a special shoe is needed point to the fact that walking is our natural form of locomotion and that the foot is well constructed for it. The rebuttal is that the foot did not evolve to walk on hard streets and sidewalks. This author suggests that it is probably wise to invest in a walking shoe for the protection it affords, if, walking is pursued as a form of regular exercise. It is best to be safe than sorry.

The features of a good walking shoe are similar to those of a good jogging shoe with one major difference. Walking shoes should be more flexible under the forefoot bending 45 to 55 degrees at this point. Jogging shoes usually bend approximately 30 degrees under the forefoot.[20] Stiff walking shoes can lead to lower leg soreness and injury. Other features to look for include a heel counter for stability, well cushioned heel for shock absorption, breathable uppers, and a well-fitting toe box.

The only disadvantage connected with the many forms of walking is that walking is not a total conditioner—but then few activities are. Walking should be supplemented with flexibility and strength development exercises.

Skating (Ice and Roller). Both ice and roller skating have the potential to provide a cardiorespiratory training effect. As with many of the other activities, these must be performed continuously for optimal benefit. Both of these activities were highly rated by the PCPFS panel and are particularly popular among young people. Skating may not appeal to older adults because of the fear of falling and injury. Compared to many other activities, the cost of equipment is relatively inexpensive. Skating contributes to all of the components of fitness, but a good stretching program should be maintained. These activities do not contribute to upper body strength.

Rebound Running. Rebound running employs a mini-trampoline with a bed large enough to accommodate jogging in place (see Fig. 12.8). The effectiveness of this mode of exercise has been investigated by several researchers. Katch and his associates studied the energy cost of rebound running in 12 healthy sedentary subjects who ranged in age from 19 to 56.[21] They found the intensity of rebound running to be equal to jogging a very slow 13 to 15 minute mile pace. The subjects were unable to raise their heart rates above 116 beats per minute. Cooper equates rebound running to a 12- to 13-minute mile pace.[22] Gettman concluded that it is difficult to raise the energy cost of rebound running because the mini-tramp does much of the work by catapulting the runner into the air.[23]

In a paper presented to the American College of Sports Medicine in 1983, Gerberich reported that ten women subjects who exercised by rebound running

FIGURE 12.8

Rebound Running

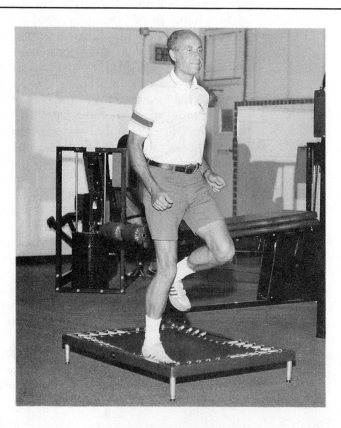

for 30 minutes per day for 12 weeks improved their maximal oxygen consumption by only 4.5 percent.[24] Atterbom found that a high stepping rate (120 steps per minute) increased the aerobic benefits of rebound running but only male subjects were able to sustain this rate.[25] The female subjects, who probably are the major users of rebound joggers, consistently fell behind the metronome and tended to "ride" the mini-tramp.

More study is needed but the early data indicate that these devices may have some merit for sedentary people. Higher levels of fitness can only be achieved through more vigorous activities. Rebound running may be a good way for sedentary people to develop the fitness needed to progress to jogging.

Currently under study is the combined effect of using hand-held weights while exercising on the mini-tramp. Male subjects, ages 15 to 43, jogged at a rate of 120-foot strikes per minute with a required foot lift 6 inches above the rim of the mini-tramp.[26] They jogged without weights and then while pumping one-, two-, and three-pound weights to heights of two and three feet. All combinations of weights and pumping heights, resulted in higher oxygen utilization and higher heart rates than rebounding without weights.

The price of mini-tramps has declined steadily during the last few years making it affordable to more people. They can be used indoors and out. These devices are minimally effective in training the aerobic system and they do not enhance strength or flexibility.

Stair Climbing. Interest in stair climbing as a fitness activity increased when the results of the Harvard Alumni study were made public. Stair climbing was one of several activities which contributed to longevity in this study.[27] Take the stairs instead of the elevator is good advice for anyone but it is particularly appropriate for those who are not interested in the normal "leisure-time exercise activities." Stair climbing combined with taking care of lawn and garden, and running errands on foot, and so forth, may contribute to longevity if participation in these activities is routine. Stair climbing becomes a physical fitness activity when the appropriate intensity, frequency, and duration are attained.

Rating Selected Sports

Sports are often categorized as either lifetime (individual and dual) or team. For adults, the emphasis on fitness development through sports in the past few years has centered upon the lifetime sports, such as racquetball (see Fig. 12.9), and tennis (see Fig. 12.10). Many team sports (soccer, basketball, speedball, ice and roller hockey) also have the potential for developing fitness, but the major impediment associated with these is the number of participants needed to play. People with similar interests and availability who are willing to participate in these activities are difficult to find. A second problem concerns the level of skill needed to achieve fitness and the satisfaction and reinforcement that comes from successful performance in these activities. A third problem is the difficulty of meeting the fitness criteria of intensity, frequency, and duration with team sports.

Lifetime sports are more amenable to fitness development than team sports because fewer players are needed. To reiterate, the philosophy expressed in this text is that fitness should be developed and maintained principally through the rhythmic and continuous activities of jogging, cycling, swimming, and so on,

FIGURE 12.9

Racquetball
One of the most popular
of the lifetime sports.

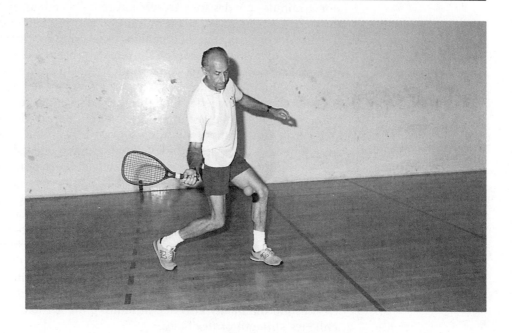

FIGURE 12.10

Tennis
This, like racquetball, is
another very popular
lifetime sport.

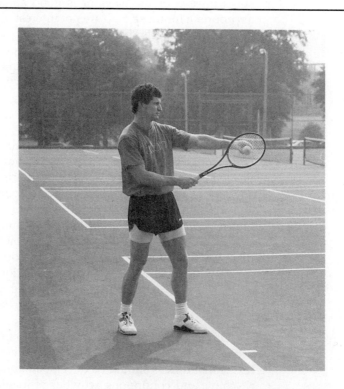

but variety may be important for sustaining the fitness program for many exercisers. Lifetime sports fit the bill very nicely by supplying a different challenge, fun, and variety. Bear in mind that optimal fitness from these activities is dependent upon the skill level of the participants and their willingness to play hard in singles competition. The tempo and pace of these activities is intermittent; that is, there are periods of activity, some of which may be very vigorous, interspersed with rest. Also consider that the orthopedic demands of these activities may be more than a sedentary beginner can tolerate. Quick stops and starts, bursts of high-intensity activity, sudden changes of direction, and rapid twists and turns place a great deal of stress upon the musculoskeletal system. Those who are physically fit are better equipped to handle the musculoskeletal and aerobic demands of active sports. Many sedentary ex-athletes attempt to "play themselves into shape" through sports. They elect this approach because they are competitive people who associate jogging and similar activities with the rigors of training for athletic competition. They also remember the ubiquitous slogan "no pain, no gain" as they were pushed by their coaches. Sports participation for fitness is particularly inappropriate for sedentary ex-athletes because their competitiveness will probably get them into trouble. They are not likely to give in during competitive play; extending themselves beyond their limits and risking injury. But after fitness has been attained with the rhythmic and continuous activities, participation in active sports once or twice a week is fine. Table 12.3 provides an estimate of the relative merit of some selected sports with regard to the components of physical fitness.

TABLE 12.3 Rating of Selected Sports*

| Sport | Cardiorespiratory Endurance | Muscular Strength and Endurance | | Flexibility | Body Composition |
		Upper Body	*Lower Body*		
Badminton	M–H	L	M–H	L	M–H
Basketball	H	L	H	M	H
Bowling	L	L–M	L	L	L
Football (touch)	L–M	L–M	M	L	L–M
Golf (no cart)	L	L	L–M	L	L–M
Handball	H	M	H	M	H
Ice hockey	H	M	H	L	H
Racquetball	H	M	H	M	H
Rugby	H	M–H	H	M	H
Soccer	H	L	H	M	H
Softball	L	L–M	L–M	L	L
Tennis	M	M	M	L–M	M
Volleyball	M	M	M	L–M	M
Wrestling	H	H	H	M–H	H

*H = High; M = Medium; L = Low. The values in this table are estimates that will vary according to the skill and motivation of the participants.

POINTS TO PONDER

1. *What are the health-related benefits associated with regular exercise?*
2. *What is the most commonly occurring injury to people who participate in aerobic dance?*
3. *What criteria would you use to select an aerobic dance class?*
4. *Compare cross-country skiing, cycling, rope skipping, swimming, and jogging on their contribution to cardiorespiratory endurance.*
5. *What are some of the characteristics of a good jogging shoe? What is the major difference between a jogging shoe and a walking shoe?*
6. *Describe some of the techniques that might be used to increase the aerobic demand of walking.*
7. *How would you rate rebound running as a means for developing cardiorespiratory endurance? How does it compare to stair climbing?*
8. *Describe the problems involved when people attempt to play themselves into shape by participating in sports activities.*

Rating Selected Exercise Equipment

The manufacture and sale of physical fitness equipment has become very big business. There are so many different pieces of equipment on the market that selecting the proper one can be a confusing experience. Consumers must guard against slick advertising and a smooth sales pitch that might lure them to select the wrong equipment for their needs.

Having equipment in the home makes exercising very convenient. Part of the problem of exercise compliance is the physical act of transporting oneself to a club or facility for exercise. Home equipment allows one to exercise in a comfortable and safe environment free of traffic hassles.

Equipment provides motivation for exercise. Unfortunately, the novelty wears off quite rapidly and unless one is sincere about achieving physical fitness, the equipment will end up in a closet or attic. It would be interesting to know how much unused fitness equipment is stored in homes throughout the United States—probably enough to restock the market. Many prospective exercisers purchase equipment with the idea that this is the stimulus that they need—the panacea they have been searching for—that will make exercise interesting, exciting, and keep them compliant. But if exercise equipment is to contribute to fitness it will require those three ingredients which many fitness seekers are attempting to avoid: time, effort, and patience. There is no machine that can develop fitness *for* you. The truth is that equipment is not necessary for physical fitness.

Exercise devices fall into one of two categories: active and passive. Active equipment is preferred because it requires the participant to supply the muscle and aerobic power to perform. Passive devices do the work for you and do not build fitness.

Active Devices

Rebound Joggers (Mini-Tramps). The merits of rebound jogging were discussed earlier in this chapter. These devices may suffice for introducing sedentary people to exercise, but they are ineffective in providing a workout for those who are fit. A high stepping rate of two steps per second is necessary to improve fitness, but this is unattainable for many people. Rebound joggers are poor devices for the attainment of fitness but their potential is enhanced when participants swing hand-held weights.

Rowing Machines. Rowing machines are excellent devices that exercise the arms, shoulders, back, legs, and the aerobic system. The seat slides backward as you pull on the oars and push with your legs and slides forward as you return the oars to the starting position. The oars on today's rowing machines are operated by gas cylinders whose resistance can be changed to conform to almost any level of fitness. A good, sturdy rower will last for many years and when not being used is small enough to store in a closet.

Ski Machines. Several models of indoor ski machines are available and each differs in the manner in which they stress the arms and legs. Basic models cost $60 to $400 and provide no feedback regarding the intensity of exercise. Deluxe models cost as much as $1000 and have built-in electronic monitors that display total minutes of exercise, miles per hour, and miles traveled.

Simulated cross-country skiing on these devices places less stress on the joints than impact exercises such as jogging, aerobic dancing, walking, and court games. Resistance can be adjusted for both arms and legs which make these excellent devices for the development of cardiorespiratory and muscular endurance. One of the best of these simulators, the Nordic Track, was used by 22 sedentary women (ages 20 to 40) for 20 to 40 minutes, four times per week for 19 weeks.[28] Their Max VO_2 improved by 12 percent which compares favorably with stationary cycling and rowing.

These machines simulate the action of cross-country skiing and develop the cardiorespiratory and muscular endurance specifically required for participation in this sport. These devices provide excellent off-season training for cross-country devotees. However, people who are not cross-country skiers will probably quickly tire of this form of exercise. The movements required will seem foreign to the nonskier and coordinating the movements will take some effort. Used correctly, many muscles are exercised simultaneously, the cardiorespiratory system is stressed, and many kcals are consumed in the process. Stretching exercises for upper and lower body are important.

Stair Climbing Devices. Manufacturers have developed stair climbing simulators (Figure 12.11) for the purpose of exercise for physical fitness. In one study, 15 women (ages 25 to 48) exercised on a stair treadmill ergometer at 75 percent of Max VO_2 for 30 minutes, three times per week for 12 weeks.[29] The women improved significantly in Max VO_2 and the amount of improvement was comparable to that of walking, jogging, and cycling.

These devices are quite expensive and can run as high as $7000. For this reason, they are usually found in health clubs and other exercise facilities.

People with arthritis or knee instabilities may not be able to use stair climbers. However, these devices are being used to rehabilitate some types of chronic low-back problems. Stair climbing should be supplemented with stretching and strength developing exercises.

FIGURE 12.11

A Stair Climbing Device

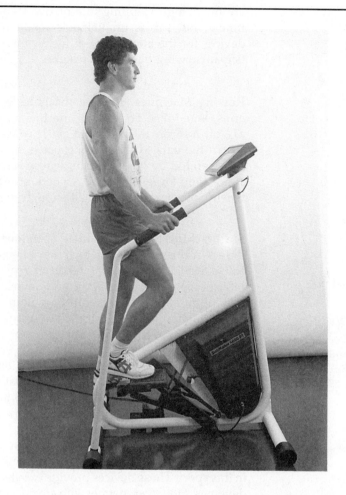

Stationary Bikes. A good stationary bike should weigh more than 50 pounds for sturdiness and durability, be equipped with a speedometer, odometer, and some means of adjusting pedaling, and have an adjustable seat which adapts to different leg length. Bicycle ergometers are more expensive than the department store variety of exercise bikes. Ergometers measure the amount of work and allow you to quantify improvement. Ergometers are relatively expensive, beginning at approximately $375. But fitness may be developed with a good quality department store stationary bike. Be sure that you test ride the bike and pay attention to the smoothness of the flywheel as it spins against varied resistance.

Treadmills. These are excellent devices for walking, jogging, sprinting or any combination of the three. The motor driven treadmills (see Fig. 12.12), are preferred over the nonmotorized type because the speed and incline can be set to elicit the target heart rate. A second advantage is that walking, jogging, and running can be performed in an upright posture with a normal gait. It is difficult to ambulate normally on nonmotorized treadmills because you must push backward against the belt to move it over the rollers. The required gait deviates

FIGURE 12.12

One of the Many Types
of Motorized Treadmills

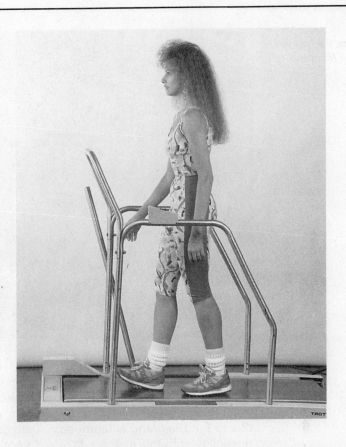

enough from a natural gait that consistent use of these types of treadmills is unusual. A good motorized treadmill for home use sells for approximately $2000 while the nonmotorized types sell for about $600.

Weight Machines. Weight machines are excellent for developing muscular strength and endurance, and, if the exercises are used as part of a "circuit" they may also contribute to improving aerobic capacity. Weight machines come in a variety of forms (see Fig. 12.13), from single-station devices costing about $400 to multistation complexes costing several thousand dollars. These machines are safe, convenient, and easy to use.

Free weights (dumbbells and barbells) are inexpensive. A good set of free weights totalling 175 to 200 pounds can be purchased for less than $100.

Passive Devices

Body Wraps. Some exclusive health clubs and salons feature body wrapping as a means of promoting weight loss. The body wrap gurus claim that a single treatment will result in a total loss of 4 to 12 inches. The procedure is quite involved. First the client is measured at given sites and then wrapped from neck to ankles with tapes soaked in a solution reputed to hasten the loss of weight. Then the individual puts on a rubberized suit that is tied tightly around the

FIGURE 12.13

**Bench Press Performed
on a Weight Machine**

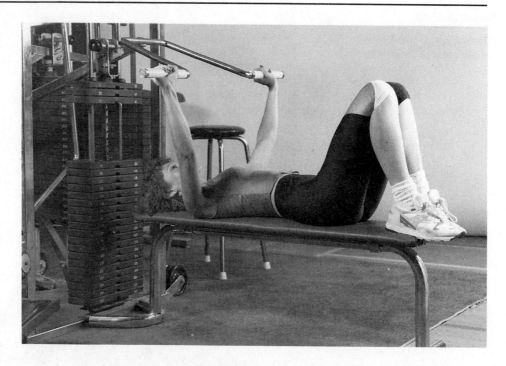

wrists, ankles and neck to keep heat from escaping. At this point the client sits in a lounge chair for an hour while covered with a blanket.

The weight loss and difference in pre- and posttreatment measurements is due to fluid loss and is temporary. Dehydration and heat illness are a distinct possibility with this method. Wraps do not promote permanent weight loss and are potentially hazardous.

Constricting Bands. Constricting bands are smaller versions of body wraps (see Fig. 12.14). These are placed around a specific body part, such as the waist, which is to be trimmed. The result is a reduction in girth, but as with the wraps, the loss is fluid and it is temporary. The Food and Drug Administration tested an early version of the constricting bands and found that they were not effective in promoting tissue loss but they did impede blood flowing from the legs to the heart. The downward pressure of blood on the leg veins stimulated the development of varicose veins. These devices are ineffective and hazardous.

Electric Bicycles. Electric bicycles are advertised as fitness development equipment (see Fig. 12.15). The typical electric bike features several types of rhythmic movements that occur simultaneously. The pedals rotate, the handlebars move back and forth, and the seat moves up and down. All of this motion is powered by an electrical current; the bike is plugged in to an electrical outlet and the power switch is turned on. The workout is minimal because the individual simply hangs on and goes with the flow. To receive a bona fide workout with this equipment, the rider should attempt to resist the motion of the pedals and handlebars. This usually proves to be much too inconvenient for practitioners, and as a result the electric cycle is ineffective in producing a training effect either aerobically or muscularly. The electric bicycle is an expensive piece of equipment.

FIGURE 12.14

Attempting to Spot Reduce with a Constricting Band

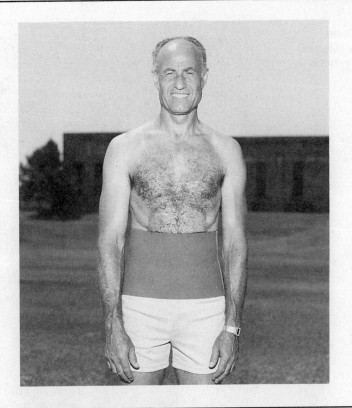

FIGURE 12.15

Electric Bicycle

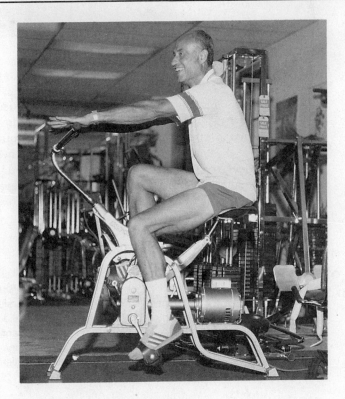

FIGURE 12.16

Inversion Boots
A more sophisticated
method for inverted
hanging.

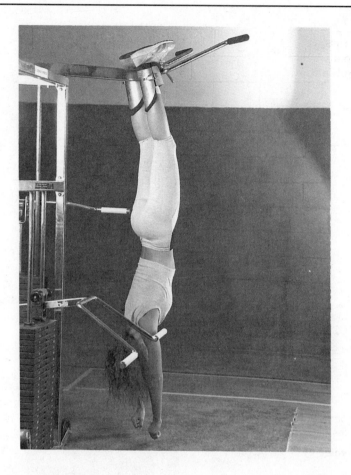

Inversion Boots. Inversion boots are strapped around the ankles and allow participants to hang upside down (see Fig. 12.16). They are reputed to stretch the spine, cure hemorrhoids, improve muscle tone, mental function and mood, and relieve stress. Promoters of these devices suggest hanging upside down two to three times per day for three to four minutes each.

Le Marr and his associates studied the effects of complete inversion on 50 healthy young subjects with normal blood pressures.[30] These researchers found that blood pressure was significantly elevated for the entire three minutes of inversion, and there was a significant decrease in heart rate, resulting in a variety of cardiac arrhythmias.

Hazards of Gravity Inversion Boots

Ronald Klatz (Chicago) writes in the Oct-83 issue of the Western Journal of Medicine on the hazards of hanging by your ankles. Studies at the Chicago College of Osteopathic Medicine indicated that gravity inversion therapy can be very hazardous for patients with glaucoma, hypertension, carotid narrowing, spinal instability, heart failure, persons on aspirin or other anticoagulant therapy, those over 55 and those with a family history of CVA. Why? The inversion therapy caused dangerous increases in blood pressure in normal individuals. Systolic retinal arterial pressure rose from

45 (resting) to 118 (during inversion). Intraoccular pressure rose from 18 to 33. These changes greatly increase the risk for the population groups mentioned above.

COMMENT: I always knew that "Inversion boots" were silly and expensive; now we know they are dangerous too!

Bassler, T. J. "Hazards of Gravity Inversion Boots" *AMJA Newsletter*, p7, 1984.

Some users of inversion boots perform sit-ups while in the inverted position. This does not appear to be a healthy practice because inversion increases the blood pressure and so does exercise. Doing both together is unwise. Also, sit-ups in the inverted position have damaged the peroneal nerve that runs down the outer portion of the lower legs, causing a loss of feeling in the feet. Inversion boots are potentially dangerous when used by hypertensives or by those who exercise in this position.

Massage. There is no known method to knead, beat, slap, or rub fat off the body. Massage is useless for weight loss, except for the masseur or masseuse, since he or she does all of the work. Massage is great for relaxation and it sometimes feels good to be pampered, but its role in weight loss or fitness is negligible.

Plastic and Rubberized Suits. Plastic and rubberized suits, and all other non-porous clothing, create a microenvironment between them and the skin which prevents the evaporation of sweat. When these garments are worn during exercise, they deprive the body of its most effective form of removing heat generated by exercise. These are worn for the purpose of accelerating weight loss, but of course the lost weight is fluid and will be replaced soon after exercise ends and fluids are consumed.

These garments promote a significant amount of sweating, which can lead to dehydration and heat illness. The risk increases when they are worn during exercise in hot weather, but they are potentially dangerous in any kind of weather. As the body heats up, the blood vessels near the skin dilate to accept more blood in an effort to cool the body. But the nonporous garments prevent the evaporation of sweat and cooling does not occur. The shunting of blood to the surface vessels reduces the supply going to the muscles, which, in turn, forces the heart to pump harder. Exercise continued under these conditions will lead to heat illness and possible death. These nonporous garments should never be used!

Passive motion machines will bend and twist and move your body but they do not work your muscles.
—Lawrence Lamb

Roller Machines. These devices can still be found in some health clubs and spas. The machines consist of a series of rollers that rotate over various body sites and are supposed to liquify the fat beneath for faster removal during exercise (see Fig. 12.17). Physiologically, fat does not liquify and spot reduction does not work. The individual does not burn many extra calories while being "rolled," so these machines contribute very little to weight loss. In addition, they may be hazardous for those who have varicose veins or other circulatory disorders. The best advice is to forget the roller machines.

FIGURE 12.17

Roller Machines

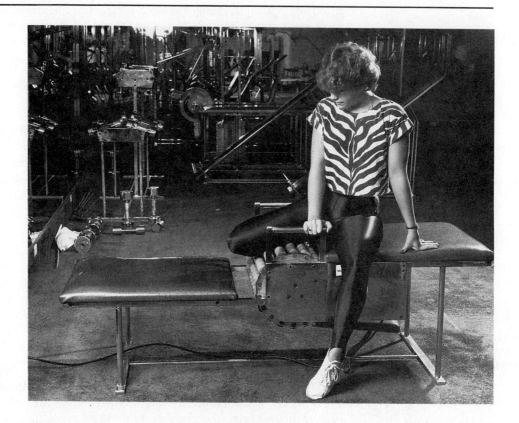

Steam Rooms, Saunas, and Hot Tubs. The temperature in steamrooms is kept between 110 and 130 degrees, and because of the nature of the heat source, the humidity is also extremely high. Sweating is accelerated, but under the high humidity, it cannot evaporate to cool the bather. A steam bath should never be taken immediately after exercise because the heat generated during the workout cannot be removed. The exerciser has lost body fluid during the workout and a steam bath immediately after will exacerbate the loss. This is a dangerous practice. Steam baths do not contribute to tissue loss and are not effective in promoting lasting weight loss.

The sauna features high temperatures but very low humidity. Sweat evaporates but the high heat and high sweat rate dictates that a sauna should not be used immediately following exercise. Many health benefits have been claimed for regular sauna use, including circulatory improvement, stress reduction, and the removal of poisons from the body. The sauna does speed subcutaneous circulation during and immediately afterward but there are probably no long-term effects. Those who are tense are often able to relax in the sauna but the long-term effects are unknown. The body does not cleanse or detoxify itself by sweating. In fact, sweating promotes the loss of such valuable life-supporting substances as sodium, potassium, vitamins, and fluid. The sauna and steam bath are not effective weight loss techniques.

The hot environments associated with steam and sauna bathing can result in dehydration and cardiovascular stress. "The shunting of massive amounts of blood to the skin can increase cardiac output by 50 to 75 percent with a 60 percent increase in pulse rate."[31] The healthy body can tolerate this stress for a short time, however, people with cardiovascular limitations would do well to avoid the risk.

Hot tubs have become popular in health clubs and in the home as deck accouterment. They are often used immediately after exercise in much the same way as people use the steam and sauna. The problems are similar plus it is difficult to maintain a bacteria-free environment particularly if it is heavily used as in a health club.

Steam, sauna, and hot tub use is beneficial as a treatment for sore and stiff muscles. These devices may also be of some benefit to arthritics, and they may help one to feel relaxed.

Vibrators. Vibrators consist of a wide belt attached to an electric motor. The belt is placed around a body part that is to be reduced and the motor is activated (see Fig. 12.18). Allegedly, the belt vibrates to shake fat from the body. These devices are a waste of money and do not contribute to weight loss. Using the vibrator for 15 minutes every day for a full year burns enough energy to lose one pound of fat.

FIGURE 12.18

Vibrating Belt

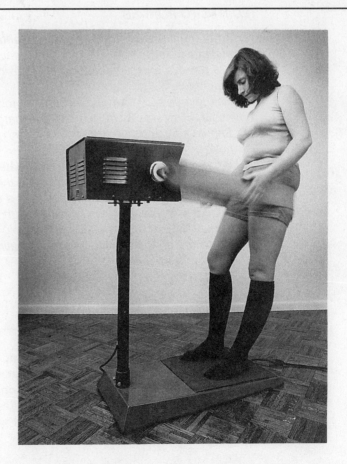

Some Advice on Equipment

Devices that require effort and allow the participant to apply the principles of fitness development are fine provided these principles are used. But the no-effort approaches to fitness and weight control are futile. Gadgets and gimmicks that promise fitness and weight loss effortlessly in just a few minutes a day are a sham. The ways of acquiring fitness and weight loss are well-known and well-documented: they require time, patience, and effort. Those who are willing to pursue this approach achieve their goals and often change their lifetime habits as well. Newly acquired energy, a feeling of well-being, an improved silhouette, and healthy changes in the risks associated with the chronic diseases are the rewards of an active life. If you are sedentary, get involved in exercise, but do it safely by following the guidelines in this text. When faced with a seemingly herculian task, the Chinese—those paragons of patience—are fond of saying that a journey of 1000 miles begins with one small step. The journey cannot be completed unless you are willing to take that first step. Afterwards, persistance and patience are necessary to complete the journey. This is the philosophy needed for a successful venture in becoming physically fit. It may seem to be a formidable task, but millions have achieved it one step at a time. If you are currently pursuing the active life, congratulations!

Perhaps this text will play a role in reinforcing your continued participation.

POINTS TO PONDER

1. *What are the advantages and disadvantages of relying upon exercise equipment for the development and maintenance of physical fitness?*
2. *Are passive exercises and passive devices effective in promoting fitness and weight loss?*
3. *Hanging upside down for a couple of minutes each day is good for one's health. How would you react to this statement?*
4. *Should sit-ups be performed when one is hanging upside down? Why or why not?*
5. *What are some of the hazards associated with wearing plastic and rubberized suits while exercising? Do these promote lasting weight loss?*
6. *What is the major difference between a steam and sauna bath?*
7. *Should one take a steam or sauna bath immediately after exercise? Why?*
8. *Should the hot tub be used immediately after exercise?*
9. *Comment on the effectiveness of vibrating belts and roller machines for promoting weight loss.*

Chapter Highlights

The results of exercise are short-lived and begin to wane 48 to 72 hours after the last workout. Exercise must be diligently pursued if it is to contribute to fitness and health. Consistent participation leads to an increase in energy level, modification of many of the risk factors associated with the chronic diseases, and promotes a feeling of buoyancy and well-being.

Rhythmic and continuous activities include aerobic dancing, cross-country skiing, cycling, jogging, rebound running, rope jumping, rowing, skating (ice and roller), swimming, and walking. Sports can also contribute to physical fitness.

Exercise equipment is categorized as being active or passive. Active equipment includes rebound joggers (mini-tramps), rowing machines, stationary bikes, treadmills, and weight machines. The passive devices include body wraps, constricting bands, electric bicycles, inversion boots, massage, plastic and rubberized suits, roller machines, steam and sauna baths, and vibrators. Most of the active devices have the potential to substantially improve fitness, but the passive devices are essentially a waste of time and money.

References

1. D. S. Siscovick et al., "The Incidence of Primary Cardiac Arrest During Vigorous Exercise," *New England Journal of Medicine*, 311, (1984): 874.

2. N. M. Kaplan, "Joggers May Live Longer," *The Journal of the American Medical Association*, 252, (1984): 528.

3. D. H. Richie et al., "Aerobic Dance Injuries: A Retrospective Study of Instructors and Participants," *The Physician and Sportsmedicine*, 13, (1985): 130.

4. J. G. Garrick et al., "The Epidemiology of Aerobic Dance Injuries," *American Journal of Sports Medicine*, 14, (1986): 67.

5. Y. Mutoh et al., "Aerobic Dance Injuries Among Instructors and Students," *The Physician and Sportsmedicine*, 16, (1988): 80.

6. "The Best All-Around Exercise" *University of California, Berkely Wellness Letter*, 5, (Dec. 1988): 6.

7. K. E. Powell et al., "An Epidemiological Perspective on the Causes of Running Injuries," *The Physician and Sportsmedicine*, 14, (1986): 100.

8. S. D. Walter et al., "Training Habits and Injury Experience in Distance Runners: Age- and Sex- Related Factors," *The Physician and Sportsmedicine*, 16, (1988): 101.

9. J. A. Baker, "Comparison of Rope Skipping and Jogging as Methods of Improving Cardiovascular Efficiency of College Men," *Research Quarterly*, 39, (1968): 240.

10. M. T. Buyze et al., "Comparative Training Responses to Rope Skipping and Jogging," *The Physician and Sportsmedicine*, 14, (1986): 65.

11. C. Foster et al., "World-Record Rope Skipping Performance," *The Physician and Sportsmedicine*, 8, (1980): 65.

12. American College of Sports Medicine, *Guidelines for Exercise Testing and Prescription*, Philadelphia: Lea and Febiger, 1986.

13. W. H. Martin III et al., "Cardiovascular Adaptations to Intense Swim Training in Sedentary Middle-Aged Men and Women," *Circulation*, 75, (1987): 323.

14. T. E. Auble et al., "Aerobic Requirements for Moving Handweights Through Various Ranges of Motion While Walking," *The Physician and Sportsmedicine*, 15, (1987): 133.

15. S. L. Makalous et al., "Energy Expenditure During Walking with Hand Weights," *The Physician and Sportsmedicine*, 16, (1988): 139.

16. V. DeBenedette, "Keeping Pace with the Many Forms of Walking," *The Physician and Sportsmedicine*, 16, (1988): 145.

17. J. F. Miller et al., "Intensity and Energy Cost of Weighted Walking vs. Running for Men and Women," *Journal of Applied Physiology*, 62, (1987): 1497.

18. J. Porcari et al., "Is Fast Walking an Adequate Aerobic Training Stimulus for 30- to 69-Year-Old Men and Women?" *The Physician and Sportsmedicine*, 15, (1987): 119.

19. L. Barnes, "Do Exercise Walkers Need Special Walking Shoes?" *The Physician and Sportsmedicine*, 15, (1987): 213.

20. E. H. DeSimone and W. A. Rossi, "Picking the Best of the New Crop," *The Walking Magazine*, (August/September, 1988): 56.

21. V. L. Katch et al., "Energy Cost of Rebound Running," *Research Quarterly in Exercise and Sport*, 52, (1981): 269.

22. K. H. Cooper, *The Aerobics Program for Total Well-Being*, New York: Bantam Books, 1982.

23. L. R. Gettman, "Aerobic Points for Stationary Cycling," *Aerobics Newsletter*, (May, 1981).

24. S. G. Gerberich et al., "Analysis of the Acute Effects of Rebound Exercise," *Medicine and Science in Sports and Exercise*, 16, (1984): 175 (Abstract).

25. H. A. Atterbom and T. A. MacLean, "Aerobic Benefits of Rebound Jogging," *Annals of Sports Medicine,* 1, (1983): 113.

26. J. F. Smith et al., "Exercise Intensity Increase by Addition of Handheld Weights to Rebounding Exercise," *American Journal of Sports Medicine,* (In review).

27. R. S. Paffenbarger et al., "Physical Activity, All-Cause Mortality and Longevity of College Alumni," *New England Journal of Medicine,* 31, (1986): 605.

28. D. J. Jacobsen et al., "The Effects of Simulated Cross-Country Skiing on Physical Fitness and Blood Lipid Levels," *Medicine and Science in Sports and Exercise,* 18, (1986): 510 (Abstract).

29. D. Verstraete et al., "Stairclimbing As a Training Modality for Women," *Medicine and Science in Sports and Exercise,* 18, (1986): 528 (Abstract).

30. J. D. LeMarr et al., "Cardiorespiratory Responses to Inversion," *The Physician and Sportsmedicine,* 11, (1983): 51.

31. B. Stamford, "Saunas, Steam Rooms, and Hot Tubs," *The Physician and Sportsmedicine,* 17, (1989): 188.

Appendix A
Fast-Food Nutrients

TABLE A-1 Main Meal Items in Calories, Fat, and Sodium

Breakfast Items	Calories	Fat (tsp)	Sodium (mg)
Grapefruit or orange juice, 6 oz.	80	0	2
English muffin w/butter (McDonald's)	186	1	310
Arby's butter croissant (Arby's)	220	2	225
Scrambled eggs (McDonald's)	180	3	205
Omelet w/mush., onion, green pepper (Wendy's)	210	3	200
Biscuit (Roy Rogers)	231	3	575
Breakfast Jack (Jack-Box)	307	3	871
Egg McMuffin (McDonald's)	340	4	885
Mushroom & swiss croissant (Arby's)	340	5	630
Crescent roll (Roy Rogers)	287	5	547
Omelet-ham, cheese & mushroom (Wendy's)	290	5	570
French toast, 2 slices (Wendy's)	400	4	850
Biscuit w/egg (Hardee's)	383	5	819
Bacon & egg croissant (Arby's)	420	6	550
Pancake platter w/ham (Roy Rogers)	506	4	1264
Breakfast crescent sandwich (Roy Rogers)	401	6	867
Sausage biscuit (Hardee's)	413	6	864
Sausage McMuffin (McDonald's)	427	6	942
Steak & egg biscuit (Hardee's)	527	7	973
Ham & egg biscuit (Hardee's)	458	6	1585
Sausage & egg croissant (Arby's)	530	10	745
Sausage McMuffin w/egg (McDonald's)	517	7	1044

Breakfast Items (Continued)	Calories	Fat (tsp)	Sodium (mg)
Biscuit with sausage (*McDonald's*)	467	7	1147
Sausage & egg biscuit (*Hardee's*)	521	8	1033
Pancake platter w/sausage (*Roy Rogers*)	608	7	1167
Biscuit w/bacon, egg, cheese (*McDonald's*)	483	7	1269
Egg & biscuit platter w/sausage (*Roy Rogers*)	550	9	1059
Sausage crescent (*Jack-Box*)	584	10	1012
Biscuit w/sausage and egg (*McDonald's*)	585	9	1301
Brkfst crescent sandwich w/ham (*Roy Rogers*)	557	9	1192
Scrambled eggs breakfast (*Jack-Box*)	720	10	1110

Chicken	Calories	Fat (tsp)	Sodium (mg)
Original Recipe drumstick (*Ky. Fd. Chkn.*)	117	1	207
Litely breaded chicken (*D'Lites*)	170	2	430
Original Recipe wing (*Ky. Fd. Chkn.*)	136	2	302
Fried chicken leg (*Church's*)	147	2	286
Chicken sandwich multi-grain bun (*Wendy's*)	320	2	500
Roasted chicken breast (*Arby's*)	254	2	930
Original Recipe breast (*Ky. Fd. Chkn.*)	199	3	558
Chicken filet sandwich (*D'Lites*)	280	3	760
Original Recipe thigh (*Ky. Fd. Chkn.*)	257	4	566
Chicken breast (*Roy Rogers*)	324	4	601
Fried breast (*Church's*)	278	4	560
Kentucky Nuggets (6) (*Ky. Fd. Chkn.*)	282	4	810
Chicken McNuggets (6) (*McDonald's*)	323	5	512
Fried wing (*Church's*)	303	4	583
Fried thigh (*Church's*)	305	5	448
Chicken filet sandwich (*Hardee's*)	510	6	360
Extra Crispy thigh (*Ky. Fd. Chkn.*)	343	5	549
Turkey club sandwich (*Hardee's*)	426	5	1185
Chicken breast filet sand. (*Ky. Fd. Chkn.*)	436	5	1093

Chicken (Continued)	Calories	Fat (tsp)	Sodium (mg)
Chicken breast & wing (*Roy Rogers*)	466	6	867
Chicken salad croissant (*Arby's*)	460	8	725
Chicken club sandwich (*Arby's*)	620	7	1300
Chicken Supreme (*Jack-Box*)	601	8	1582
Specialty chicken sandwich (*Burger King*)	690	10	775

Fish	Calories	Fat (tsp)	Sodium (mg)
Chilled shrimp, 1 piece (*L. J. Silver*)	6	0	19
Battered shrimp, 1 piece (*L. J. Silver*)	47	1	154
Baked fish w/sauce (*L. J. Silver*)	151	0	361
Catfish, one 3/4 ounce piece (*Church's*)	67	1	151
1/4-pound fish filet sandwich (*D'Lites*)	390	5	520
Fisherman's filet (*Hardee's*)	469	5	1013
Whaler sandwich (*Burger King*)	540	5	745
Moby Jack (*Jack-Box*)	444	6	820
Filet-o-Fish (*McDonald's*)	435	6	799
Whaler sandwich w/cheese (*Burger King*)	590	6	885

Meat Item	Calories	Fat (tsp)	Sodium (mg)
Burgers			
Jr. D'Lite (*D'Lites*)	200	2	210
Hamburger, kid's meal (*Wendy's*)	200	2	265
Hamburger (*McDonald's*)	263	3	506
Hamburger (*Burger King*)	310	3	560
Hamburger (*Hardee's*)	305	3	682
Happy Star hamburger (*Carl's Jr.*)	330	3	670
Hamburger, multi-grain bun (*Wendy's*)	340	4	290
Cheeseburger (*McDonald's*)	318	4	743
Cheeseburger (*Burger King*)	360	4	705
Bacon cheeseburger (*D'Lites*)	370	4	730
Whopper Jr. (*Burger King*)	370	4	545
Double D'Lite (*D'Lites*)	450	5	290
Cheeseburger (*Hardee's*)	335	4	789
Double hamburger (*Burger King*)	430	5	585

Meat Item (Continued)	Calories	Fat (tsp)	Sodium (mg)
Whopper Jr. w/cheese (*Burger King*)	410	5	685
Quarter-Pounder (*McDonald's*)	427	5	718
Hamburger (*Roy Rogers*)	456	6	495
Jumbo Jack (*Jack-Box*)	485	6	905
Mushroom 'n' Swiss burger (*Hardee's*)	512	5	1051
Big Deluxe (*Hardee's*)	546	6	1083
Bacon cheeseburger, white bun (*Wendy's*)	460	6	860
Quarter-Pounder w/cheese (*McDonald's*)	525	7	1220
Big Mac (*McDonald's*)	570	8	979
Bacon double-cheeseburger (*Burger King*)	600	8	985
Whopper (*Burger King*)	670	9	975
Cheeseburger (*Roy Rogers*)	463	8	1404
McD-L-T (*McDonald's*)	680	10	1030
RR-Bar Burger (*Roy Rogers*)	611	9	1826
Whopper w/cheese (*Burger King*)	760	10	1260
Bacon Cheeseburger Supreme (*Jack-Box*)	724	10	1307
Double-beef Whopper (*Burger King*)	890	12	1015
Double-beef Whopper w/cheese (*Burger King*)	980	14	1295
Triple cheeseburger (*Wendy's*)	1040	15	1848
Roast Beef Sandwiches			
Junior roast beef (*Arby's*)	220	2	530
Roast beef sandwich (*Roy Rogers*)	317	2	785
Regular roast beef (*Arby's*)	350	3	880
Roast beef sandwich (*Hardee's*)	377	4	1030
Roast beef sand w/cheese (*Roy Rogers*)	424	4	1694
Large roast beef w/cheese (*Roy Rogers*)	467	5	1953
Super roast beef (*Arby's*)	620	6	1420
Bac'n cheddar deluxe (*Arby's*)	561	8	1375
Ham Sandwiches			
Hot ham 'n cheese (*D'Lites*)	280	2	1160
Hot ham 'n cheese (*Hardee's*)	376	3	1067
Hot ham 'n cheese sandwich (*Arby's*)	353	3	1655
Ham biscuit (*Hardee's*)	349	4	1415
Specialty ham & cheese (*Burger King*)	550	7	1550

Miscellaneous (Continued)	Calories	Fat (tsp)	Sodium (mg)
Reduced cal. Italian dressing (1 Tbsp.) (*Wendy's*)	25	0	180
Cole slaw (*Ky. Fd. Chkn.*)	121	2	225
Thousand island dressing (1 Tbsp.) (*Wendy's*)	70	1	115
Pick-up window side salad (*Wendy's*)	110	1	540
12″ cheese pizza, 2 slices (*Domino's*)	340	1	660
Potato salad (*Roy Rogers*)	107	1	696
Regular taco (*Jack-Box*)	191	2	406
Club Pita (*Jack-Box*)	284	2	953
Chili, 8 oz. (*Wendy's*)	260	2	1070
Macaroni (*Roy Rogers*)	186	2	603
Vegetarian D'Lite (*D'Lites*)	270	3	610
Chef salad (*Hardee's*)	277	4	517
16″ pepperoni pizza, 2 slices (*Domino's*)	440	3	1080
Onion rings (*Burger King*)	270	4	450
Taco salad (*Wendy's*)	390	4	1100
Hot dog (*Hardee's*)	346	5	744
Veal parmigiana (*Burger King*)	580	6	805
Pasta seafood salad (*Jack-Box*)	394	5	1570
Shrimp salad (*Hardee's*)	362	7	941
Seafood salad (*L.J. Silver*)	471	7	993

Potatoes	Calories	Fat (tsp)	Sodium (mg)
Baked and others			
Baked potato (*several*)	215	0	10
Mashed potatoes (*Ky. Fd. Chkn.*)	64	0	268
Potato skins, per skin (*D'Lites*)	90	1	174
Potato w/margarine (*Roy Rogers*)	274	2	161
Mexiskins, per skin (*D'Lites*)	99	2	227
Hash brown potatoes (*McDonald's*)	125	2	325
Potato cakes (2) (*Arby's*)	201	3	476
Potato w/chicken a la king (*Wendy's*)	350	1	820
Hash rounds (*Hardee's*)	200	3	310
Potato w/broccoli & cheddar (*D'Lites*)	410	4	820
Potato w/chili & cheese (*Wendy's*)	510	5	610
Potato w/sour cream & chives (*Wendy's*)	460	5	230

Potatoes (Continued)	Calories	Fat (tsp)	Sodium (mg)
Mexican potato (*D'Lites*)	510	4	1000
Broccoli & cheddar potato (*Arby's*)	541	5	475
Mushroom & cheese potato (*Arby's*)	510	5	640
Potato w/taco beef & cheese (*Roy Rogers*)	463	5	726
Potato w/stroganoff & sour cream (*Wendy's*)	490	5	910
Home fries (*Wendy's*)	360	5	745
Taco potato (*Arby's*)	620	6	1060
Potato w/cheese (*Wendy's*)	590	8	450
Potato w/bacon & cheese (*Wendy's*)	570	7	1180
Deluxe potato (*Arby's*)	650	9	480
Fries			
Kentucky fries (*Ky. Fd. Chkn.*)	184	2	174
Fries, regular (*McDonald's*)	220	3	109
Fryes, bigger better (*L.J. Silver*)	247	3	6
French fries, regular (*D'Lites*)	260	3	100
French fries, small (*Hardee's*)	239	3	121
French fries, regular (*Burger King*)	210	3	230
French fries (*Arby's*)	211	2	39
French fries, regular (*Wendy's*)	280	3	95
French fries, large (*Hardee's*)	381	5	192

Adapted from: Center for Science in Public Interest, 1501 16th St., NW, Washington, DC. 20036. First Printing 1986.

TABLE A-2 Desserts and Dairy Products by Calories, Fat, Sodium, and Sugar

Desserts	Calories	Fat (tsp)	Sodium (mg)	Sugar (tsp)
Chocolate D'Lite (D'Lites)	203	1	70	5
Soft serve with cone (McDonald's)	185	1	109	4
Strawberry sundae (McDonald's)	320	2	90	9
Caramel sundae (McDonald's)	361	2	145	10
Lemon meringue pie (L. J. Silver)	200	1	254	5
Brownie (Roy Rogers)	264	3	150	5
McDonaldland cookies (McDonald's)	308	2	358	6
Hot fudge sundae (Roy Rogers)	337	3	186	9
Frosty dairy dessert, 12 oz. (Wendy's)	400	3	220	10
Apple turnover (Hardee's)	282	3	310	5
Big cookie (Hardee's)	278	3	258	5
Apple pie (Burger King)	330	3	385	4
Cherry pie (McDonald's)	260	3	427	4
Chocolaty chip cookies (McDonald's)	342	4	313	5
Danish (Wendy's)	360	4	340	2
Blueberry turnover (Arby's)	340	5	255	6
Strawberry shortcake (Roy Rogers)	447	4	674	7
Pecan pie (L. J. Silver)	446	5	435	10
Apple turnover (Jack-Box)	410	5	350	7

Shakes, Milk	Calories	Fat (tsp)	Sodium (mg)	Sugar (tsp)
Milk, 2.0% butterfat (McDonald's)	86	1	125	0
Whole milk (several)	150	2	125	0
Milk shake, average (Jack-Box)	323	2	147	9
Milk shake (Hardee's)	391	2	74	11
Milk shake, average (McDonald's)	367	2	236	10
Milk shake, average (Roy Rogers)	326	2	278	9
Milk shake, average (Arby's)	368	2	275	10
Milk shake, average (Burger King)	340	2	300	9

Adapted from: Center for Science in Public Interest, 150116th St., NW, Washington, DC. 20036. First Printing 1986.

Appendix B
Nutrients of Selected Foods

TABLE B-1 Selected Foods by kcal, Protein, Fat, and Carbohydrates

Food	Weight g	oz	Approximate Measure and Description	kcal	Protein g	Fat g	Carbohydrate g
Alcoholic beverages (located in Table B.2)							
Apples, raw	150	5.3	1 apple, about 3 per lb.	70	tr	tr	18
Apple, baked	130	4.6	1 medium apple, 2½ in. dia.	120	tr	tr	30
Apple brown betty	115	4.0	½ cup	175	2	4	34
Apple juice (sweet cider)	124	4.3	½ cup, bottled or canned	60	tr	tr	15
Apple pie (*see* pies)							
Applesauce, canned sweetened	128	4.5	½ cup	115	tr	tr	31
Apricots, fresh, raw (as purchased)	114	4.0	3 apricots, about 12 per lb.	55	1	tr	14
Apricots, canned	130	4.6	½ cup or 4 medium halves, 2 tbsp. juice (syrup pack)	110	1	tr	29
Apricots, dried, stewed	108	3.8	½ cup (scant) or 8 halves, 2 tbsp. juice, sweetened	135	2	tr	34
Apricot nectar (peach and pear nectar have similar values)	125	4.4	½ cup	70	1	tr	19
Asparagus, cooked, green	73	2.6	½ cup, 1½- to 2-in. lengths	15	2	tr	3
Avocado, raw (as purchased)	142	5.0	½ avocado, 3⅛ in. dia., pitted and peeled	185	3	19	7
Bacon, broiled or fried	15	0.5	2 slices, cooked crisp (20 slices per lb., raw)	90	5	8	1
Bacon, Canadian, cooked	43	1.5	3 slices, cooked crisp	100	18	12	tr
Bananas, raw (as purchased)	175	6.1	1 medium banana	100	1	tr	26
Bavarian cream, orange	99	3.5	½ cup	210	2	10	30
Bean sprouts, mung, cooked	63	2.2	½ cup, drained	18	2	tr	4
Beans, green snap, cooked	63	2.2	½ cup	15	1	tr	4
Beans, dry, green lima, cooked	144	5.0	¾ cup	195	12	1	37
Beans, immature, green lima, cooked	85	2.8	½ cup	95	7	1	17
Beans, dry, red kidney, canned	191	6.7	¾ cup	173	11	1	32
Beans, dry, white, canned with tomato sauce, without pork	196	6.9	¾ cup	233	12	1	45
Beans, dry, white, canned with tomato sauce and pork	191	6.7	¾ cup	233	12	5	37
Beef, corned, canned	85	3.0	3 slices, 3 × 2 × ¼ in.	185	22	10	0
Beef, corned hash, canned	85	3.0	½ cup (approx.)	155	7	10	9
Beef, dried or chipped	57	2.0	4 thin slices, 4 × 5 in.	115	19	4	0
Beef, hamburger, broiled	85	3.0	1 patty, 3 in. dia. (regular ground beef)	245	21	17	0

Food	Weight g	Weight oz	Approximate Measure and Description	kcal	Protein g	Fat g	Carbohydrate g
Beef, heart, braised	85	3.0	2 round slices, $2\frac{1}{2}$ in. dia., $\frac{1}{2}$ in. thick	160	27	5	1
Beef liver (*see* liver)							
Beef loaf (*see* meat loaf)							
Beef potpie, baked	227	7.9	1 pie, $4\frac{1}{4}$ in. dia.	560	23	33	43
Beef, pot roast, cooked	85	3.0	1 piece, $4 \times 3\frac{3}{4} \times \frac{1}{2}$ in.	245	23	16	0
Beef roast, oven-cooked	85	3.0	2 slices, $6 \times 3\frac{1}{4} \times \frac{1}{8}$ in., relatively lean	165	25	7	0
Beef steak, broiled	85	3.0	1 piece, $3\frac{1}{2} \times 2 \times \frac{3}{4}$ in., relatively fat, no bone	330	20	27	0
Beef stroganoff, cooked	130	4.6	$\frac{1}{2}$ cup	250	17	18	6
Beef tongue, braised	85	3.0	7 slices, $2\frac{1}{4} \times 2\frac{1}{4} \times \frac{1}{8}$ in.	210	18	14	tr
Beets, cooked	85	3.0	$\frac{1}{2}$ cup, diced	28	1	tr	6
Beverages, alcoholic (*see* p. 316)							
Beverages, cola-type	185	6.5	about $\frac{3}{4}$ cup	75	0	0	19
Beverages, ginger ale	240	8.4	1 cup	75	0	0	19
Biscuits, baking powder	28	1.0	1 biscuit, 2 in. dia. (enriched flour)	105	2	5	13
Blackberries, raw	72	2.5	$\frac{1}{2}$ cup	45	1	1	10
Blueberries, raw	70	2.5	$\frac{1}{2}$ cup	45	1	1	11
Bluefish, cooked	85	3.0	1 piece, $3\frac{1}{2} \times 2 \times \frac{1}{2}$ in.	135	22	4	0
Bologna (*see* sausage)							
Bouillon cubes	4	0.1	1 cube, $\frac{5}{8}$ in.	5	1	tr	tr
Bran flakes	26	0.9	$\frac{3}{4}$ cup, 40% bran, (thiamin and iron added)	80	3	1	21
Bread, Boston brown	48	1.7	1 slice, $3 \times \frac{3}{4}$ in.	100	3	1	22
Bread, cracked wheat	25	0.9	1 slice, 18 slices per lb. loaf	65	2	1	13
Bread, French or Vienna	20	0.7	1 slice, $3\frac{1}{4} \times 2 \times 1$ in. (enriched flour)	60	2	1	11
Bread, Italian	20	0.7	1 slice, $3\frac{1}{4} \times 2 \times 1$ in. (enriched flour)	55	2	tr	11
Bread, light rye	25	0.9	1 slice, 18 slices per lb. loaf ($\frac{1}{3}$ rye, $\frac{2}{3}$ wheat)	60	2	tr	13
Bread, pumpernickel	34	1.2	1 slice, $3\frac{1}{4} \times 2 \times 1$ in. (dark rye flour)	85	3	0	19
Bread, raisin	25	0.9	1 slice, 18 slices per lb. loaf	65	2	1	13
Bread, white firm crumb (enriched)	23	0.8	1 slice, 20 slices per lb. loaf	65	2	1	12
Bread, white soft crumb (enriched)	25	0.9	1 slice, 18 slices per lb. loaf	70	2	1	13
Bread, white soft crumb (enriched), toasted	22	0.8	1 slice, 18 slices per lb. loaf	70	2	1	13
Bread, white soft crumb (unenriched)	25	0.9	1 slice, 18 slices per lb. loaf	70	2	1	13
Bread, whole wheat firm crumb	25	0.9	1 slice, 18 slices per lb. loaf	60	3	1	12
Bread crumbs	25	0.9	$\frac{1}{4}$ cup, dry grated	98	3	1	18
Broccoli, cooked	78	2.7	$\frac{1}{2}$ cup, stalks cut into $\frac{1}{2}$-in. pieces	20	3	1	4
Brussels sprouts, cooked	78	2.7	$\frac{1}{2}$ cup or 5 medium sprouts	28	4	1	5
Buns (*see* rolls)							
Butter	14	0.5	1 tbsp or $\frac{1}{8}$ stick	100	tr	12	tr
Cabbage, cooked	73	2.6	$\frac{1}{2}$ cup, cooked short time in little water	15	1	tr	3
Cabbage, raw	45	1.6	$\frac{1}{2}$ cup, finely shredded	10	1	tr	3
Cabbage, raw, Chinese	38	1.3	$\frac{1}{2}$ cup, 1-in. pieces	5	1	tr	1
Cake, angel food (from mix)	53	1.9	1 piece, $\frac{1}{12}$ of 10-in.-dia. cake	135	3	tr	32
Cake, Boston cream pie	69	2.4	1 piece, $\frac{1}{12}$ of 8-in.-dia. pie (unenriched flour)	210	4	6	34

Food	Weight g	Weight oz	Approximate Measure and Description	kcal	Protein g	Fat g	Carbohydrate g
Cake, plain chocolate-iced cupcake (from mix)	36	1.3	1 cupcake, $2\frac{1}{2}$ in. dia.	130	2	5	21
Cake, plain uniced cupcakes (from mix)	25	0.9	1 cupcake, $2\frac{1}{2}$ in. dia.	90	1	3	14
Cake, 2-layer devil's food with chocolate icing (from mix)	69	2.4	1 piece (mix), $\frac{1}{16}$ of 9-in.-dia. cake	235	3	9	40
Cake, fruit, dark	15	0.5	1 slice, $\frac{1}{30}$ of 8-in.-long loaf (enriched flour)	55	1	2	9
Cake, pound	30	1.1	1 slice, $2\frac{3}{4} \times 3 \times \frac{5}{8}$ in. (unenriched flour)	140	2	9	14
Cake, sponge	66	1.4	1 piece, $\frac{1}{12}$ of 10-in.-dia. cake (unenriched)	195	5	4	36
Cake, 2-layer white with chocolate icing	71	2.5	1 piece, $\frac{1}{16}$ of 9-in.-dia. cake	250	3	8	45
Candy, caramels	28	1.0	4 small	115	1	3	22
Candy, plain chocolate	28	1.0	1 bar, $3\frac{3}{4} \times 1\frac{1}{2} \times \frac{1}{4}$ in.	145	2	9	16
Candy, chocolate with almonds	51	1.8	1 bar, $5\frac{1}{3} \times 1\frac{7}{8} \times \frac{1}{3}$ in.	265	4	19	25
Candy, chocolate creams	28	1.0	2 pieces, $1\frac{1}{4}$ in. dia. (base), $\frac{5}{8}$ in. thick	110	1	4	20
Candy, chocolate fudge	28	1.0	1 piece, $1\frac{1}{4} \times 1\frac{1}{4} \times 1$ in.	115	1	4	21
Candy, hard	28	1.0	6 pieces, 1 in. dia., $\frac{1}{4}$ in. thick	110	0	tr	28
Candy, peanut brittle	28	1.0	1 piece, $3\frac{1}{4} \times 2\frac{1}{2} \times \frac{1}{4}$ in.	125	2	4	21
Cantaloupes	385	13.5	$\frac{1}{2}$ melon, 5 in. dia.	60	1	tr	14
Carrots, raw grated	55	1.9	$\frac{1}{2}$ cup grated	23	1	tr	6
Carrots, raw whole or strips	50	1.8	1 carrot, $5\frac{1}{2}$ in. long, or 25 thin strips	20	1	tr	5
Carrots, cooked	73	2.6	$\frac{1}{2}$ cup diced	23	1	tr	5
Catsup, tomato (*see* tomato)							
Cauliflower, cooked	60	2.1	$\frac{1}{2}$ cup flowerets	13	2	tr	3
Celery, raw diced	50	1.8	$\frac{1}{2}$ cup	8	1	tr	2
Celery, raw whole	40	1.4	1 stalk, large outer, 8 in. long	5	tr	tr	2
Cheese, blue (Roquefort type)	28	1.0	$\frac{3}{4}$-in. sector or 3 tbsp	105	6	9	1
Cheese, cheddar (American), cubed	28	1.0	1 cube, $1\frac{1}{8}$ in.	115	6	10	2
Cheese, cheddar (American), grated	7	0.3	1 tbsp	30	2	2	tr
Cheese, creamed cottage	61	2.1	$\frac{1}{4}$ cup (made from skim milk)	65	8	3	2
Cheese, uncreamed cottage	28	1.0	2 tbsp (made from skim milk)	25	5	tr	1
Cheese, cream	16	0.5	1 tbsp	60	1	6	tr
Cheese, Swiss (domestic)	28	1.0	1 slice, $7 \times 4 \times \frac{1}{8}$ in.	105	8	8	1
Cheese foods, cheddar	28	1.0	2 round slices, $1\frac{5}{8}$ in. dia., $\frac{1}{4}$ in. thick or 2 tbsp	90	6	6	2
Cheese sauce	60	2.1	$\frac{1}{4}$ cup	110	5	9	4
Cheese soufflé	79	2.8	$\frac{3}{4}$ cup	200	10	16	7
Cheesecake	162	5.7	$\frac{1}{10}$ of 9-in.-dia. cake	400	15	23	35
Cherries, raw sweet	130	4.6	1 cup with stems	80	2	tr	20
Cherries, raw West Indian (acerola)	11	0.4	2 medium cherries	3	—	—	1
Chick peas, dry raw (garbanzos)	105	3.7	$\frac{1}{2}$ cup	380	22	5	64
Chicken, broiled	85	3.0	3 slices, flesh only	115	20	2	0
Chicken, canned	85	3.0	$\frac{1}{3}$ cup boned meat	170	18	10	0
Chicken, creamed	99	3.5	$\frac{1}{2}$ cup	222	20	12	6
Chicken breast, fried	94	3.3	$\frac{1}{2}$ breast with bone	155	25	5	1
Chicken drumstick, fried	59	2.1	1 drumstick with bone	90	12	4	tr
Chicken pie (*see* poultry potpie)							
Chili con carne with beans, canned	188	6.5	$\frac{3}{4}$ cup	250	14	11	23
Chili con carne without beans, canned	191	6.7	$\frac{3}{4}$ cup	383	20	29	11
Chili powder	15	0.5	1 tbsp hot red peppers, dried and ground	50	2	2	8

Food	Weight g	Weight oz	Approximate Measure and Description	kcal	Protein g	Fat g	Carbohydrate g
Chili sauce	17	0.6	1 tbsp, mainly tomatoes	20	tr	tr	4
Chocolate, bitter (baking chocolate)	28	1.0	1 square	145	3	15	8
Chocolate candy (*see* candy)							
Chocolate-flavored milk drink	250	8.8	1 cup (made with skim milk)	190	8	6	27
Chocolate morsels	15	0.5	30 morsels or $1\frac{1}{2}$ tbsp	80	1	4	10
Chocolate syrup	40	1.4	2 tbsp	80	tr	tr	22
Chop suey, cooked	122	4.3	$\frac{3}{4}$ cup	325	19	20	16
Clams, canned	85	3.0	$\frac{1}{2}$ cup or 3 medium clams	45	7	1	2
Cocoa, beverage	182	6.3	$\frac{3}{4}$ cup (made with milk)	176	7	8	20
Coconut, dried shredded, sweetened	16	0.6	$\frac{1}{4}$ cup	85	1	6	8
Coconut, fresh shredded	33	1.2	$\frac{1}{4}$ cup	113	1	12	3
Codfish, dried	51	1.8	$\frac{1}{2}$ cup	190	41	2	0
Coffee cake, frosted	79	2.8	1 piece, 3 × 3 × $1\frac{1}{4}$ in.	260	4	11	37
Cole slaw	60	2.1	$\frac{1}{2}$ cup	50	1	4	5
Cookies, brownies	26	0.9	1 piece, $1\frac{7}{8}$ × $1\frac{7}{8}$ × $\frac{5}{8}$ in.	145	2	9	17
Cookies, chocolate chip	11	0.4	1 cookie, $2\frac{1}{4}$ in. dia.	60	1	3	7
Cookies, coconut bar chews	11	0.4	1 cookie, 3 × $\frac{7}{8}$ × $\frac{1}{3}$ in.	55	tr	2	9
Cookies, oatmeal with raisins and nuts	11	0.4	1 cookie, $2\frac{1}{8}$ in. dia.	65	1	4	6
Cookies, sugar, plain	9	0.3	1 cookie, $2\frac{1}{2}$ in. dia.	40	1	2	6
Corn, sweet, cooked	140	4.9	1 ear, 5 in. long	70	3	1	16
Corn, sweet, canned	128	4.5	$\frac{1}{2}$ cup, solids and liquid	85	3	1	20
Corn grits, cooked	163	5.7	$\frac{2}{3}$ cup, enriched and degermed	85	2	tr	18
Corn muffins	40	1.4	1 muffin, $2\frac{3}{8}$ in. dia., enriched flour and enriched degermed meal	125	3	4	19
Corned beef (*see* beef)							
Corned beef hash (*see* beef)							
Cornflakes	33	1.2	$1\frac{1}{3}$ cup (added nutrients)	133	3	tr	28
Cornmeal, dry	138	4.8	1 cup, white or yellow, enriched and degermed	500	11	2	108
Cow peas (*see* peas)							
Crabmeat, canned	85	3.0	$\frac{1}{2}$ cup flakes	85	15	2	1
Crackers, graham, plain	14	0.6	2 medium or 4 small	55	1	1	10
Crackers, saltines	8	0.3	2 crackers, 2 in. square	35	1	1	6
Cranberry juice, canned	125	4.4	$\frac{1}{2}$ cup or 1 small glass, ascorbic acid added	85	tr	tr	21
Cranberry sauce, canned	69	2.4	$\frac{1}{4}$ cup, strained and sweetened	85	tr	tr	21
Cream, coffee (light cream)	15	0.5	1 tbsp	30	1	3	1
Cream, half-and-half	15	0.5	1 tbsp	20	1	2	1
Cream, heavy, whipping	15	0.5	1 tbsp, unwhipped (volume doubled when whipped)	55	tr	6	1
Creamer, coffee (imitation cream)	2	—	1 tsp powder	10	tr	1	1
Cucumber, raw	50	1.8	6 slices, pared, $\frac{1}{8}$ in. thick	5	tr	tr	2
Custard, baked	124	4.3	$\frac{1}{2}$ cup	143	7	7	14
Dates, pitted	45	1.6	$\frac{1}{4}$ cup or 8 dates	123	1	tr	33
Dessert topping, whipped	11	0.4	2 tbsp (low-calorie, with nonfat dry milk)	17	1	—	3
Doughnuts, cake-type	32	1.1	1 (enriched flour)	125	1	6	16
Egg, raw, boiled, or poached	50	1.8	1 whole egg	80	6	6	tr
Egg white, raw	33	1.2	1 egg white	15	4	tr	tr
Egg yolk, raw	17	0.6	1 egg yolk	60	3	5	tr
Eggs, creamed	113	4.0	$\frac{1}{2}$ cup (1 egg in $\frac{1}{4}$ cup white sauce)	190	9	14	7
Eggs, fried	54	1.9	1 egg, cooked in 1 tsp fat	115	6	10	tr
Eggs, scrambled	64	2.2	1 egg, with milk and fat	110	7	8	1

Food	Weight g	Weight oz	Approximate Measure and Description	kcal	Protein g	Fat g	Carbohydrate g
Endive, curly, raw	57	2.0	3 leaves (includes escarole)	10	1	tr	2
Farina, cooked	163	5.7	⅔ cup (quick, enriched)	70	2	tr	14
Fats, cooking, lard	13	0.5	1 tbsp solid fat	115	0	13	0
Fats, cooking, vegetable	13	0.5	1 tbsp solid fat	110	0	13	0
Figs, dried	21	0.7	1 large fig, 1 × 2 in.	60	1	tr	15
Figs, fresh raw	114	4.0	3 small, 1½ in. dia.	90	1	tr	23
Fish (*see* various kinds of fish)							
Fish, creamed (tuna, salmon, or other, in white sauce)	136	4.8	½ cup	220	20	13	8
Fish sticks, breaded, cooked	114	4.0	5 sticks, each 3.8 × 1.0 × 0.5 in.	200	19	10	8
Frankfurter, heated	56	2.0	1 frankfurter	170	7	15	1
French toast, fried	79	2.8	1 slice (enriched bread)	180	6	12	14
Fruit balls, raw (dried apricots, dates, nuts)	11	0.4	1 ball, 1 in. dia.	45	1	1	8
Fruit cocktail, canned	128	4.5	½ cup, with heavy syrup	98	1	tr	25
Gelatin, plain, dry	7	0.3	1 tbsp (1 envelope)	25	6	tr	0
Gelatin dessert, plain	120	4.2	½ cup, ready to eat	70	2	0	17
Gingerbread	63	2.2	1 piece (mix), ⅑ of 8-in.-square cake	175	2	4	32
Grapefruit, white, raw (as purchased)	241	8.4	½ medium, 3¾ in. dia.	45	1	tr	12
Grapefruit, white, canned	125	4.4	½ cup, syrup pack	88	1	tr	22
Grapefruit juice, canned	124	4.3	½ cup, unsweetened	50	1	tr	12
Grapefruit juice, dehydrated crystals	124	4.3	½ cup or 1 small glass, prepared, ready to serve	50	1	tr	12
Grapes, raw American-type	153	5.4	1 cup or 1 medium bunch (slip skin, as Concord)	65	1	1	15
Grapes, raw European-type	160	5.6	1 cup or 40 grapes (adherent skin, as Tokay)	95	1	tr	25
Grape juice, canned	127	4.4	½ cup	83	1	tr	21
Greens, collards, cooked	95	3.3	½ cup	28	3	1	5
Greens, dandelion, cooked	90	3.2	½ cup	30	2	1	6
Greens, kale, cooked	55	1.9	½ cup, leaves and stems	15	2	1	2
Greens, mustard, cooked	70	2.5	½ cup	18	2	1	3
Greens, spinach, cooked	90	3.2	½ cup	20	3	1	3
Greens, turnip, cooked	73	2.6	½ cup	15	2	tr	3
Guavas, raw	82	2.8	1 guava	50	1	tr	12
Haddock, fried	85	3.0	1 fillet, 4 × 2½ × ½ in.	140	17	5	5
Ham, boiled	57	2.0	1 slice, 6¼ × 3¾ × ⅛ in.	135	11	10	0
Ham, cured, roasted	85	3.0	2 slices, 5½ × 3¾ × ⅛ in.	245	18	19	0
Ham, luncheon, canned	57	2.0	2 tbsp, spiced or unspiced	165	8	14	1
Hamburger (*see* beef, hamburger)							
Honey, strained	21	0.7	1 tbsp	65	tr	0	17
Hot dog (*see* frankfurter)							
Ice cream, plain	50	1.8	1 container, 3 fluid oz (factory packed)	95	2	5	10
Ice cream, plain brick	71	2.5	1 slice, ⅛ of qt brick	145	3	9	15
Ice milk	66	2.3	½ cup	100	3	4	15
Jams, jellies, preserves	20	0.7	1 tbsp	55	tr	tr	14
Kale (*see* greens)							

Food	Weight		Approximate Measure and Description	kcal	Protein g	Fat g	Carbohydrate g
	g	oz					
Lamb chop, cooked	137	4.8	1 thick chop with bone	400	25	33	0
Lamb, leg, roasted	85	3.0	2 slices, 3 × 3¼ × ⅛ in., lean and fat, no bone	235	22	16	0
Lard (see fats, cooking)							
Lemon juice, fresh	15	0.5	1 tbsp	5	tr	tr	1
Lemonade	248	8.7	1 cup (made from frozen, sweetened concentrate)	110	tr	tr	28
Lentils, dry, cooked	100	3.5	½ cup	120	9	tr	22
Lettuce, headed, raw	454	16.0	1 head (compact, as iceberg), 4¾ in. dia.	60	4	tr	13
Lettuce, loose leaf, raw	50	1.8	2 large leaves or 4 small leaves	10	1	tr	2
Lime juice, canned	62	2.2	¼ cup	15	tr	tr	6
Liver, beef, fried	57	2.0	1 slice, 5 × 2 × ⅓ in.	130	15	6	3
Liver, calf, fried	74	2.6	1 slice, 5 × 2 × ½ in.	230	15	15	4
Liver, chicken, fried	85	3.0	3 medium livers	235	20	15	5
Liver, pork, fried	70	2.5	1 slice, 3¾ × 1¾ × ½ in.	225	17	15	3
Macaroni, cooked	105	3.7	¾ cup (enriched)	115	4	1	24
Macaroni and cheese, baked	150	5.3	¾ cup (enriched macaroni)	325	13	17	30
Mackerel, broiled	85	3.0	1 piece	200	19	13	0
Mangoes, raw	198	7.0	1 medium mango	90	1	—	23
Margarine	14	0.5	1 tbsp or ⅛ stick (fortified with vitamin A)	100	tr	12	tr
Marshmallows	9	0.3	1, 1¼ in. dia.	25	tr	0	8
Meat loaf, beef, baked	77	2.7	1 slice, 3¾ × 2¼ × ¾ in.	240	19	17	3
Milk, dry skim (nonfat)	17	0.6	¼ cup powder, instant	61	6	tr	9
Milk, dry whole	26	0.9	¼ cup powder	129	7	7	10
Milk, evaporated, canned	126	4.4	½ cup, undiluted and unsweetened	173	9	10	12
Milk, fluid, skim or buttermilk	245	8.6	1 cup (½ pt)	90	9	tr	12
Milk, fluid, whole	244	8.5	1 cup (½ pt), 3.5% fat	160	9	9	12
Milk, malted, plain	353	12.4	1 fountain size glass (about 1½ cup)	368	17	15	42
Milkshake, chocolate	342	12.0	1 fountain size glass	420	11	18	58
Molasses, cane, black-strap	20	0.7	1 tbsp, 3rd extraction	45	—	—	11
Molasses, cane, light	20	0.7	1 tbsp, 1st extraction	50	—	—	13
Muffins, plain	40	1.4	1 muffin, 2¾ in. dia. (enriched white flour)	120	3	4	17
Mushrooms, canned	122	4.3	½ cup, solids and liquid	20	3	tr	3
Noodles, egg, cooked	120	4.2	¾ cup (enriched)	150	5	2	28
Nuts, almonds	36	1.3	¼ cup shelled	213	7	19	7
Nuts, cashew, roasted	35	1.2	¼ cup	196	6	16	10
Nuts, peanuts (see peanuts, roasted)							
Nuts, pecan halves	27	0.9	¼ cup	185	3	19	4
Nuts, walnut halves	25	0.9	¼ cup, English or Persian	163	4	16	4
Oatmeal or rolled oats, cooked	160	5.6	⅔ cup (regular or quick-cooking)	87	3	1	15
Oils, salad or cooking	14	0.5	1 tbsp	125	0	14	0
Okra, cooked	43	1.5	4 pods, 3 × ⅝ in.	13	1	tr	3
Olives, green	16	0.6	4 medium or 3 large	15	tr	2	tr
Olives, ripe	10	0.4	3 small or 2 large	15	tr	2	tr
Onions, raw	110	3.9	1 onion, 2½ in. dia.	40	2	tr	10
Onions, cooked	105	3.7	½ cup or 5 onions, 1¼ in. dia.	30	2	tr	7
Onions, young green	50	1.8	6 small, without tops	20	1	tr	5
Oranges	180	6.3	1 orange, 2⅝ in. dia. (all commercial varieties)	65	1	tr	16
Orange juice, canned unsweetened	125	4.4	½ cup or 1 small glass	60	1	1	13
Orange juice, dehydrated crystals	124	4.3	½ cup or 1 small glass, prepared, ready to serve	60	1	tr	14

Food	Weight g	Weight oz	Approximate Measure and Description	kcal	Protein g	Fat g	Carbohydrate g
Orange juice, fresh	124	4.3	½ cup or 1 small glass (all varieties)	55	1	tr	15
Orange juice, frozen concentrate	125	4.4	½ cup or 1 small glass, diluted, ready to serve	60	1	tr	14
Oysters, raw	120	4.2	½ cup or 8–10 oysters	80	10	2	4
Oyster stew, milk	230	8.1	1 cup with 3–4 oysters	200	11	12	11
Pancakes, wheat	27	0.9	1 griddle cake, 4 in. dia. (enriched flour)	60	2	2	9
Papayas, raw	91	3.2	½ cup in ½-in. cubes	35	1	tr	9
Parsley, raw	4	0.1	1 tbsp chopped	tr	tr	tr	tr
Parsnips, cooked	77	2.7	½ cup	50	1	1	12
Peaches, canned halves or slices	129	4.5	½ cup, solids and liquid, syrup-pack	100	1	tr	26
Peaches, canned whole	123	4.3	½ cup, solids liquid (water pack)	38	1	tr	10
Peaches, raw sliced	84	2.9	½ cup fresh or frozen	33	1	tr	8
Peaches, raw whole	114	4.0	1 peach, 2 in. dia.	35	1	tr	10
Peanuts, roasted	36	1.3	¼ cup halves, salted	210	9	18	7
Peanut butter	32	1.1	2 tbsp	190	8	16	6
Pears, canned	117	4.1	2 medium halves with 2 tbsp juice (syrup pack)	90	tr	tr	23
Pears, raw (as purchased)	182	6.3	1 pear, 3 × 2½ in. dia.	100	1	1	25
Peas, cowpeas, dry, cooked (blackeye peas or frijoles)	124	4.3	½ cup	95	7	1	17
Peas, green, cooked	80	2.8	½ cup	58	5	1	10
Peas, pigeon, dry raw (gandules)	99	3.5	6 tbsp	310	22	2	50
Peas, split, dry cooked	125	4.4	½ cup	145	10	1	26
Peppers, green, stuffed	113	4.0	1 medium pepper, cooked with meat stuffing	200	12	14	12
Peppers, hot red (*see* chili powder)							
Peppers, pimentos, canned	38	1.3	1 medium pod	10	tr	tr	2
Peppers, raw sweet green	74	2.6	1 medium pod without stem	15	1	tr	4
Peppers, raw sweet red	60	2.1	1 medium pod without stem and seeds	20	1	tr	4
Perch, ocean, fried	85	3.0	1 piece, 4 × 3 × ½ in.	195	16	11	6
Persimmons, raw (Japanese)	125	4.4	1 fruit, 2½ in. dia.	75	1	tr	20
Pickle relish	15	0.5	1 tbsp	20	tr	tr	5
Pickles, cucumber, bread and butter	42	1.5	6 slices, ¼ × 1½ in. dia.	30	tr	tr	7
Pickles, cucumber, dill	65	2.3	1 large pickel, 3¾ × 1¼ in.	10	1	tr	1
Pickles, cucumber, sweet	15	0.5	1 pickle, 2½ × ¾ in. dia.	20	tr	tr	6
Pie, apple	135	4.7	4-in. sector or ⅐ of 9-in.-dia. pie (unenriched flour)	350	3	15	51
Pie, cherry	135	4.7	4-in. sector of ⅐ of 9-in.-dia. pie (unenriched flour)	350	4	15	52
Pie, custard	130	4.6	4-in. sector or ⅐ of 9-in.-dia. pie (unenriched flour)	285	8	14	30
Pie, lemon meringue	120	4.2	4-in. sector or ⅐ of 9-in.-dia. pie (unenriched flour)	305	4	12	45
Pie, mince	135	4.7	4-in. sector or ⅐ of 9-in.-dia. pie (unenriched flour)	365	3	16	56
Pie, pumpkin	130	4.6	4-in. sector or ⅐ of 9-in.-dia. pie (unenriched flour)	275	5	15	32
Pineapple, canned crushed	130	4.6	½ cup (syrup packed)	100	1	tr	25
Pineapple, canned slices	122	4.3	1 large or 2 small slices, 2 tbsp juice (syrup pack)	90	tr	tr	24
Pineapple, raw	70	2.5	½ cup, diced	38	1	tr	10
Pineapple juice, canned	125	4.4	½ cup or 1 small glass	68	1	tr	17

Food	Weight g	Weight oz	Approximate Measure and Description	kcal	Protein g	Fat g	Carbohydrate g
Pizza (cheese)	75	2.6	5½-in. sector or ⅛ of 14-in.-dia. pie	185	7	6	27
Plantain, raw, green	100	3.5	1 baking banana, 6 in.	135	1	—	32
Plums, canned	128	4.5	½ cup or 3 plums with 2 tbsp juice (syrup pack)	100	1	tr	27
Plums, raw	60	2.1	1 plum, 2 in. diameter	25	tr	tr	7
Popcorn, popped	9	0.3	1 cup (oil and salt) added	40	1	2	5
Pork chop, cooked	99	3.5	1 thick chop, trimmed, with bone	260	16	21	0
Pork roast, cooked	85	3.0	2 slices, 5 × 4 × ⅛ in.	310	21	24	0
Potato chips	20	0.7	10 medium chips, 2 in. dia.	115	1	8	10
Potatoes, baked	99	3.5	1 medium potato, about 3 per pound raw	90	3	tr	21
Potatoes, boiled	122	4.3	1 potato, peeled before boiling	80	2	tr	18
Potatoes, French fried	57	2.0	10 pieces, 2 × ½ × ½ in., cooked in deep fat	155	2	7	20
Potatoes, mashed	98	3.4	½ cup (milk and butter added)	95	2	4	12
Poultry (chicken or turkey) potpie	227	7.9	1 indiv. pie, 4¼ in. dia.	535	23	31	42
Pretzels	3	0.1	5, 3⅛-in. sticks	10	tr	tr	2
Prunes, dried, cooked	105	3.7	5 medium prunes with 2 tbsp juice, sweetened	160	1	tr	42
Prune juice, canned	128	4.5	½ cup or 1 small glass	100	1	tr	25
Pudding, chocolate blanc mange	130	4.6	½ cup	190	6	8	26
Pudding, cornstarch (plain blanc mange)	124	4.3	½ cup	140	5	5	20
Pudding, rice with raisins (old-fashioned)	136	4.8	½ cup	300	8	8	52
Pudding, tapioca	74	2.6	½ cup	140	5	5	12
Radishes, raw	40	1.4	4 small	5	tr	tr	1
Raisins, seedless	10	0.4	1 tbsp pressed down	30	tr	tr	8
Raspberries, raw, red	62	2.2	½ cup	35	1	1	9
Rhubarb, cooked	136	4.8	½ cup (sugar added)	190	1	tr	50
Rice, parboiled, cooked	131	4.6	¾ cup (enriched)	140	3	tr	31
Rice, puffed	15	0.5	1 cup (nutrients added)	60	1	tr	13
Rice flakes	30	1.1	1 cup (nutrients added)	115	2	tr	26
Rolls, bagel (egg)	55	1.9	1 roll, 3 in. dia.	165	6	2	28
Rolls, barbecue bun	40	1.3	1 bun, 3½ in. dia. (enriched)	120	3	2	21
Rolls, hard	52	1.8	1 round roll	160	5	2	31
Rolls, plain, white	28	1.0	1 commercial pan roll (enriched flour)	85	2	2	15
Rolls, sweet, pan	43	1.5	1 roll	135	4	4	21
Rutabagas, cooked	77	2.7	½ cup	25	1	tr	6
Salad, chicken	125	4.4	½ cup, with mayonnaise	280	25	19	1
Salad, egg	128	4.5	½ cup, with mayonnaise	190	6	18	1
Salad, fresh fruit (orange, apple, banana, grapes)	125	4.4	½ cup, with French dressing	130	—	6	21
Salad, jellied, vegetable	122	4.3	½ cup, no dressing	70	3	—	16
Salad, lettuce	130	4.6	¼ solid head, with French dressing	80	1	6	5
Salad, potato	139	4.9	½ cup, with mayonnaise	185	2	12	17
Salad, tomato aspic	119	4.2	½ cup, no dressing	45	5	0	7
Salad, tuna fish	102	3.6	½ cup, with mayonnaise	250	21	18	1
Salad dressing, blue cheese	15	0.5	1 tbsp	75	1	8	1
Salad dressing, boiled	16	0.6	1 tbsp, home-made	25	1	2	2
Salad dressing, commercial	15	0.5	1 tbsp, mayonnaise-type	65	tr	6	2
Salad dressing, French	16	0.6	1 tbsp	65	tr	6	3

Food	Weight g	Weight oz	Approximate Measure and Description	kcal	Protein g	Fat g	Carbohydrate g
Salad dressing, low-calorie	26	0.9	2 tbsp (cottage cheese, nonfat dry milk, no oil)	17	2	0	2
Salad dressing, mayonnaise	14	0.5	1 tbsp	100	tr	11	tr
Salad dressing, Thousand Island	16	0.6	1 tbsp	80	tr	8	3
Salmon, boiled or baked	119	4.2	1 steak, 4 × 3 × ½ in.	200	34	7	tr
Salmon, pink, canned	85	3.0	½ cup	120	17	5	0
Salmon loaf	113	4.0	½ cup or 1 slice, 4 × 1¼ × 1¼ in.	235	29	10	5
Sardines, canned oil	57	2.0	5 small fish, 3 × 1 × ¼ in.	120	13	6	0
Sauce, chocolate	40	1.4	2 tbsp	75	1	4	9
Sauce, custard	31	1.1	2 tbsp (low calorie, with nonfat dry milk)	45	2	1	7
Sauce, hard	17	0.6	1 tbsp	90	—	6	11
Sauce, hollandaise (mock)	26	0.9	2 tbsp	75	2	7	3
Sauce, lemon	28	1.0	2 tbsp	40	0	1	8
Sauerkraut, canned	118	4.1	½ cup, solids and liquid	25	1	tr	5
Sausage, bologna	57	2.0	2 slices, 4.1 × 0.1 in.	173	7	16	1
Sausage, frankfurters (see frankfurters)							
Sausage, liverwurst	57	2.0	3 slices, 2½ in. dia. ¼ in. thick	150	10	12	1
Sausage, pork, cooked	26	0.9	2 small patties or links	125	5	11	tr
Sausage, Vienna	16	0.6	1 canned sausage, about 2 in. long	40	2	3	tr
Shad, baked	85	3.0	1 piece, 4 × 3 × ½ in.	170	20	10	0
Sherbet, orange	97	3.4	½ cup	130	1	1	30
Shrimp, canned	85	3.0	½ cup, meat only	100	21	1	1
Syrup, table blends	21	0.7	1 tbsp, light and dark	60	0	0	15
Soup, bean with pork, canned	250	8.8	1 cup, ready to serve	170	8	6	22
Soup, beef broth, bouillon, consommé, canned	240	8.4	1 cup, ready to serve	30	5	0	3
Soup, chicken noodle, canned	250	8.8	1 cup, ready to serve	65	4	2	8
Soup, clam chowder, canned	255	8.9	1 cup, ready to serve	85	2	3	13
Soup, cream of vegetable (e.g., tomato, mushroom), canned	240	8.4	1 cup, ready to serve	135	2	10	10
Soup, minestrone, canned	245	8.6	1 cup, ready to serve	105	5	3	14
Soup, tomato, canned	245	8.6	1 cup, ready to serve	90	2	3	16
Soup, vegetable, canned	250	8.8	1 cup, ready to serve	80	3	2	14
Spaghetti, cooked	105	3.7	¾ cup (enriched)	115	4	1	24
Spaghetti, in tomato sauce, with cheese	188	6.5	¾ cup	200	7	7	28
Spaghetti, in tomato sauce, with meat balls	186	6.5	¾ cup	250	15	9	30
Spinach (see greens)							
Squash, summer, cooked	105	3.7	½ cup, diced	15	1	tr	4
Squash, winter, baked	103	3.6	½ cup, mashed	65	2	1	16
Stew, beef and vegetable	176	6.2	¾ cup	160	11	8	11
Strawberries, raw	75	2.6	½ cup, capped	30	1	1	7
Sugar, brown	14	0.5	1 tbsp firmly packed	50	0	0	13
Sugar, granulated	11	0.4	1 tbsp (beef or cane)	40	0	0	11
Sugar, lump	6	0.2	1 domino, 1⅛ × ¾ × ⅜ in.	25	0	0	6
Sugar, powdered	8	0.3	1 tbsp	30	0	0	8
Sweet potatoes, baked	110	3.9	1 medium potato, about 6 oz raw	155	2	1	36
Sweet potatoes, candied	175	6.1	1 potato, 3½ × 2¼ in.	295	2	6	60
Tangerine	116	4.1	1 medium tangerine, 2⅜ in. dia.	40	1	tr	10
Tartar sauce (see salad dressing, mayonnaise)							
Toast, melba	6	0.2	1 slice, 3¾ × 1¾ in.	20	1	tr	4
Tomato catsup	15	0.5	1 tbsp	15	tr	tr	4

Food	Weight		Approximate Measure and Description	kcal	Protein g	Fat g	Carbohydrate g
	g	oz					
Tomato juice, canned	122	4.3	½ cup or 1 small glass	23	1	tr	5
Tomatoes, canned	121	4.2	½ cup	25	1	1	5
Tomatoes, raw	200	7.0	1 tomato, about 3 in. dia., 2⅛ in. high	40	2	tr	9
Topping, whipped	4	0.1	1 tbsp, pressurized	10	tr	1	tr
Tortillas	20	0.7	1 tortilla, 5 in. dia.	50	1	1	10
Tuna fish, canned in oil	85	3.0	½ cup, drained solids	170	24	7	0
Tuna salad (see salad, tuna fish)							
Turnip greens (see greens)							
Turnips, cooked	78	2.7	½ cup, diced	18	1	tr	4
Veal cutlet, breaded (wiener schnitzel)	136	4.8	2 slices, 2½ × 2½ × ¾ in.	315	26	21	5
Veal cutlet, broiled	85	3.0	1 cutlet, 3¾ × 3 × ½ in.	185	23	9	—
Veal roast, cooked	85	3.0	2 slices, 3 × 2½ × ¼ in.	230	23	14	0
Vinegar	15	0.5	1 tbsp	2	0	—	1
Waffles	75	2.6	1 waffle, 7 in. dia. (enriched flour)	210	7	7	28
Watermelon, raw	925	32.4	1 wedge, 4 × 8 in., with rind	115	2	1	27
Welsh rarebit	125	4.4	½ cup	330	19	26	6
Wheat flour, white enriched	115	4.0	1 cup, sifted	420	12	1	88
Wheat flour, white unenriched	110	3.9	1 cup, sifted	400	12	1	84
Wheat flour, whole wheat	120	4.2	1 cup, hard wheat	400	16	2	85
Wheat germ	9	0.3	2 tbsp	30	2	1	4
Wheat flakes	30	1.1	1 cup (nutrients added)	105	3	tr	24
Wheat, shredded	25	0.9	1 biscuit, 4 × 2¼ in.	90	2	1	20
White sauce (medium)	65	2.3	¼ cup	110	3	8	6
Yeast, brewers, dry	8	0.3	1 tbsp	25	3	tr	3
Yeast, compressed	28	1.0	one 1-oz cake	25	3	tr	3
Yeast, dry active	28	1.0	four ¼-oz packages	80	12	tr	12
Yogurt, plain	245	8.6	1 cup (made from partially skimmed milk)	125	8	4	13

Adapted from C. F. Adams, *Nutritive Value of American Foods* (Washington, D.C.: U.S. Dept. of Agriculture, 1975).

TABLE B-2   Caloric Content of Selected Alcoholic Beverages

Beverage	Amount	Number of Calories
Beer	8-oz glass	100
Eggnog, holiday variety, made with whiskey and rum	½ cup	225
Whiskey, gin, rum, and vodka		
100 proof	1 jigger (1½ oz)	125
90 proof	1 jigger (1½ oz)	110
86 proof	1 jigger (1½ oz)	105
80 proof	1 jigger (1½ oz)	100
70 proof	1 jigger (1½ oz)	85
Wines		
table wines (such as chablis, claret, Rhine wine, and sauterne)	1 wine glass (about 3 oz)	75
dessert wines (such as muscatel, port, sherry, or Tokay)	1 wine glass (about 3 oz)	125

Adapted from C. F. Adams, *Nutritive Value of American Foods* (Washington, D.C.: U.S. Dept. of Agriculture, 1975).

Glossary

Active warm-up: Dynamic movements for the purpose of readying the body for activity. *(Ch. 6)*

Acute disease: A severe disease of short duration. *(Ch. 1)*

Adenosine diphosphate (ADP): A complex, high-energy compound from which ATP is resynthesized. *(Ch. 6)*

Adenosine triphosphate (ATP): A complex, high-energy compound stored in the cells from which the body derives its energy. *(Ch. 6)*

Adherence: Long-term participation. *(Ch. 5)*

Adipose tissue: Fat cells. *(Ch. 11)*

Aerobic: Literally means "with oxygen." *(Ch. 6)*

Aerobic capacity: The maximal ability to take in, deliver, and use oxygen; also referred to as cardiorespiratory endurance or max VO$_2$. *(Ch. 7)*

Agility: The ability to rapidly change direction while maintaining dynamic balance. *(Ch. 1)*

Agonist muscle: The muscle that contracts to produce a specific movement; the prime mover. *(Ch. 8)*

Alveoli: Tiny air sacs in the lungs that are richly perfused with blood. Gaseous exchange between the lungs and blood occurs at these sites. *(Ch. 7)*

Amenorrhea: Failure to menstruate. *(Chs. 4, 11)*

Amino acids: The building blocks of proteins. *(Ch. 10)*

Anabolic steroid: A drug with tissue-building or growth-stimulating properties. *(Ch. 8)*

Anaerobic: Literally means "without oxygen." *(Ch. 6)*

Anaerobic threshold: That point where exercise cannot be totally sustained by the aerobic processes. Anaerobic processes contribute to the production of ATP and lactic acid begins to accumulate in the blood. *(Ch. 6)*

Androgen: Male sex hormone produced in the testes and to a limited extent, from the adrenal cortex. *(Ch. 8)*

Android obesity: Male pattern of fat deposition in the abdominal region. *(Ch. 11)*

Anorexia nervosa: A psychological and emotional disorder characterized by excessive underweight. *(Ch. 11)*

Antagonist muscle: The muscle that stretches in response to the contraction of the agonist muscle. *(Ch. 8)*

Aorta: Largest artery in the body. *(Ch. 2)*

Arterial-venous O$_2$ Difference (a-vo$_2$ diff): The difference between the oxygen (O$_2$) content of arterial and mixed venous blood. *(Chs. 2, 7)*

Asthma: Widespread narrowing of the airways of the lungs due in varying degrees to spasm of smooth muscle, edema of the mucosa, and mucus in the bronchi and bronchioles. *(Ch. 4)*

Atherosclerosis: A progressive disease which results in the narrowing of arterial channels due to the build-up of plaque. *(Ch. 2)*

Balance: Involves the maintenance of a desired body position either statically or dynamically. Also referred to as equilibrium. *(Ch. 1)*

Baroreceptors: Sensory nerve endings which respond to stretching of the walls in which they are embedded. *(Ch. 6)*

Basal metabolic rate (BMR): The energy required to sustain life while in a fasted and rested state. *(Ch. 11)*

Blood lactate: A metabolite that produces fatigue; results from incomplete breakdown of sugar. *(Ch. 5)*

Blood platelets: Blood cells which are involved in preventing blood loss. They are important components in clot formation. *(Ch. 2)*

Blood pressure: The force that the blood exerts against the walls of the blood vessels. *(Ch. 3)*

Body composition: The amount of lean versus fat tissue in the body. *(Ch. 7)*

Bulimarexia nervosa: An eating disorder characterized by episodes of secretive binge eating followed by purging. *(Ch. 11)*

Burnout: A loss of energy, creativity, and direction. *(Ch. 5)*

Cancer: A large group of disorders that are characterized by abnormal cellular growth. *(Ch. 4)*

Carbon monoxide: A colorless, odorless gas formed by the incomplete oxidation of carbon and highly poisonous when inhaled. *(Ch. 3)*

Carbohydrate: An organic compound composed of one or more sugars that are derived from plant sources. *(Ch. 10)*

Carbohydrate loading: A method of overfilling the glycogen stores used by endurance athletes. *(Ch. 10)*

Cardiac muscle: Specialized muscle tissue found only in the heart. *(Ch. 8)*

Cardiac output: The amount of blood pumped by the heart in one minute *(Ch. 7)*

Cardiovascular disease: A complex of diseases of the heart and circulatory system. *(Ch. 1)*

Cardiovascular endurance: The ability to take in, deliver, and extract oxygen for physical work. *(Ch. 1)*

Cerebrovascular accidents: Diseases of the blood vessels to the brain or in the brain which result in a stroke. *(Ch. 2)*

Cholesterol: An organic substance, it is the most abundant steroid in animal tissues, especially in bile and gallstones. Elevated blood cholesterol is a primary risk factor for heart disease. *(Ch. 3)*

Chronic disease: A long-lasting and/or frequently occurring disease. *(Ch. 1)*

Chronological age: An individual's calendar age. *(Ch. 1)*

Chylomicrons: Large, buoyant particles which are the primary transporters of triglycerides in the fasting state. *(Ch. 3)*

Circuit training: A series of 6 to 10 exercises performed in sequence and as rapidly as one's fitness level allows. *(Ch. 8)*

Concentric contraction: That phase of muscular contraction in which the muscle shortens. *(Ch. 8)*

Conduction: Transference of heat from one object to another by means of physical contact. *(Ch. 6)*

Congenital heart disease: Heart defects which exist at birth and occur when the heart or its structures or the blood vessels near the heart fail to develop normally before birth. *(Ch. 2)*

Convection: Transfer of heat from the body to a moving gas or liquid. *(Ch. 6)*

Coordination: The integration of body parts resulting in smooth, fluid motion. *(Ch. 1)*

Coronary collateral circulation: The development of auxiliary blood vessels, to enhance blood flow to cardiac muscle. *(Ch. 7)*

Cortical bone: The dense, hard outer layer of bone such as that which appears in the shafts of the long bones of the arms and legs. *(Ch. 4)*

Creatine phosphate (CP): A chemical that donates its phosphate to ADP for the resynthesis of ATP. *(Ch. 6)*

Cross-training: Selection and participation in more than one physical activity on a consistent basis. *(Ch. 6)*

Crude fiber: The fiber that remains in food after it has been treated with harsh chemicals during laboratory analysis. *(Ch. 10)*

Dehydration: Excessive loss of body fluids. *(Ch. 6)*

Diabetes mellitus: A metabolic disorder in which the ability to oxidize carbohydrates is more or less completely lost due to faulty pancreatic activity and consequent disturbance of normal insulin mechanisims. This is often accompanied by resistance of receptor cells to insulin. *(Ch. 3)*

Diastolic blood pressure: The lowest pressure of arterial blood against the walls of the vessels or heart during diastole. *(Ch. 3)*

Dietary fiber: The fiber that remains after food is digested in the human body. *(Ch. 10)*

Disaccharide: A combination of two simple sugars. *(Ch. 10)*

Distress: Normal stress that has become chronic. *(Ch. 3)*

Double product (RPP): Heart rate multiplied by systolic blood pressure; it is an estimate of the oxygen required by the heart during aerobic exercise. *(Ch. 7)*

Dynamic stretching: Also known as ballistic stretching, it employs bouncing and bobbing to stretch muscles. *(Ch. 9)*

Eccentric contraction: That phase of a muscular contraction in which the muscle lengthens. *(Ch. 8)*

Electrolyte: Any solution that conducts an electrical current through its ions. *(Ch. 6)*

Endogenous cholesterol: Cholesterol which is manufactured within the body. *(Ch. 3)*

Endorphins: One of a family of opioid-like polypeptides originally isolated in the brain but now found in many parts of the body. In the brain they bind to the same receptors that bind exogenous opiates. *(Ch. 3)*

Erythrocytes: The red blood cells which transport oxygen from the lungs to the various tissues of the body and carbon dioxide from the tissues to the lungs. *(Ch.2)*

Eustress: Good stress; occurs when one accepts and successfully handles a challenge. *(Ch. 3)*

Evaporation: The loss of heat by changing a liquid to a vapor. *(Ch. 6)*

Exogenous cholesterol: Cholesterol which is received through the Diet. *(Ch. 3)*

Extrinsic reward: Any positive reinforcement emanating from an outside source, i.e., friends, coaches, etc., that increases the strength of a response. (external reward) *(Ch. 5)*

Fast-twitch muscle fiber: A type of muscle fiber which contracts rapidly but fatigues rapidly. Also referred to as "white" muscle fibers. *(Ch. 8)*

Fats: Organic compounds that are composed of glycerol and fatty acids. *(Ch. 10)*

Fiber: The indigestible polysaccharides that are found in the stems, leaves, and seeds of plants. *(Ch. 10)*

Flexibility: The range of motion about a joint or series of joints. *(Chs. 1, 9)*

Flexometer: An instrument for measuring static flexibility. *(Ch. 9)*

Glycogen: The stored form of sugar. *(Ch. 6)*

Goal: Something toward which effort or movement is directed; an end or objective to be achieved. *(Ch. 5)*

Goniometer: A protractor-like device used to measure static flexibility. *(Ch. 9)*

Gynoid obesity: Female pattern of fat deposition in the thighs and gluteal areas. *(Ch. 11)*

Health age: An individual's biological age. *(Ch. 1)*

Health-related fitness: A type of fitness that enhances one's health. *(Ch. 1)*

Heat exhaustion: A condition characterized by a build-up of body heat. Symptoms include dizziness, fainting, rapid pulse, and cool skin. *(Ch. 6)*

Heat stroke: The most dangerous of the heat stress illnesses. Symptoms include a temperature of 106 F and above, absence of sweating, dry skin, and often delirium, convulsions, and loss of consciousness. *(Ch. 6)*

Hemoglobin: Iron pigment of the red cells that combines with O2. *(Ch. 6)*

HDL-cholesterol: A lipoprotein which transports cholesterol from the blood to the liver for degradation and removal (good cholesterol). *(Ch. 3)*

Hydrostatic weighing: A method for determining specific gravity and percent body fat by underwater weighing. *(Ch. 11)*

Hyperplasia: An increase in size due to an increase in the number of cells. *(Ch. 8)*

Hypertension: Medical term for high blood pressure. *(Ch. 2)*

Hyperthermia: Overheating; abnormally high body temperature. *(Ch. 6)*

Hypertrophy: An increase in size due to an increase in the thickness of fibers. *(Ch. 8)*

Hypokinesis: Lack of physical activity. *(Ch. 3)*

Hypothermia: Abnormally low body temperature. *(Ch. 6)*

Insoluable fiber: Include cellulose, lignin, and hemicellulose. Insoluable fibers add bulk to the contents of the intestine accelerating the passage of food remnants through the digestive tract. These reduce the risk of colon cancer as well as other diseases of the digestive tract. *(Ch. 10)*

Intrinsic reward: Reinforcement coming from within; the degree of satisfaction derived from participation in the absence of some visible reward (internal reward). *(Ch. 5)*

Isokinetic contraction: A dynamic contraction in which the muscles generate force against a variable resistance that moves at a constant rate of speed. *(Ch. 8)*

Isometric contraction: A static contraction in which the muscles generate force against an immovable object with no observable shortening. *(Ch. 8)*

Isotonic contraction: A dynamic contraction in which the muscles generate force against a constant resistance; movement occurs as the muscles shorten and lengthen with each repetition. *(Ch. 8)*

Kilocalories: The amount of energy found in food, it is the quantity of heat needed to raise the temperature of one kilogram of water one degree centigrade. *(Ch. 10)*

Lactic acid: A fatiguing metabolite resulting from the incomplete breakdown of sugar. *(Ch. 6)*

LDL-cholesterol: A lipoprotein which transports cholesterol to the tissues; it is involved in the atherosclerotic process (bad cholesterol). *(Ch. 3)*

Leukocytes: White blood cells that protect the body against invading microorganisms and remove dead cells and debris from the body. *(Ch. 2)*

Locomotor movement: Movements which bring about a change in location and include walking, jogging, climbing, cycling, and swimming, to name but a few. *(Ch. 8)*

Lordosis: Swayback; abnormal curvature of the low back. *(Ch. 8)*

Mean arterial blood pressure (MAP): The average pressure in the large arteries of the body. *(Ch. 3)*

Metabolism: The sum of the chemical reactions and processes that supply the energy used by the body. *(Ch. 7)*

Metastasis: The spread of cancer from the original site to other sites in the body. *(Ch. 4)*

Minerals: Inorganic substances that exist freely in nature. *(Ch. 10)*

Mitochondria: The cells powerhouse in which ATP is produced aerobically. *(Ch. 6)*

Monosaccharide: Simple sugars such as table sugar, honey, molasses, etc. *(Ch. 10)*

Morbidity: The sick rate or ratio of sick to well in a population. *(Ch. 3)*

Motivation: The internal mechanisms and external stimuli that arouse and direct behavior. *(Ch. 5)*

Motor unit: A motor nerve and all of the muscle fibers that it innervates. *(Ch. 8)*

Muscular endurance: The ability of a muscle to sustain repeated contractions. *(Chs. 1, 8)*

Muscular strength: The maximum amount of force that a muscle can exert in a single contraction. *(Ch. 1)*

Myocardial infarction: A heart attack. The term literally means "death of heart muscle." *(Ch. 2)*

Myocardium: Heart muscle. *(Ch. 2)*

Neoplasm: Growth of new tissue (tumor). *(Ch. 4)*

Nicotine: A stimulant and poisonous drug found in tobacco products. *(Ch. 3)*

Non-locomotor movement: Movements that take place around the axis of the body. The subject remains in one place creating dynamic movement by means of stretching, bending, stooping, pushing, pulling, and twisting, to name but a few. *(Ch. 8)*

Obesity: Excessive body fat—23 to 24 percent or greater for males; 30 percent or greater for females. *(Ch. 3)*

Oligomenorrhea: Scanty menses: *(Ch. 4)*

Osteoarthritis: A degenerative joint disease characterized by the deterioration of articular cartilage particularly in the weight bearing joints. Often referred to a "wear and tear" arthritis. *(Ch. 4)*

Osteoporosis: Reduction in the quantity of bone due to demineralization and atrophy of skeletal tissue. *(Ch. 4)*

Overload: Periodically stressing the body with greater loads than those that are usually experienced. *(Ch. 8)*

Overweight: Excess body weight irrespective of body composition. *(Ch. 3)*

O₂ debt: The amount of oxygen needed in recovery from exercise, above that normally required during rest. *(Ch. 7)*

O₂ deficit: Occurs at the beginning of exercise when the body does not supply all of the oxygen needed to support exercise. *(Ch. 7)*

Passive warm-up: Inactive means of preparing for physical activity; may include massage and dry and wet heat. *(Ch. 6)*

Performance-related fitness: A type of fitness that allows one to perform physical skills with a high degree of proficiency. *(Ch. 1)*

Periodization: A way to provide variety in training; The training period is divided into different cycles in which the volume is periodically reduced and the intensity is concomitantly increased. *(Ch. 8)*

Phospholipids: Similar to a triglyceride except that one of the fatty acids is replaced by a phosphorous-containing acid. *(Ch. 10)*

Placebo effect: Healing that results from a person's belief in the efficacy of a pill, treatment, or other measures when there is no known medicinal value in the substances taken or treatments given. *(Ch. 3)*

Polysaccharides: The joining of three or more simple sugars to form starch and glycogen. *(Ch. 10)*

Positive reinforcement: A reward; increases the strength of a response or responses. *(Ch. 5)*

Power: A function of work divided by the time that it takes to perform the work. *(Ch. 1)*

Proprioceptive neuromuscular facilitation (PNF): A group of stretching techniques involving the alternation of contraction and relaxation of various muscles. *(Ch. 6)*

Protein: A food substance formed from amino acids. *(Ch. 10)*

Radiation: Transfer of heat from the body to the atmosphere by electromagnetic waves. *(Ch. 6)*

Reaction time: The elapsed time between the presentation of a stimulus and its response—also called response latency. *(Ch. 1)*

Residual volume: The air remaining in the lungs following a maximal expiration. *(Ch. 7)*

Resting metabolic rate (RMR): The conditions for measuring BMR are difficult to achieve and when they are approximated the term Resting Metabolic Rate is used. It is an approximation of the energy required to sustain life while in the resting state. *(Ch. 11)*

Risk factor profile: A questionnaire that assesses family history and lifestyle patterns to identify risk factors associated with physical and psychological diseases. *(Ch. 1)*

Saturated fats: Found primarily in animal flesh and dairy products. Chemically, they carry the maximum number of hydrogen atoms. *(Ch. 10)*

Self-concept: The set of peoples' beliefs about and evaluations of themselves as persons. *(Ch. 5)*

Skeletal muscle: Voluntary muscles whose attachments to the bones of the skeletal system provide the basis for human movement. *(Ch. 8)*

Skinfold measurement: A method for determining percent body fat by measuring a pinch of skin at selected sites with a skinfold caliper. *(Ch. 11)*

Slow-twitch muscle fiber: A type of muscle fiber that contracts slowly but is difficult to fatigue; referred to as "red" muscle fibers. *(Ch. 8)*

Smooth muscle: Located in the blood vessels and digestive system; not under conscious or voluntary control. *(Ch. 8)*

Soluable fiber: Pectin, gums, and other substances add bulk to the contents of the stomach. These lower blood cholesterol levels. *(Ch. 10)*

Speed: Performance of a movement in the shortest amount of time - also known as velocity. *(Ch. 1)*

Static stretching: Stretching that employs slow movements and positions that are held for 15 to 30 seconds. *(Ch. 9)*

Sterol: One of the three major fats with a structure similar to cholesterol. *(Ch. 10)*

Stimulus: Any energy impinging upon an organism that results in a response. *(Ch. 5)*

Strength: The force exerted by a muscle or muscle group in a single maximal contraction. *(Ch. 8)*

Stretch reflex: The myotatic reflex that responds to stretching of the muscle tissues. *(Ch. 9)*

Stroke volume: The amount of blood pumped by the heart with each beat. *(Ch. 7)*

Systolic blood pressure: The greatest pressure in the blood vessels or heart during a cardiac cycle as the result of systole. *(Ch. 3)*

Testosterone: A sex hormone appearing in much higher concentrations in males than females. *(Ch. 8)*

Thermogenic effect of food (TEF): The energy required to digest and absorb food. *(Ch. 11)*

Tidal volume: The amount of air inhaled and exhaled with each breath. *(Ch. 7)*

Trabecular bone: Spongy bone, not as dense as cortical bone. *(Ch. 4)*

Triglycerides: Consist of three fatty acids attached to a glycerol molecole. *(Ch. 3, 10)*

Unsaturated fats: Fatty acids in which one or more points is free of hydrogen atoms. *(Ch. 10)*

Valsalva maneuver: Occurs when individuals lift heavy weights and hold their breath. The glottis closes and intrathoracic pressure increases, hindering the flow of blood to the heart. *(Ch. 8)*

Ventilation: The amount of air inhaled and exhaled per minute. *(Ch. 7)*

Very-low calorie diet: Diets which contain 800 kcals per day or less. *(Ch. 11)*

Vital capacity: The amount of air that can be expired after a maximum inhalation. *(Ch. 7)*

Vitamins: Organic compounds found in food that are essential to normal metabolism. *(Ch. 10)*

VLDL-cholesterol: Lipoproteins which are the primary transporters of endogenous triglycerides in the fasting state. *(Ch. 3)*

Weight cycling: Repeated cycles of weight loss followed by weight gain. *(Ch. 11)*

Wellness: A dynamic and multifaceted approach to optimal health that centers upon individuals taking responsibility for their health status. *(Ch. 1)*

Index